Pediatric Radiology   THE REQUISITES

SERIES EDITOR   **James H. Thrall,** MD
                       Radiologist-in-Chief
                       Department of Radiology
                       Massachusetts General Hospital
                       Boston, Massachusetts

OTHER VOLUMES IN THE REQUISITES SERIES   Gastrointestinal Radiology

Neuroradiology

Nuclear Medicine

Cardiac Radiology

Genitourinary Radiology

Thoracic Radiology

Ultrasound

Musculoskeletal Radiology

Mammography

Pediatric Radiology

JOHAN G. BLICKMAN, MD
Associate Professor of Radiology
Harvard Medical School
Chief, Pediatric Imaging
Massachusetts General Hospital
Boston, Massachusetts

with 382 illustrations

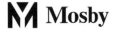 Mosby

St. Louis Baltimore Boston Chicago London Madrid
Philadelphia Sydney Toronto

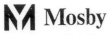

Mosby

Dedicated to Publishing Excellence

Publisher: George S. Stamathis
Editor-in-Chief: Anne S. Patterson
Editor: Robert J. Farrell
Developmental Editor: Maura K. Leib
Project Manager: Carol Sullivan Wiseman
Production Editor: Florence Achenbach
Manuscript Editor: Marilyn K. Wynd
Series Designer: Susan Lane
Design Manager: Betty Schulz

Printed in the United States of America
Composition by Digital Prepress, Inc.
Printing/binding by Maple-Vail Book Manufacturing Group

Mosby–Year Book, Inc.
11830 Westline Industrial Drive
St. Louis, Missouri 63146

Library of Congress Cataloging in Publication Data

Blickman, Johan G.
  Pediatric radiology: the requisites / Johan G. Blickman
    p. cm.
  "Requisites in radiology series"–Foreword.
  Includes bibliographical references and index.
  ISBN 0-8016-7435-2
  1. Pediatric radiology. II. Title.
III. Series: Requisites series.
  (DNLM: 1. Diagnostic Imaging–in infancy and childhood. WN 240
B648p 1993)
RJ51.R3b55 1993
618.92' 007'57–dc20
DNLM/DLC   93-29224
for Library of Congress   CIP

95 96 97 / 9 8 7 6 5 4 3 2

To
Corinne

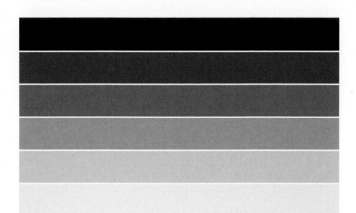

Foreword

Pediatric Radiology: The Requisites is the second book in an ongoing series designed to provide core material in major subspecialty areas of radiology for residents during their initial training and for the practicing radiologist seeking a concise review.

Dr. Blickman has done yeoman work in capturing the philosophy of the "requisites" in his text. At the chapter level, Dr. Blickman has organized his book by organ systems. Within each chapter, key strategic observations concerning approach and imaging philosophy are presented and then followed in a logical fashion by discussions of disease categories and, finally, specific entities.

A unifying theme throughout the book is the importance of the pediatric patient and the correct selection of imaging study. This is aimed at clarifying and simplifying the diagnostic algorithms but, very importantly, is also aimed at keeping radiation dose as low as possible to pediatric patients. Dr. Blickman emphasizes that children are not simply "small" adults and points out for the reader when test selection is different in the pediatric age group versus adults. This again is critical information for optimum patient care and minimization of radiation exposure.

With the focus on high technology cross-sectional imaging techniques in the last decade, plain radiography has not received the attention that many of us feel it still requires in training programs. Dr. Blickman has done on outstanding job in balancing the old with the new in a comprehensive and integrated approach to the patient.

I believe the resident in radiology will find *Pediatric Radiology: The Requisites* to be a concise and valuable approach introduction to the subject. Residents, fellows, and practicing radiologists should also find this a manageable text for basic review. I further hope that pediatricians and pediatric surgeons, as well as their resident and fellowship trainees interested in pediatric imaging, will find this to be a user friendly text to forward their understanding of pediatric radiology.

In some sense, people entering training in radiology are forced to "start over" in terms of their medical knowledge base. The fundamental principles of basic science and clinical medicine are a necessary background for training in radiology. However, the actual knowledge and skills required for correctly analyzing radiologic images and drawing diagnostic inference are left almost entirely to the residency training period. Thus, a resident entering a subspecialty rotation in a radiology training program has the formidable task of going from a minimal knowledge base of the subspecialty specifics to a working knowledge in a very short period of time.

This observation was the basis for creating the *Requisites in Radiology* series. One book specifically written for each of the major subspecialty areas is planned. The length of each book will be dictated by the material requiring coverage, but the goal is to provide the resident with a text that might be reasonably read within several days at the beginning of each subspecialty rotation and perhaps reread several times during initial and subsequent rotations. The books are not intended to be exhaustive but should provide the basic conceptual, factual, and interpretive material required for clinical practice. Each book is being written by a nationally recognized authority in the respective subspecialty area and, as a completely new series, each author has the opportunity to present material in the context of today's contemporary practice of radiology rather than grafting information about new imaging modalities and strategic approaches to text material originally developed for conventional radiography.

I congratulate Dr. Blickman on this valuable addition to the *Requisites in Radiology* series.

James H. Thrall, MD

Radiologist-in-Chief
Massachusetts General Hospital
Professor of Radiology
Harvard Medical School

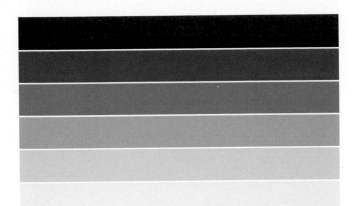

Acknowledgments

It is true that when one sets out to write a book it becomes readily apparent that the task is much larger than initially anticipated. In conjunction, one discovers that, although one is the sole author of record, the writing cannot be accomplished without the help of many.

First, this book is intended for the resident starting out in pediatric radiology. The radiology residents at the Massachusetts General Hospital and those rotating from New England Deaconess Hospital were indispensable in formulating the composition and contents of this book. Many proofread and offered constructive criticism. My gratitude to them is enormous.

Second, it became painfully obvious during this writing that in fact one's knowledge is, in many areas, limited. I was therefore fortunate to have several giants, all former teachers, available to critique chapters in their areas of expertise. The chest and skeletal chapters were reviewed by Dr. John Kirkpatrick, my mentor and Radiologists-in-Chief emeritus at Children's Hospital, Boston. The GI and GU chapters were evaluated by my colleague Dr. Robert Bramson. The cardiac section was corrected by Dr. Ken Fellows, Radiologist-in-Chief, Children's Hospital of Philadelphia. Finally, as the amount of pediatric neuro-imaging is limited at my institution, I turned to Dr. Patrick Barnes, Chief of Neuro-imaging at Children's Hospital in Boston, to co-author the CNS chapter. Felix Chew (skeletal) and Stephen Miller (cardiac), colleagues at Massachusetts General Hospital, also gave many helpful suggestions.
I am indebted to all.

Third, my two pediatric radiology colleagues deserve my gratitude for tolerating my frequent questions, requests for illustrations (a tremendous debt to Dr. Carlo Buonomo), and moments of despair (especially Dr. Bramson).

None of this, however, would have been possible without the perseverance, talents, and enthusiasm of my trusted right hand and administrative assistant Sherry Brec. Each and every utterance was typed, edited, and polished by her in superb fashion.

Also, thanks go to the editorial staff at Mosby, in particular Maura Leib, as well as to the Radiologist-in-Chief at Massachusetts General Hospital, Dr. James Thrall, for the opportunity to contribute to The Requisites series.

Finally, my parents deserve credit for their ever-present support, and Corinne, Patrick, and Christopher for their patience.

May all these efforts bear fruit in laying a solid foundation of pediatric imaging in each and every radiology resident.

J.G.B.

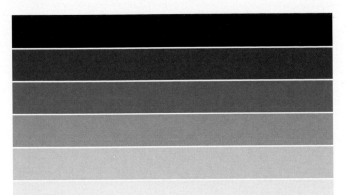

Contents

CHAPTER 1

Pediatric Imaging

In the past 35 years pediatric radiology has evolved so that it fully merits status as a subspecialty. Radiologists in training are examined at the end of their 4 years of studying pediatric imaging, and pediatric radiology is also one of the first subspecialties that offers a certificate of additional qualification (CAQ). Teaching pediatric radiology presents some unique challenges. First, it is difficult to quantify what must be known by a general radiologist about pediatric imaging. In addition, retaining that knowledge is a real challenge. Also, many general radiologists and technologists are not comfortable dealing with infants or young children. Therefore the practice of pediatric imaging demands special attention, knowledge, and understanding.

This book is designed with the neophyte radiology resident in mind and hopes to answer the question of what one could reasonably read and retain during a rotation through pediatric radiology.

The radiology resident must go from little or no knowledge of pediatric radiology to a more-or-less working knowledge in a short training interval. The radiologist-in-training must also understand pediatric disease processes, their diagnosis, therapy, and follow-up. Consequently how each of the clinical phases from initial diagnosis through therapy and follow-up can be assessed most efficiently by the different imaging modalities is the ultimate challenge of pediatric imaging and is the major focus of this book.

Although pediatric radiology is a problem-oriented specialty, an organ system approach is used in this book as a tool for presenting the essentials and as a method for systematic review. Pediatric radiologists must know general radiology, embryology, and basic pediatrics. In addition, meticulous attention to indications for diagnostic studies, standards of practice, and sensitivity to radiation dosage is just as much a part of pediatric imaging as in other radiologic subspecialties.

The book is divided into five main chapters. Within each chapter, that area's imaging techniques as they pertain to pediatric patients are briefly reviewed. Emphasis then is placed on the anatomic and embryologic aspects of each individual region because congenital lesions are an essential part of the differential diagnostic possibilities.

Each organ system is discussed in a logical anatomic sequence. Within this framework, the most common imaging approaches and clinical highlights are presented. When applicable, pathology rounds out the discussion. Practical differential diagnostic possibilities are given that help guide the process of interpretation. Further reading suggestions are made at the end of each chapter. General pediatric imaging reference texts are listed first, with pertinent page numbers. Review and classic articles follow that should enhance the understanding of specific and common pediatric imaging topics.

Some general observations are useful to assist in the efficient and practical performance of basic pediatric imaging. These observations also follow the organ system outline of the ensuing chapters.

Regarding the pediatric chest, newer imaging is not necessarily better. Expensive cross-sectional imaging such as computed tomography (CT) and magnetic resonance imaging (MRI) often require sedating the child. A conventional radiographic or fluoroscopic examination may be satisfactory without the added risk and exposure of a CT scan.

Imaging findings in the pediatric chest are influenced by (immature) physiology that differs from that of adults. The anatomic presence of the thymus also affects the overall image. First and foremost, to arrive at a proper interpretation, an acceptable technically adequate radiograph must be obtained. To achieve this objective, proper immobilization of the child is of paramount importance because it decreases length and

1

retake rate of the study. Techniques in use include the Pigg-o-stat, a device that envelops the infants. It creates both anxiety on the part of the infant and the parents and artifacts that may create anxiety on the part of the interpreter. Another option is the Tame-EM immobilizer that uses Velcro bands applied around the arms and the legs, a choice that is easier on all people involved. The Pigg-o-stat restraining device allows for upright imaging; sandbags and Tame-EM devices do not. In most instances sandbags, adhesive tape, foam rubber wedges, or towels accomplish the immobilization cheaply and effectively.

Fluoroscopy of the chest is quicker and easier to interpret than inspiratory and expiratory or oblique radiographs. This should be kept in mind if conventional chest radiographs do not answer clinical questions about the presence or absence of a check-valve airway obstruction (foreign body), retropharyngeal pathology, or in the elucidation of mediastinal contour. Horizontal beam (decubitus) radiographs are seldom necessary to answer diagnostic dilemmas in the pediatric chest.

It is imperative when imaging the gastrointestinal tract, as well as the genitourinary tract, to review prior examinations and pertinent clinical information. More important yet is to prepare the patient and parents before entering the imaging suite. During the introduction to child and parents, one must again verify the indication for the study and establish rapport to ensure a cooperative patient for an efficient study. This process also assesses whether parents will be a help or a hindrance if they accompany the child during the examination. The overwhelming majority of children benefit from the presence of the parent in the room, both to help with positioning and to reassure the child.

During fluoroscopy immobilization can be achieved by having a technologist at the head of the fluoroscopy table while the imager holds the child at the knees. Some prefer using a cradle device. "Papoosing" the child with towels or Ace bandages also works well. No matter which technique is used, during fluoroscopy the right hand of the radiologist should not let go of the patient being examined. "One hand for the fluoroscopy unit, one for the patient" should be your motto.

All upper gastrointestinal tract studies should include fluoroscopic observation of the respiratory motion of the diaphragm. The contour and motion of the mediastinum should also be assessed. With the administration of contrast material, assessment of the swallowing mechanism in the lateral position and an evaluation of the anatomic integrity from the oral cavity to the ligament of Treitz should be standard. A small bowel follow-through study generally is not necessary for children less than age 9 years except in the workup of patients for malabsorption.

In cases requiring contrast enema, bowel preparation is dependent on the clinical scenario. Children with potential Hirschsprung disease, for instance, should not be prepared, for the cleansing process could obscure a possible transition zone.

In skeletal radiology obtaining comparison views is recommended only if the observer is confused by the appearance of an epiphysis or ossification center on a certain projection, and should never be obtained on a routine basis.

Radiographs of a hip should always include an evaluation of the entire pelvis. If the pelvis is to be imaged in both a frog lateral and a neutral (AP) projection, one of the exposures should be accompanied by proper gonadal shielding.

Regarding the cervical spine, odontoid views may be difficult to obtain in young children. Fluoroscopy of the area is preferred over repeated attempts or tomography. For children less than the age of 12 years, coned-down views of the skeleton in general are not recommended, particularly in the L5 to S1 region. Oblique views of the spine also are not routinely obtained in children. MR and CT are the modalties of choice in cases in which the standard anteroposterior (AP) and lateral views do not supply adequate information. Concomitantly, in the lumbo-sacral region these views represent the single highest gonadal dose and thus should be avoided whenever possible. A skeletal series to determine child abuse should include at the minimum AP and lateral views of the skull and entire spine and an AP view of the chest, abdomen, and extremities, including the hands. Skeletal maturation is assessed on a single AP view of either hand and wrist in children more than 1 year of age. In infants less than 1 year of age, a single view of the knee suffices.

Cross-sectional imaging deserves special attention in the pediatric age group. Patients seldom require sedation for ultrasound examinations, but particularly active children may require immobilization. In general, children 4 months to 4 years of age should be sedated for CT and MRI. The slice thickness and slice interval must be adjusted from case to case, which is why there is no such thing as a routine cross-sectional imaging study in the pediatric age group. All studies should be monitored by a radiologist. The use of oral contrast is almost always mandatory on CT studies of the abdomen and pelvis, whereas the use of intravenous contrast should be considered routine, especially in cases of abdominal trauma.

Tailored imaging is stressed throughout this book. To achieve this, the imaging team should be familiar with the indications for and limitations of the various imaging modalities, the inherent risks, and expected diagnostic yield. These criteria require communication with the referring physician both before and after the imaging procedure. It requires a *team* effort to render optimum care to children of all ages.

CHAPTER 2

Chest

Imaging Techniques

Conventional Radiographs
Tomography
    Conventional
    Computed
Magnetic Resonance Imaging
Radionuclide Scanning
Ultrasound

Conventional Radiographs

Conventional radiographs of the chest frequently are done with the patient supine in those less than 3 years of age. There is no appreciable difference in magnification between the anteroposterior (AP) supine and the erect AP or posteroanterior (PA) view of the chest in the child less than age 4 years, assuming equal tube or film distance. Proper immobilization is mandatory.

The conventional examination may be expanded by horizontal beam, decubitus, or high-kV technique films. Common clinical indications include quantification of pleural fluid, or determination of the presence and size of a pneumothorax. Frequently in the pediatric patient the use of fluoroscopy is invaluable in assessing the sequelae of check-valve bronchial obstruction and is preferred over inspiration/expiration films or oblique views. In addition, fluoroscopy allows for more accurate localization of some lesions and for dynamic observation of the thymus, hemidiaphragm, mediastinum, and airways (Fig. 2-1).

The gonadal dosage for an AP and lateral view of the chest with proper coning and gonadal shielding is approximately 1 mR. Bronchography is sometimes use-

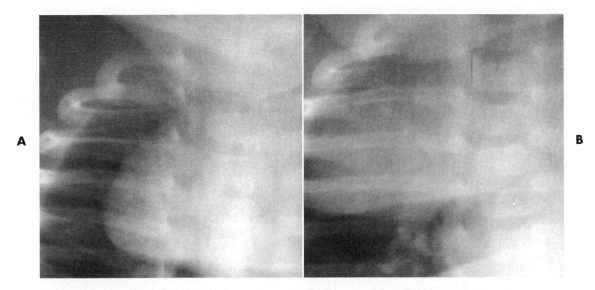

Fig. 2-1 Inspiratory (**A**) and expiratory (**B**) views of thymus confirm its change in shape with respiration.

ful and may elucidate confusing features of a bronchoscopy. High-resolution, thin-section computerized
tomography (CT) has virtually replaced this modality.

Tomography

Conventional tomography is seldom used in the
pediatric age group. Skin dose exceeds 5 rads and
greater detail is obtained by CT.

High-resolution, thin-section *CT* has replaced older
techniques such as 55° oblique tomography for looking
at lung and mediastinal anatomy. It usually requires
sedation in children 4 months to 4 years of age. The
incident radiation skin dose is approximately 2 rad for a
complete examination of the chest.

Tracheal, major bronchial, subpleural, pleural, and
chest wall lesions are evaluated particularly well by CT.
CT is a sensitive and specific modality for detecting pulmonary metastatic disease, and if magnetic resonance
imaging (MRI) is not available, with the aid of subarachnoid contrast instillation, for the evaluation of posterior
mediastinal masses.

Magnetic Resonance Imaging

Gated MRI and magnetic resonance angiography
(MRA) are becoming more widely used in the evaluation of mediastinal vasculature and in the determination
of the extent of masses and may soon make conventional angiography of the pediatric chest obsolete. The
modality is also well suited for characterization of bronchopulmonary foregut malformations. Congenital cardiac lesions and anomalies of the great vessels and of
vascular lesions of the lung clearly comprise the future
realm of MRI.

Radionuclide Imaging

Radionuclide scanning may be used to evaluate for
pulmonary embolism, cardiac structure and function
and inflammatory/neoplastic lesions. These are exten-
sively covered in other volumes in this Requisite
series. Pulmonary embolus is rare in the pediatric population.

Ultrasound

Doppler ultrasound (US) allows evaluation of intravascular access lines, patency of vessels, and/or clot
formation. Cardiac structure and function also can be
assessed exquisitely without the use of contrast or ionizing radiation.

The character of pleural disease, the thymus, and
diaphragmatic motion may be evaluated quickly and
reliably at the bedside by conventional US.

Development of the Lungs and Airway

Structural Development
Functional Development

Structural Development

During the fourth week of gestation, the trachea
first appears as a ventral diverticulum arising from the
foregut. At 5 weeks of gestation, the lobar bronchi
appear, and at 6 weeks, all subsegmental bronchi are
present. By the sixteenth week, all airway branches
are present and contain air sacs, but no alveoli are present. These sacs proliferate during the remainder of
gestation. The right upper lobe bronchus may arise
from the trachea ("pig" bronchus) in .1% of all newborns.

With the first few breaths of life, complete aeration
of the normal newborn chest is accomplished. This
breathing effort has been practiced by the fetus, as can
be seen on prenatal US. This intrauterine fetal respiratory activity occurs at a varied rate and low volume.

Alveoli develop after birth from the air sacs, increasing in number until the age of 8 years. Alveolar size
then increases until growth of the chest wall is complete. Concomitantly, the preacinar vessels (pulmonary arteries and veins) follow the development of
the airway; the intraacinar bronchial vessels follow that
of the alveoli (Table 2-1). The first differentiation of
tracheal cartilage occurs during the fourth week of gestation, and distinct rings of cartilage are present along
the trachea and main bronchi by 11 weeks. The development of cartilage lags behind the branching of the
airways; therefore it does not extend to the periphery
of the airway. The submucosal glands are even slower
to appear than cartilage. Insults (e.g., viruses) to the
lungs in young children affect primarily the terminal
and respiratory bronchioles.

**Table 2-1   Spectrum of pulmonary developmental
anomalies in relation to the pulmonary vasculature
development**

Lung anatomy and vasculature	Resultant condition
Normal lung Abnormal vasculature	Aplastic or hypoplastic lung Arteriovenous malformation Scimitar syndrome
↕	
Abnormal lung Abnormal vasculature	Intralobar or extralobar sequestration (Cystic) adenomatoid malformation
↕	
Abnormal lung Normal vasculature	Bronchogenic cyst Congenital lobar emphysema

Functional Development

The pediatric tracheobronchial tree is not a miniature adult tracheobronchial tree. During development its structure and function are still maturing. The laryngeal tissues are softer and more flaccid and the aryepiglottic folds and arytenoid folds larger and more loosely attached to the underlying cartilage than in adults. Anatomically, the overall size of the peripheral airways is smaller. Physiologically, there is more mucus production per square millimeter in the pediatric airway, and the composition of the mucus differs from that of an adult. The immune system is not as well developed yet; likewise the collateral air circulation through Kohn's pores and the channels of Lambert is not fully operational until 1 year of age, resulting in greater susceptibility to irritants of all kinds and swelling of the interstitium, with increased mucus production. This combination of events may lead the terminal bronchioles either to collapse because of their increased weight or be obstructed by the copious mucus, resulting in "disordered aeration": areas of hyperinflation (air trapping) and atelectasis (hypoaeration).

Physiologically therefore the respiratory cycles of a healthy infant, as compared with those in one suffering from peripheral airway disease, are markedly different. In children with diffuse peripheral airway disease (bronchiolitis) the tidal volume is smaller, and residual volume is significantly higher than normal, resulting in air trapping. This air trapping in severe cases may approach total lung capacity. On radiographs this condition is manifested by hyperinflation, associated with thick (thus visible) bronchial walls and areas of atelectasis. This "peribronchial cuffing" best is seen on the lateral radiograph. The radiographs may also reveal flattened diaphragms, anterior bowing of the sternum, and more "horizontal" ribs (Fig. 2-2).

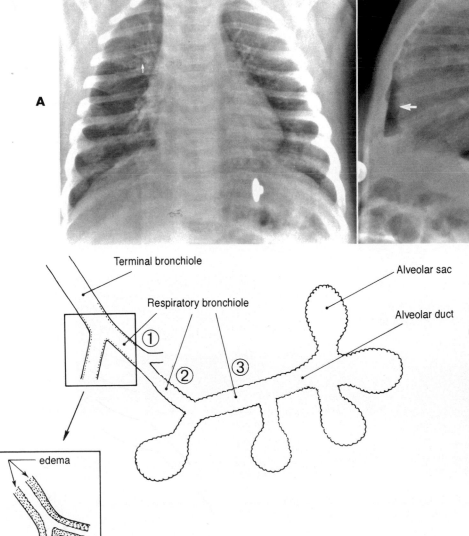

Fig. 2-2 **A**, PA and, **B**, lateral chest radiographs demonstrate flattening of diaphragms and anterior bowing of sternum consistent with hyperinflation: lung is seen "anterior" to the heart (*large arrow*). Increased interstitial markings and evidence of disordered aeration are exemplified by mild hyperinflation of right lower lobe and decreased aeration in right upper lobe (*small arrow*). **C**, Diagram illustrating difference between pediatric and adult airways. Peribronchial thickening caused by edema narrows the effective diameter of the airway, necessitating increased effort at breathing.

UPPER AIRWAY

Pharynx

Normal and variants   The pharynx is divided into the nasopharynx, oropharynx, and hypopharynx. Important nonosseous structures include the components of Waldeyer's ring: the adenoids, the palatine and lingual tonsils, and the retropharyngeal soft tissues. The retropharyngeal soft tissues extend from the adenoids, which are visible by 3 to 6 months of age, to the origin of the esophagus at the level of C4-5. Prominent adenoids become pathologic when they encroach on the nasopharyngeal airway (Fig. 2-3). The palatine tonsils are outlined by air and thus visible on a lateral radiograph only with marked dilation of the hypopharynx. The lingual tonsils are occasionally radiographically visible at the base of the tongue. Measurements of these structures are neither reliable nor useful.

Congenital anomalies   The most common anomaly of the upper airway, choanal atresia, occurs in one of 5000 live births. It is usually present bilaterally and consists of a bony obstruction to air flow in 90% of cases, with membranous obstruction accounting for the other 10%. It is commonly associated with craniofacial anomalies, a tracheoesophageal fistula, and congenital heart disease (CHD). Because neonates are obligate nose breathers, newborns with choanal atresia are seen clinically with respiratory distress immediately after birth. Respiratory distress can be severe if bilateral atresia is present. CT should reveal enlargement of the vomer and fusion of the bony aspects of the pterygoid process and palatine bone (see Fig. 6-10).

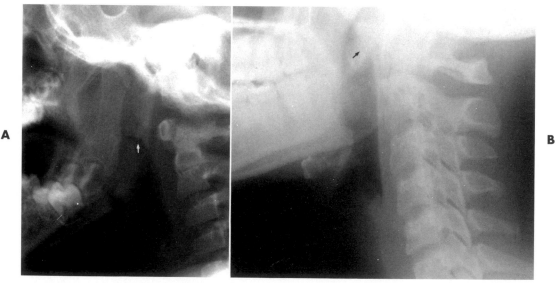

Fig. 2-3   **A,** Adenoidal tissue encroaching on the nasopharyngeal airway (*arrow*). **B,** Normal lateral neck radiograph with the normal adenoidal "pad" (*arrow*).

Tracheobronchomegaly (Mounier-Kuhn syndrome) is of unknown etiology and is rare in children, but a similar disorder has been noted in premature infants, possibly secondary to long-term respirator therapy.

Inflammatory lesions A retropharyngeal abscess is usually seen in children less than 1 year of age, and the most common causative organisms are group B streptococci or staphylococci from the oropharynx. Clinical presentation consists of fever, stiff neck, and dysphagia. Cervical adenopathy is common. Because prevertebral lymph nodes drain the posterior nasal structures, the nasopharynx, and lymphatic tissue in the neck, this is the likely route of infection. On conventional radiographs the presence of air in the retropharyngeal space strongly suggests a retropharyngeal abscess. Dissection of air cephalad from the pleura or mediastinum caused by air block phenomenon of trauma can mimic this finding. After the patient has been properly positioned, lateral fluoroscopy may confirm fixed soft tissue swelling and straightening or reversal of the normal lordotic cervical spine. This fixed soft tissue swelling separates it from the normal respiratory changes of the prevertebral soft tissues seen during inspiration and expiration in the infant. The inflammatory changes may, in turn, result in pseudosubluxation of the C2 or C3 (C3 or C4 less common) vertebra as a result of reversal of the normal lordotic curve.

The differential diagnosis of fixed retropharyngeal soft tissue fullness includes lymphadenopathy, trauma from nasogastric or endotracheal intubation, hemorrhage (hemophilia), neuroblastoma, lymphoma/leukemia, or, rarely, congenital hypothyroidism.

CT imaging is better suited to determine the character and extent of the lesion and may assist in treatment planning (Fig. 2-4).

Larynx

Normal and variants The larynx extends from the base of the tongue to the trachea and is composed of three major cartilaginous structures: the epiglottis, the thyroid cartilage, and cricoid cartilage. There are, in addition, three small paired cartilaginous structures: the arytenoid, cuneiform, and corniculate cartilages. A practical anatomic division of the larynx consists of three regions: (1) a supraglottic region, which contains the epiglottis, aryepiglottic folds, and false vocal cords; (2) a glottic portion, which contains the laryngeal ventricle and the true vocal cords; and (3) a subglottic region, which is immediately distal to the true vocal cords and extends to the lower cricoid cartilage. Calcification in respiratory cartilage, although very rare in children, is pathologic. These rare conditions include chondrodysplasia punctata and relapsing polychondritis.

Other anatomic hallmarks include the hyoid bone, body, and horns, which may be ossified at birth. The horns are oriented in such a way that they "point" to the epiglottis on a conventional lateral radiograph of the neck.

The width of the retropharyngeal soft tissues between C1 and C4-5 should never exceed one half the width of the accompanying vertebral body in children less than 3 years of age. In the first years of life the nor-

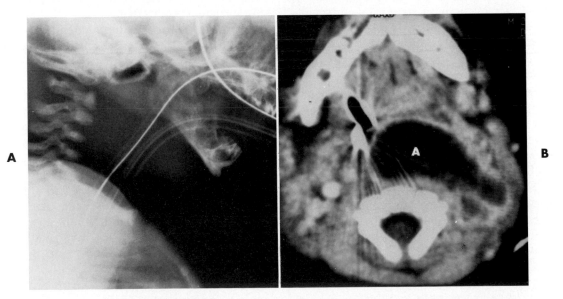

Fig. 2-4   **A,** Lateral radiograph of the neck demonstrates a soft tissue mass encroaching on the airway and esophagus. **B,** CT demonstrates the abscess cavity (A) displacing the nasogastric and endotracheal tube laterally.

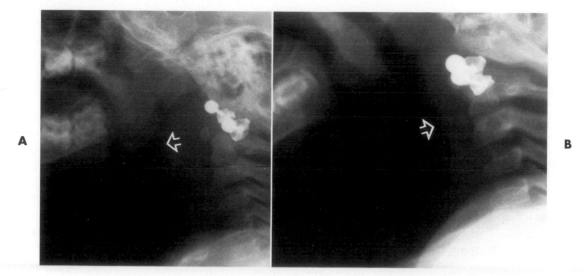

Fig. 2-5   **A,** Arrow demonstrates the prevertebral soft tissue widening on expiration that disappears on inspiration (**B**).

mal respiratory excursion of these soft tissues may mimc a mass. This respiratory motion with widening of the prevertebral soft tissues on expiration can be distinguished from pathologic conditions easily with fluoroscopy (Fig. 2-5).

Supraglottic area

Developmental lesions Developmental lesions are often midline or off-midline structures that present as a mass. Sixty-five percent occur below the level of the hyoid bone, often embedded in the strap muscles. Centrally the differential diagnosis includes a dermoid, thyroglossal duct cyst, or a remula (epithelial retention cyst). Laterally located masses include brachial cleft cysts, hemangiomas, and lymphangiomas (or cystic hygromas). All may occur with significant upper airway obstruction. Two thirds of cystic hygromas that present at birth occur in the posterior cervical triangle. Extension of this lesion into the mediastinum occurs in 10% of cases (Fig. 2-6). Brachial cleft cysts occur in the anterior cervical triangle, most commonly at the angle of the jaw. They are often infected on presentation. Conventional imaging may delineate air, fat, or calcium in these structures.

CT delineates the character of these masses better and assesses bone destruction, whereas MRI has better tissue plane resolution. The most common appearance of these masses is cystic, with a rim of enhancing tissue. The presence of thyroid tissue can be determined by scintigraphy. US may be useful, but its findings are seldom characteristic.

Laryngomalacia (supraglottic hypermobility syndrome) Laryngomalacia is a common cause of inspiratory stridor in the first year of life. It is self-limiting and is characterized by infolding of the aryepiglottic folds, with inspiration leading to collapse and obstruction of the airway (hypermobility). As the arytenoid tissues strengthen and become more firmly attached to the underlying cartilage by 1 to 2 years of age, the hypermobility and resultant stridor resolve spontaneously. This is one of the very few conditions in which stridor improves with increasing activity of the child.

Hereditary angioneurotic edema This autosomal dominant inherited disease is characterized by the deficiency of a C1 esterase inhibitor, which results in vascular damage, increasing permeability, and resultant edema. It affects the airway usually in the first decade and produces stridor in 50% of cases. The stridor can be life threatening. The gastrointestinal (GI) tract or extremities can also be involved in patients suffering from angioneurotic edema.

Acute epiglottitis Acute epiglottitis is most often caused by Haemophilus influenzae type B, and the child initially presents with a high fever, dysphagia, and a sore throat. Clinically the child assumes a bold upright position with the head held forward and the tongue protruding (and panic-stricken eyes)—all the result of the rapidly progressive respiratory obstruction. Peak incidence occurs from 3 to 6 years of age. The condition is treated by intubation, with verification of the diagnosis by endoscopy. Imaging should not be done with the child in a recumbent position or without accompanying qualified personnel. The lateral soft tissue radiograph of the neck will show an enlarged hypopharynx that is caused by a reflex—the tongue goes up, the larynx goes down, and the retropharyngeal soft tissues flatten. In addition, the epiglottis swells and the aryepiglottic folds thicken, with the latter finding the real cause for the stridor and dysphagia. The valleculae are barely identifiable because of the soft tissue swelling of the epiglottis or aryepiglottic

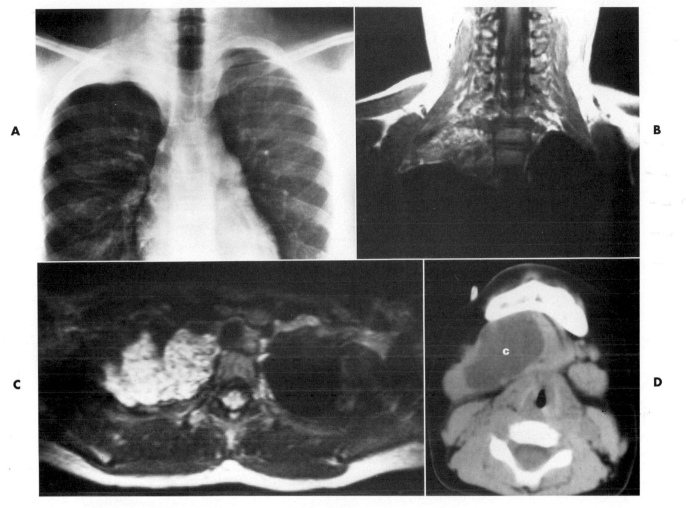

Fig. 2-6 **Cystic hygroma.** **A,** Frontal chest radiograph a reveals right apical soft tissue mass without bony erosion, displacing the trachea to the left. Coronal T1 (**B**) and axial T2 (**C**) MR images delineate the cystic character and extent of this lesion. **D,** CT demonstrating a cystic hygroma (**c**) in a different patient.

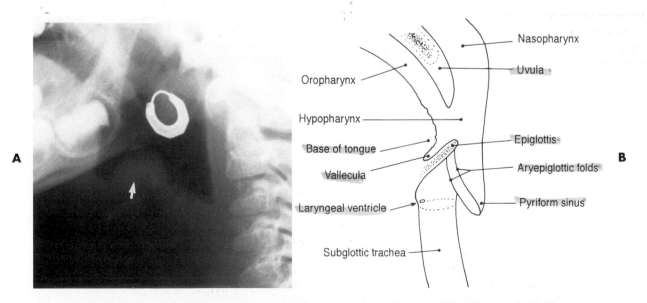

Fig. 2-7 **A,** Lateral radiograph of neck demonstrates the "thumb sign" of acute epiglottitis (*arrow*). Note horns of hyoid bone pointing to the general area of the epiglottis. **B,** Normal anatomy of the upper airway.

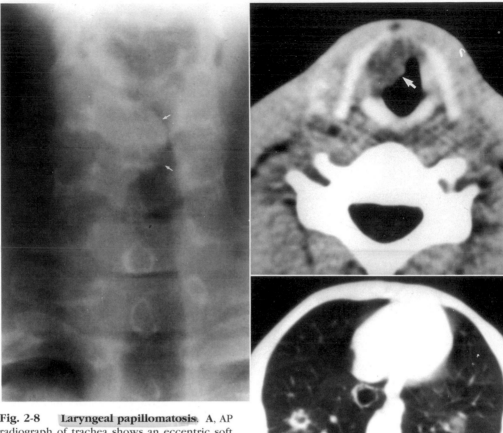

Fig. 2-8   Laryngeal papillomatosis. A, AP radiograph of trachea shows an eccentric soft tissue mass (*arrows*) encroaching on the air column from the right. CT better illustrates the character and extent of this soft tissue lesion (*arrow*) (**B**) and the "metastatic" lesions in the lung (**C**).

folds. Radiographically, this may result in the "thumb" sign (Fig. 2-7). Approximately one fourth of children will also have accompanying subglottic edema indistinguishable from croup.

The differential diagnosis includes angioneurotic edema, epiglottic cysts, or a hematoma secondary to trauma or hemophilia.

Neoplasms   Neoplasms are very uncommon.

Juvenile angiofibroma is a benign, vascular, locally invasive mass located posteriorly in the nasal cavity. It occurs almost exclusively in adolescent boys. It often presents initially with epistaxis (95%) or nasal obstruction (80%). Conventional radiographs of the sinus show anterior bowing of the posterior wall of the maxillary antrum, displacement of the nasal septum, and/or a large soft tissue mass in the nasopharynx that can be associated with body erosion. CT and MRI accurately depict the anatomic extent of the mass and allow for staging. CT demonstrates bony involvement better, but MRI permits differentiation between sinus extension of the tumor and obstruction of the sinus by tumor (i.e.,

different echo characterization) (see Fig. 6-12). Preoperative embolization of this highly vascular structure is recommended. Recurrence rate after resection is 25% to 30%.

The most common *malignant neoplasm* is an embryonal rhabdomyosarcoma that grows rapidly and infiltrates and metastasizes widely. Hodgkin lymphoma is the second most common malignant neoplasm. MRI is the modality of choice to delineate the extent of the lesion.

Glottic region   Developmental lesions are rare and include laryngeal web, laryngocele, and laryngeal papillomatosis and most often present with stridor.

A membranous or cartilaginous *web* results from failure of recanalization of the larynx in fetal week 10. It most often involves the anterior portion of the vocal cords, and the child has crouplike symptoms.

A *laryngocele* rarely occurs but arises from the laryngeal ventricle, is air filled, and extends into the soft tissues laterally. The child presents with inspiratory stridor.

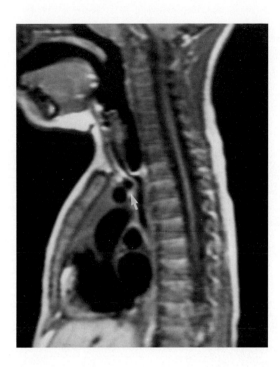

Fig. 2-9   T1 sagittal MR illustrating the innominate artery (*arrow*) causing an anterior impression of the trachea.

Papillomatosis is a clinically aggressive but histologically benign lesion that is seen in a child before age 7 to 10 years. It is the most common laryngeal tumor. The lesions may prolapse into the subglottic region or, seldom, metastasize to the lungs (Fig. 2-8). A viral cause has been suggested. Human papillomavirus and maternal condyloma acuminatum of the cervix or vagina have been reported in parents of half of these children.

Subglottic region

Tracheomalacia (soft trachea)   In the normal infant, tracheal "buckling" occurs anteriorly to the right (because the aortic arch is present on the left). The caliber of the trachea does not change. A "soft trachea" may be caused by weak supporting cartilage and/or muscles of the trachea. It can be caused by intrinsic or extrinsic causes. The latter is more common. The severity of clinical features varies, depending on the cause. Expiratory or, at times, biphasic stridor is the clinical hallmark as a result of tracheal collapse.

Primary tracheomalacia can be caused by chondromalacia, polychondritis, or prematurity or may be idiopathic. Secondary tracheomalacia usually is caused by congenital anomalies such as vascular rings or mediastinal masses.

If the innominate artery originates to the left of the trachea, a normal variant that occurs in 30% of all infants, the superior mediastinum at the level of the thoracic inlet can become crowded. The innominate artery can then compress the trachea during its oblique ascent into the mediastinum and neck. Fluoroscopy, endoscopy, CT, or MRI can all aid in establishing the degree and extent of tracheal compromise. There may be an association with esophageal atresia and tracheoesophageal fistula, which may indicate that segmental tracheomalacia (inflammation or tracheal underdevelopment) may also be present. The decision to intervene must be weighed against the fact that as the infant grows older, more room develops in the thoracic inlet and the indentation may disappear. Aortopexy has been advocated to alleviate this "crowded" superior mediastinum if symptoms warrant (Fig. 2-9).

Another vascular indentation of the trachea may be caused by a double aortic arch, which is the most common vascular ring and may be associated with congenital heart disease. It is caused by persistence of both the right and left primitive aortic arch, resulting in a true vascular ring encircling the trachea and esophagus, with characteristic impressions on both, which are readily seen using fluoroscopy with contrast (barium) in the esophagus see Fig. 3-15. The posterior indentation, because the right posterior arch is the larger of the two, is usually the most prominent.

Other conditions, including a right aortic arch, or a pulmonary "sling," occurring when the left pulmonary artery arises from the right pulmonary artery and crosses between the trachea and the esophagus and a high (cervical) aortic arch, have also been implicated as rare causes for tracheomalacia.

Primary tracheal stenosis   *Primary* tracheal steno-

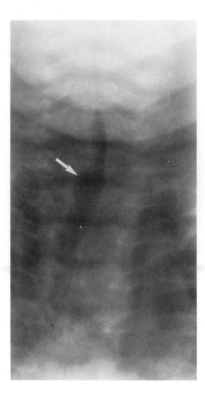

Fig. 2-10   AP radiograph of the trachea demonstrating an eccentric, asymmetric soft tissue mass encroaching on the subglottic trachea: a hemangioma (*arrow*).

sis is almost always a lethal condition caused by intact tracheal rings (i.e., rings not open posteriorly). The diagnosis usually is made with bronchoscopy, although conventional radiographs of the chest may show a narrow trachea in both directions. The condition usually is associated with vascular rings, pulmonary sling, or H-type tracheoesophageal fistulas.

Secondary tracheal stenosis Subglottic hemangioma is the most common soft tissue mass causing respiratory tract obstruction in the first 3 months of life. It is accompanied by dyspnea, a "croupy" cough, and stridor. There is a 50% association with cutaneous hemangiomas. The mass is usually eccentric and asymmetric and deforms the subglottic portion of the trachea on AP conventional radiographs (Fig. 2-10). Endoscopy is indicated to confirm the diagnosis, and laser excision is the current treatment of choice.

Acute laryngotracheobronchitis *(croup)* is the most common cause of upper airway obstruction in children. It most commonly occurs between 6 months and 3 years of age. The condition is usually viral in origin (most common offenders: parainfluenza and respiratory syncytial virus [RSV]). The child has upper respiratory symptoms, a "barking" cough, and stridor. The condition is usually self-limited to 3 to 7 days duration. It is unusual for a child with croup to require intubation and hospitalization. There is a seasonal component in children less than age 2 years, who are afflicted more frequently in fall and winter. Effective imaging (Fig. 2-11) includes a lateral soft tissue radiograph of the neck that demonstrates distention of the hypopharynx, a normal epiglottis, and (symmetric) subglottic narrowing. Because the trachea should not change in diameter from the false vocal cords to the thoracic inlet, the subglottic narrowing is obvious. This examination also allows exclusion of foreign body or retropharyngeal abscess as the cause for the symptoms. On the AP radiograph, symmetric narrowing of the subglottic region can be noted in croup but may also occur with normal respiration. Often chest radiographs obtained at the same time will reveal bronchiolitic changes, most often hyperinflation.

Foreign bodies that lodge in the airway cause a crouplike picture clinically. If it is radiopaque, identification on conventional radiographs is the rule. Fluoroscopy for nonopaque foreign bodies may demonstrate a check-valve mechanism with resultant overinflation of the involved lung segment and mediastinal shift away from the affected side on expiration. Decubitus views and an expiration film may be difficult to interpret. The affected lung, when dependent, *should* remain inflated. Endoscopic removal of the foreign body is the rule.

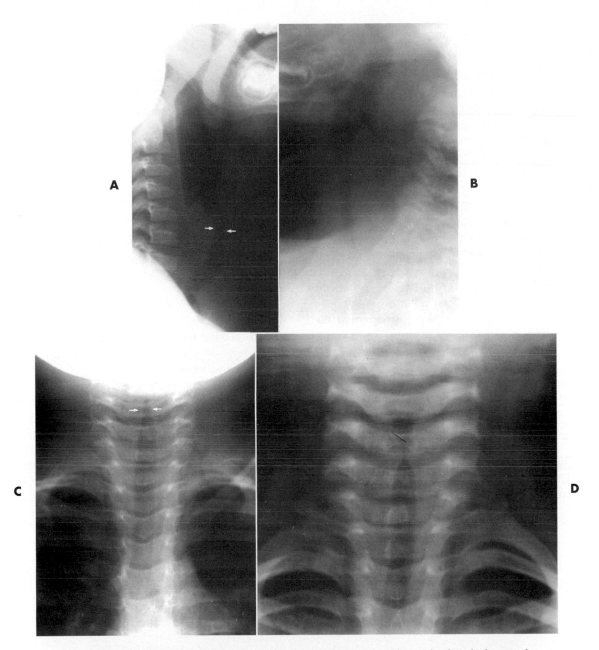

Fig. 2-11 The subglottic region. **A**, Croup: lateral soft tissue radiograph of neck shows subglottic narrowing (*arrows*). **B**, The normal subglottic trachea does not change in its anteroposterior diameter from thoracic inlet to the vocal cords. AP radiograph (**C**) reveals symmetric subglottic narrowing (*arrows*), often referred to as "steepling" in croup. **D**, The normal "bordeaux bottle" appearance of the subglottic region.

THORACIC SKELETON

Developmental Aspects
Systemic Involvement
Neoplasms

Developmental Aspects

At least five ossification centers of the sternum should be present at 6 months of life. There should be one main ossification center for the manubrium and the first sternal segment, whereas the other segments consist of variably paired centers. The first three are ossified at birth. Hypersegmentation is seen in 85% of children with Down syndrome. Early fusion is seen in 50% of children with cyanotic CHD but can be seen normally in 15% of patients. It may result in pectus carinatum (pigeon breast). Pectus excavatum (funnel breast) occurs in approximately 1% of the general population and is more common in boys than girls. Most children are asymptomatic.

The clavicle may contain a prominent rhomboid fossa in the inferior mediastinal aspect at the site where the sternoclavicular ligament attaches. In addition, its medial growth plate is the last epiphysis to close at approximately 16 years. The midclavicular nerve canal also is often identified on the inferior aspect. Absence of the clavicle is seen in cleidocranial dysostosis.

Failure of descent of the scapula (Sprengel's deformity) is accompanied by persistence of a ligament, occasionally ossified (omohyoid bone), extending from the spine to the scapula. There are often associated vertebral segmentation anomalies (Fig. 2-12), a condition known as *Klippel-Feil syndrome*. It may be associated with congenital deafness and renal agenesis.

The ribs may show segmentation abnormalities and may be fused or bifid. Proximal (medial) fractures should lead to suspicion for child abuse.

Systemic Involvement

Expansile lesions of the ribs include Langerhans' cell histiocytosis and multiple hereditary osteochondromatosis. Expansion of an entire rib may occur in secondary involvement of the ribs in systemic conditions such as hyperparathyroidism, sickle cell disease or thalassemia, and the mucopolysaccharidoses. Hyperostosis of the ribs is seen in Caffey disease, a rare entity. Erosion of the ribs may occur in neurofibromatosis (ribbon rib) and as a result of collateral circulation as a result of coarctation of the aorta.

Neoplasms

Tumors of the chest wall are extremely rare. Soft tissue masses (lipomas, fibromas, sarcomas) are slightly more common and may arise from the cutaneous or subcutaneous tissues. Tumors related to the skeletal system can be benign or malignant. The benign lesions include multiple hereditary exostoses. Langerhans' cell histocytosis have been mentioned previously. However, most skeletal tumors in children are of the malignant variety.

In the thorax, the most common first degree skeletal lesion is Ewing sarcoma. A variant of Ewing sarcoma is the primitive neuroectodermal tumor (PNET), which simulates it clinically, histologically, and radiographically. Askin first described this lesion of the thoracic wall, which contained rhabdoid elements, in adolescent girls. Metastatic disease may include neuroblastoma, Ewing sarcoma, and leukemia or lymphoma. Imaging

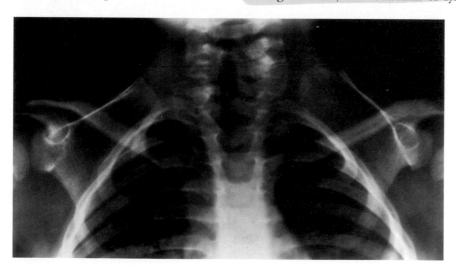

Fig. 2-12 AP radiograph of chest demonstrates segmentation anomalies of cervicothoracic junction (Klippel-Feil syndrome) and failure of descent of both scapulae (Sprengel's deformity). (See also Fig. 6-52).

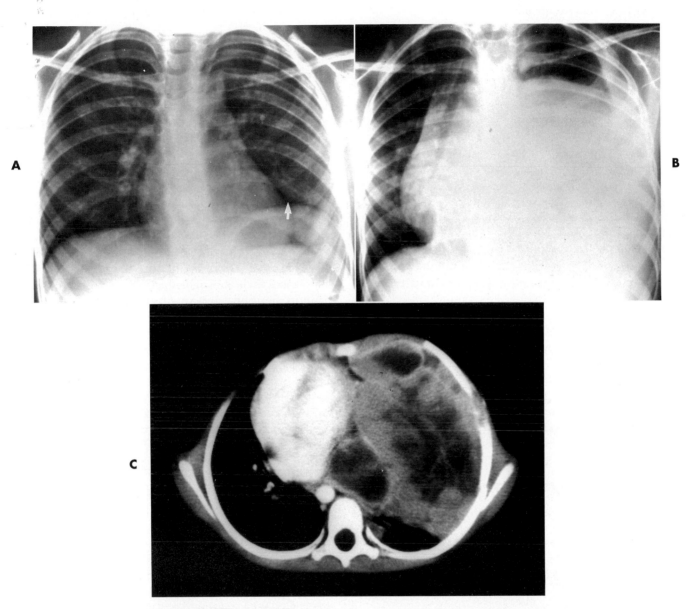

Fig. 2-13 PNET. A, AP radiograph of the chest reveals mild splinting on the left and a moth-eaten appearance of the ninth rib posteriorly (*arrow*). Three months later (**B**) a large soft tissue mass displaces the mediastinum to the right. **C,** CT demonstrates extent of lesion.

may reveal rib destruction, a pleural-based soft tissue mass, and/or a pleural effusion. CT is the modality of choice to delineate the extent (Fig. 2-13).

LUNG

Developmental Anomalies
> Primary anomalies
>> Agenesis of the lung
>> Lobar underdevelopment
> Secondary anomalies
>> Congenital diaphragmatic hernia
>> Accessory fissures and lobes
> Congenital (cystic) masses
>> Sequestration
>> Congenital cystic adenomatoid malformation
>> Congenital lobar emphysema
>> Bronchogenic cysts
>> Neurenteric cysts
>> Pulmonary arteriovenous malformation

Neonatal Chest
> Hyaline membrane disease, respiratory distress syndrome
> Transient tachypnea of the newborn (retained fetal lung liquid)
> Meconium aspiration
> Neonatal pneumonia
> Pulmonary lymphangiectasia
> Persistent fetal circulation

Inflammatory Lung Disease
> Bacterial causes
>> Chlamydia trachomatis pneumonia
>> Pertussis pneumonia
> Viral etiologies
>> Mycoplasma pneumoniae
> Mycobacterial infection
>> Tuberculosis
> Other infections
>> Pulmonary mycosis
>> Opportunistic infections
>>> *Pneumocystis carinii* infection
>>> Varicella (chickenpox)
>>> Aspergillosis
> Aspiration pneumonia
> Asthma

Cystic Lung Disease
> Cystic fibrosis
> Kartagener's syndrome
> Bronchiectasis
> Swyer-James syndrome
> Cysts
>> Solitary cysts
>> Multiple cysts
>> Bilateral cysts

Lung Neoplasms
> Malignant neoplasms
> Benign neoplasms

Miscellaneous Diffuse Interstitial Lung Diseases
> Chronic granulomatous disease of childhood
> Sarcoidosis
> AIDS
> Primary pulmonary histiocytosis X

Developmental Anomalies

Primary anomalies

Agenesis of the lung. Agenesis of the lung is a very uncommon lesion in which there is a single lung with alveolar number and size equivalent to that of two lungs. The number of airways equals that of a single lung (Fig. 2-14).

Lobar underdevelopment Agenesis (no pulmonary bud or artery), aplasia, or hypoplasia almost always involves the right lung. Hypoplasia is manifested by a decrease in volume, by a decrease in the size of the pulmonary artery, and by shift of the mediastinal structures to the right. There is usually compensatory hyperinflation (overgrowth?) of the contralateral (left) lung and loss of the (right) heart border. A retrosternal "band" may be seen in children with pulmonary hypoplasia on the lateral radiograph, believed caused by extrapleural areolar tissue taking the place of the "missing" lung tissue (Fig. 2-15). It has also been erroneously referred to as an "accessory" hemidiaphragm.

Pulmonary hypoplasia usually is an incidental and insignificant anomaly except when it is part of the scimitar syndrome (Fig. 2-16), the "pulmonary venolobar" syndrome. This syndrome comprises hypoplasia or aplasia of one or more lobes of the right lung, with partial anomalous pulmonary venous return below the diaphragm, an absent or small pulmonary artery, and occasional rib and vertebral body anomalies. It is slightly more common in girls (1.4:1) and may be inherited. On imaging, the conventional chest radiograph may reveal the anomalous vein draining medially and inferiorly into the inferior vena cava in proximity to the right hemidiaphragm. This venous structure may have the shape of a Turkish sword (scimitar) and may be associated with the tetrad of Fallot or truncus arteriosus and hemivertebrae, with resultant scoliosis. An atrial septal defect occurs in 25% of these children (see Table 2-1). The differential diagnosis of pulmonary hypoplasia includes Swyer-James syndrome, effects of radiation therapy, scoliosis, or aspiration of toxic substances with pulmonary necrosis.

Secondary anomalies

Congenital diaphragmatic hernia. Impaired development of the airways and resultant pulmonary

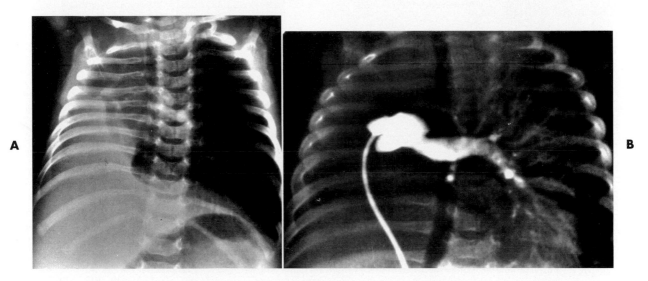

Fig. 2-14   Agenesis of the lung. **A**, An AP radiograph reveals a mediastinal shift to the right and an over-expanded left lung. **B**, Pulmonary angiogram demonstrates a normal left pulmonary artery with no evidence of a right pulmonary artery.

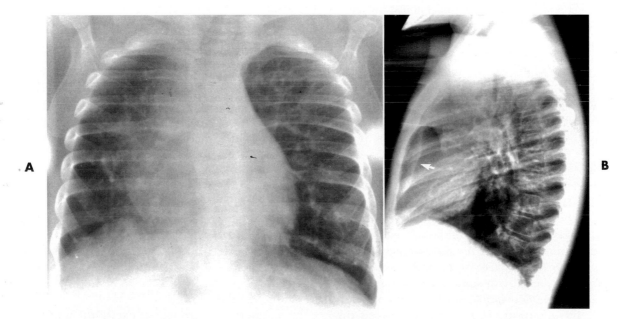

Fig. 2-15   Hypoplasia of the lung. **A**, An AP radiograph reveals shift of the mediastinum to the right due to decreased right lung volume, evidenced by increased inter-rib distance on the right as compared to the left. A retrosternal band (*arrow*) is the attempt by extrapleural areolar tissue to fill in the empty space (**B**).

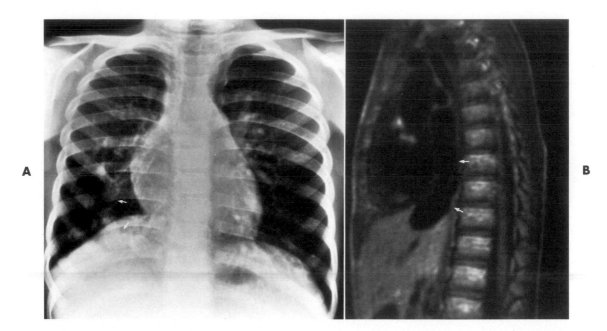

Fig. 2-16   Scimitar syndrome. **A**, AP radiograph demonstrates decreased right lung volume and a tubular structure (*arrows*) coursing inferomedially below the diaphragm. **B**, Partial anomalous pulmonary venous return is confirmed on MRI by the flow void in the anomalous venous channel (*arrows*).

hypoplasia may be caused by the mechanical presence of bowel in the thorax, which occurs through a defect in the diaphragm, the pleuroperitoneal foramen. This condition occurs in one in 2500 live births (M:F, 2:1).

Prenatal US often detects the hernia. There is hope that in utero palliation may improve the outcome for children with this condition. Postnatal conventional radiographs are also often diagnostic (Fig. 2-17), especially if swallowed air has entered the loops of the intestine.

Associated anomalies include neural tube defects (in 30%), malrotation (in 95%), and cardiovascular anomalies (in 20%). The severity of the lung hypoplasia depends on the amount of bowel in the hemithorax and on the embryological timing of the herniation.

This herniation occurs on the left side 75% of the time. Contralateral hypoplasia of the lung is frequently present, probably because of some degree of lung compression from the mediastinal shift. Extracorporeal membrane oxygenation (ECMO) has improved the prognosis only marginally. The overall mortality rate remains at approximately 50% in most centers.

Overall, a posterior Bochdalek's herniation occurs in 85% of affected children (*back* of diaphragm, *big babies*). A herniation through the foramen of Morgagni occurs in 3% to 5% (*middle* of diaphragm, *mature, miniscule baby*). These are more common on the right; the heart "protects" on the left.

Acquired hypoplasia can also be caused by bronchiolitis obliterans (in Swyer-James or MacLeod syndrome). A viral lower respiratory tract infection leads to destruction and scarring of bronchi and bronchioles, eventually resulting in a small hyperlucent lung on conventional chest radiographs (Fig. 2-18). Other causes of acquired pulmonary hypoplasia are rare and may include thromboembolism with infarction of the lung (Westermark's sign), postradiation therapy, severe dehydration, or nephrotic syndrome.

Accessory fissures and lobes   A fissure caused by the azygos vein is a common entity and results in part of the upper lobe separated from itself by the azygos vein within two layers of pleura, the so-called "azygos lobe."

The medial part of the lower lobe may be separated by a more-or-less vertical inferior fissure, creating an inferior lobe, usually on the right side behind or adjacent to the right atrium.

A superior fissure may separate the apical segment from the rest of the left lower lobe at approximately the level of the minor fissure on the right.

Congenital (cystic) masses   Masses of congenital origin can be solid, cystic, or mixed lesions that usually become clinically apparent when they become infected or cause respiratory distress.

Sequestration   Pulmonary sequestration, accessory lung, and bronchopulmonary foregut malformation

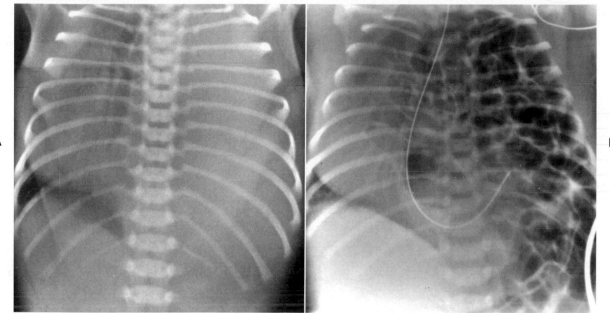

Fig. 2-17   Diaphagmatic hernia. **A,** There is a large left hemithorax mass shifting mediastinal structures to the right in a newborn with respiratory distress. After insertion of nasogastric tube, bowel contents occupying left hemithorax confirm the diagnosis (**B**).

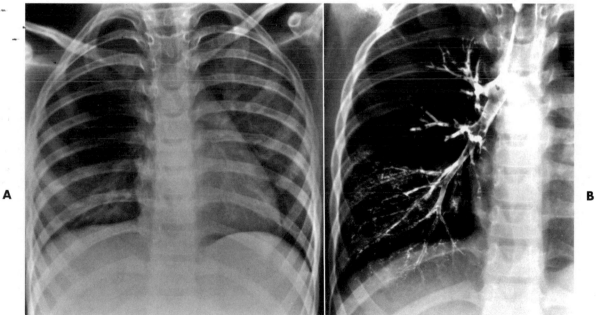

Fig. 2-18   Swyer-James syndrome. **A,** Unilateral hyperlucent right upper lung with overall low right lung volume. **B,** Bronchography confirms obliterated lung tissue in right upper and middle lobes.

probably all describe the same entity. Sequestration is defined as a congenital mass of aberrant pulmonary tissue that has no normal connection with the bronchial tree or with the pulmonary arterial system. The lung parenchyma may be normal or dysplastic. The most common vascular supply is through persistent fetal vessels with a variable venous drainage. The intralobar and extralobar variants can be differentiated most reliably on the basis of venous drainage. Intralobar drainage occurs mainly through the left atrium or pulmonary veins; extralobar drainage is mainly through the systemic venous plexus, including the inferior vena cava or azygos system. Both types usually are supplied by systemic arteries arising from the aorta or its branches, often from below the diaphragm. The majority of sequestrations are intralobar; relatively few are extralobar. Commonly, an *intralobar* sequestration is supplied by a large systemic vessel, is contained within the lung and has no separate pleural covering, occurs on the left side 60% of the time, and is initially seen in teenagers. An *extralobar* sequestration often is supplied by a small vessel, has its own pleural covering, occurs on the left side, and occurs in boys 90% of the time. It often causes symptoms in the first month of life. A sequestration is usually located in the posterior basilar segments of the lower lobes and is occasionally bilateral. Gastroenteric communication is not common. Conventional radiographs may show either recurrent lower lobe consolidation that never totally clears or cysts. MRI often delineates the vascular supply; US may do so (Fig. 2-19). Complete surgical removal to treat recurrent infection is the therapy of choice; if no symptoms are present, removal is not necessary.

Congenital cystic adenomatoid malformation

Congenital cystic adenomatoid malformation (CCAM) is characterized by anomalous fetal development of terminal respiratory structures. This results in a dysplastic, multicystic mass with a variable amount of proliferating bronchial structures. These cysts then interfere with alveolar development. A CCAM often enlarges after birth, presents in the first month of life (70%) as a cause of respiratory distress, and has an equal gender distribution. It is most often unilobar, and 90% of children with this condition present before age 1 year with increasing respiratory distress. CCAM can be divided into three types: (1) single or multiple air-filled cysts, often more than 2 cm in size (most common); (2) cysts smaller than 2 cm mixed with solid tissue; and (3) a solitary solid mass (rare). Appearance on chest radiographs depends on air replacing fluid in the cysts as they communicate with the airway. These findings may mimic staphylococcal pneumonia or diaphragmatic hernia (Fig. 2-20). Surgical lobectomy is curative in type 1; but in types 2 and 3, the lesions are large, and the prognosis parallels that of a diaphragmatic hernia in terms of morbidity and mortality (40%). Prenatal US detection has improved morbidity and mortality.

Congenital lobar emphysema

The presumed cause of congenital lobar emphysema (CLE), a progressive overdistention of a lobe, includes bronchial cartilage deficiency, dysplasia, or immaturity, which in turn may be caused either by an intrinsic cartilage anomaly or by compression by an extrinsic vascular structure or mass (e.g., bronchogenic cyst). The pulmonary tissue may be emphysematous or associated with an increase in number of alveoli. Destruction of alveolar walls may occur if infection occurs. A child with CLE presents

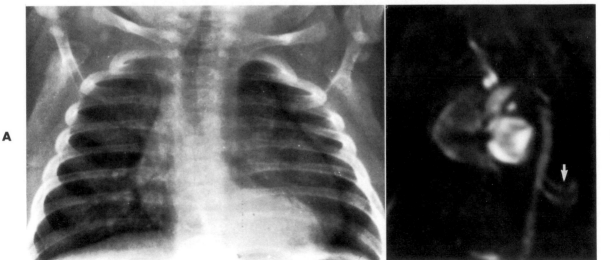

Fig. 2-19   Sequestration. **A,** Frontal radiograph demonstrates a left lower lobe consolidation that persisted more than 4 weeks despite appropriate therapy. **B,** MR angiography reveals the vascular supply of the sequestration (*arrow*) on coronal lateral projection.

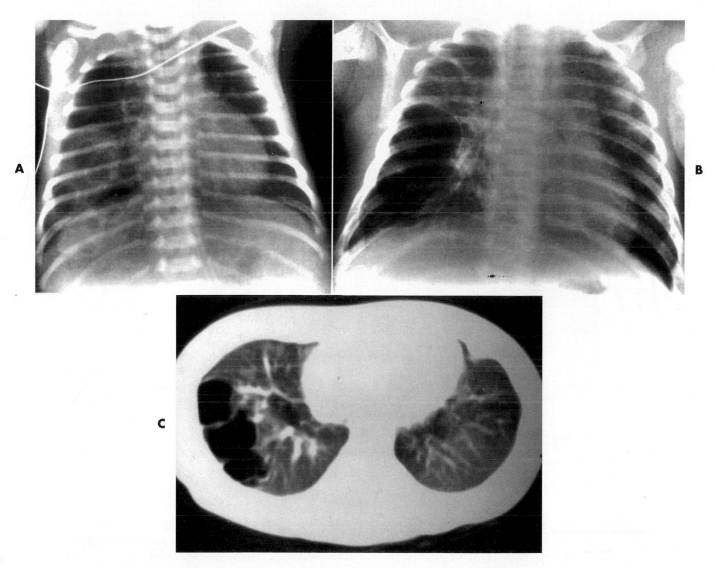

Fig. 2-20   CCAM. A, At birth, several cystic lesions, as well as solid components, are seen in the right lower lobe. One month later (**B**), multiple enlarging cysts are seen in right lower lobe, confirmed on CT (**C**). At surgery: CCAM, type I.

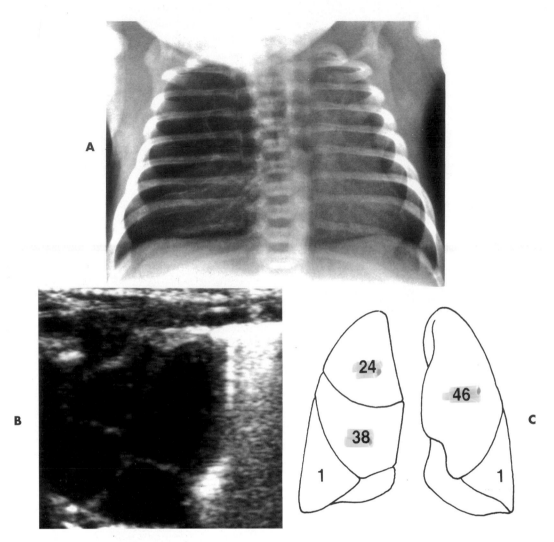

Fig. 2-21   **CLE**. **A**, AP radiograph at 2 weeks of age demonstrates hyperaerated right upper lobe with mass effect on lower lung and mediastinum causing it to shift to the left. **B**, US evaluation of this area at birth had revealed a fluid-filled lesion. **C**, Relative lobar incidence of CLE. (After Hendren WH, McKee DN: J ped surg 1:24, 1966.)

with respiratory distress in the first 6 months of life. CLE occurs in boys three times more often than girls. It involves the upper lobes in two thirds of patients, the left lobe twice as often as the right, and the right middle lobe in approximately 30% of patients (Fig. 2-21). There is an associated ventricular septal defect (VSD) or patent ductus arteriosus (PDA) in 15% of these patients. The radiograpic appearance depends on the resorption of the fetal lung fluid. The lesion thus may range from solid to reticular to hyperlucent with mass effect. Lower lobe involvement is rare (1%). Definitive treatment is surgical resection in acute cases of respiratory distress.

Bronchogenic cysts   Bronchogenic cysts are believed caused by abnormal ectopic bronchial bud-

ding during lung development. They usually do not communicate with the airway and consist of an oval or round lesion, frequently incidentally noted unless the child is in respiratory distress or the lesion becomes infected. There is an equal gender incidence. Bronchogenic cysts may contain serous or mucus material and cartilage rests and are twice as often located in the lower lobes, more common on right. Most are located in relation to the airway (often the carina). Fewer are located within the lung. This variation in location depends on the timing of the abnormal budding: an early event results in a mediastinal lesion; a late event results in an intraparenchymal lesion.

Imaging confirmed an oval or round mass that is cystic on CT and with characteristically high T2 contents

LUL > RML > RLL

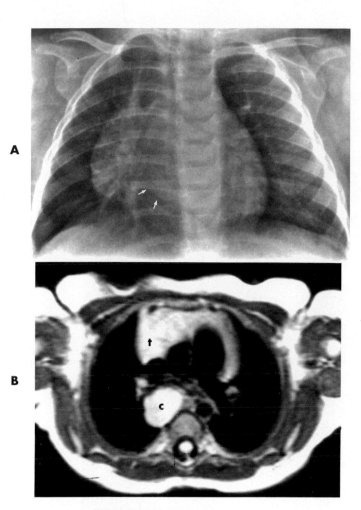

A

B

Fig. 2-22 **Brochongenic cyst**: **A**, Slightly oblique radiograph of the chest reveals a subcarinal mass (*arrows*). **B**, T2-weighted MR confirms the cystic nature (*c*). Note thymus (*t*).

on MRI (see Fig. 2-22). These lesions may grow, either because of recurrent infection or secretions. If growth and thus symptoms occur, they are often resected.

Neurenteric cysts Neurenteric cysts occur when there is failure of complete separation of the pulmonary from the notochordal (primitive neural crest) structures during the third week of gestation. Occasionally, there is communication with the enteric canal by the fibrous band or canal (neurenteric canal of Kovalevsky). Vertebral anomalies are almost always seen, including hemivertebrae, anterior spina bifida, or butterfly vertebrae. Thus a posterior mediastinal mass with dysraphic changes is pathognomonic for this lesion. More than 50% of the children with this condition present with neurologic symptoms, and imaging is definitive, with MRI showing a cyst containing fluid consistent with cerebrospinal fluid (CSF) signal.

The differential diagnostic possibilities of cystic or solid thoracic lesions include cystic, solid adenomatoid malformation; the brochopulmonary foregut malformations, including sequestration, neurenteric or bron-

chogenic cysts, as well as diaphragmatic hernia, CCAM, and congenital lobar emphysema.

Pulmonary arteriovenous malformation A pulmonary arteriovenous malformation may be single or multiple (40%), with the remaining 60% occurring in patients with herditary hemorrhagic telangiectasia (Osler-Weber-Rendu disease). The children may initially be seen with cyanosis, dyspnea, or hemoptysis, clubbing, and polycythemia. The malformations most often are in a subpleural location and are best diagnosed on CT or MRA.

Neonatal Chest

Hyaline membrane disease, respiratory distress syndrome Hyaline membrane disease (HMD) is the most common cause of respiratory distress in the neonatal period. It almost always occurs in premature infants, although infants of diabetic mothers and those born by cesarean section are occasionally at risk. The imaging findings consist of underinflated lungs resulting from generalized air sac atelectasis. In the premature infant approximately 95% of the surface of the air sacs is covered by type I pneumocytes where air exchange occurs and 5% by type II pneumocytes, which contain osmiophilic lamellar inclusion bodies that are responsible for the synthesis and storage of a lipoprotein, pulmonary surfactant. Pulmonary surfactant lowers the surface tension in the air sacs, increases pulmonary compliance, and thus decreases the work of breathing. The ability of air sacs to stay distended is also part of the "driving force" preventing pulmonary edema (Starling forces). Surfactant synthesis begins at 24 to 28 weeks gestation, and it gradually increases until full gestation. It is the lack of surfactant and resulting poor compliance of the lungs that causes debris consisting of damaged or desquamated cells, exudative necrosis, and mucus (protein seepage) to line the alveolar sacs. This lining stains like hyaline cartilage under the microscope; hence the term *hyaline membrane disease*. A decreased lecithin:sphingomyelin ratio is present in infants lacking surfactant and is a useful prenatal indicator to predict the development of HMD. Clinically, these infants are seen in the first few hours of life and weigh less than 1500 grams. Girls outnumber boys by 2:1. Respiratory distress beginning after 8 hours of life makes the presence of HMD very unlikely.

Conventional radiographs show the typical ground-glass (finely granular) appearance of the lungs, low lung volumes, poor definition of the vessels, and a bell-shaped thorax. Air bronchograms may extend to the periphery. Low lung volumes can also be seen in infants with neonatal pneumonia or pulmonary hemorrhage or edema, whereas hyperinflation in nonventilated infants virtually excludes HMD. An effusion is sel-

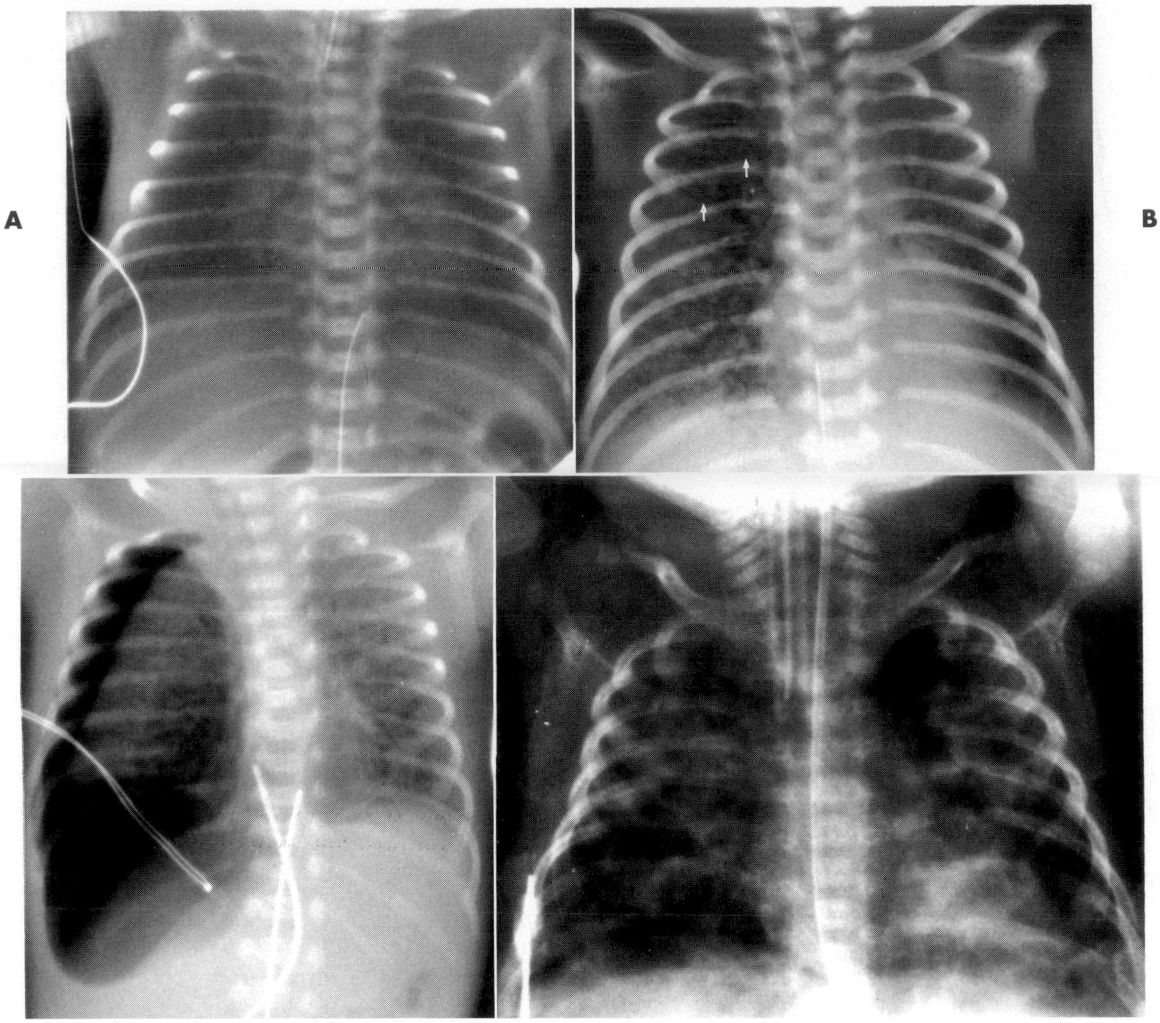

Fig. 2-23   **A,** Typical "ground-glass" appearance of the lungs in 27-week gestation infant: hyaline membrane disease (HMD) **B,** Pulmonary interstitial emphysema (*arrows*) in right hemithorax, generalized atelectasis with air bronchograms almost to the periphery on left. **C,** Right-sided pneumothorax. **D,** Dysplastic changes of pulmonary parenchyma bilaterally in a 1-month-old former 28-week gestation infant colon: bronchopulmonary dysplasia (BPD). Proper ETT level is 1 to 2 cm above the carina.

dom present, and the lung findings are generalized (Fig. 2-23). To prevent acidosis and hypoxemia, these diseased lungs must be ventilated and oxygenated to maintain open terminal air sacs and maintain arterial oxygen levels. Positive pressure ventilation (positive end-expiratory pressure [PEEP], continuous positive airway pressure [CPAP]) is often instituted through an endotracheal tube. The "classic" HMD lung with low volumes often become a hyperinflated lung at this juncture. From this moment the imaging findings of HMD are the result of the complications of therapy.

In addition to supportive therapy with oxygen and diuretics, providing exogenous surfactant replacement may result in increased pulmonary compliance and gas exchange. The effect on the chest radiography is variable. Clinical improvement, even after one administered dose, has been reported and may be evident as clearing of the lung fields on chest radiographs.

Complications of ventilatory therapy include the following. Overdistention of the air sacs in poorly compliant lungs may lead to their rupture and a subsequent leak of air into the pulmonary interstitium. This is evident as pulmonary interstitial emphysema (PIE). It may develop as early as the first 24 hours of life when it carries a poor prognosis. Usually occurring on day 2 or 3 of life, PIE is characterized by peripheral streaks or bubbles of air in the interstitium, presumably the lymphatics, and can be unilateral or bilateral and asymptomatic. The air may migrate centrally, resulting in a pneumomediastinum, or peripherally and rupture into the

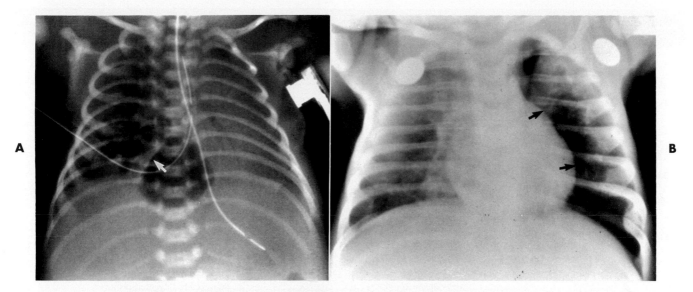

Fig. 2-24   **A,** Extraalveolar air collection outlines inferior pulmonary ligament (*arrow*). **B,** "Sharp-mediastinum" sign caused by a medial pneumothorax (*arrows*).

pleural space, resulting in a pneumothorax. Because these infants are supine and because air rises to the highest point of the thorax, a pneumothorax will be located paramediastinally, resulting in the "sharp mediastinum sign." It may also dissect along the hemidiaphragms and may dissect into the neck. The distinction from a pneumopericardium is made by recalling that pericardial air can only rise as high as the pericardial reflection at the level of the pulmonary arteries. Extraalveolar air collections may also be identified adjacent to the inferior pulmonary ligament (Fig. 2-24).

The ductus arterosus may remain patent (PDA) in these patients. This complication may become clinically evident at approximately 5 to 7 days. Increased interstitial markings caused by congestive failure secondary to persistent fetal circulation may be difficult to appreciate superimposed on the radiographic findings of HMD.

After 28 days of ventilatory support, due to the cummulative effect of the therapeutic insults to the pulmonary parenchyma, interstitial fibrosis will result. It often is accompanied by exudative necrosis and a honeycomb appearance to the lungs on chest radiographs, a condition known as *respiratory distress syndrome (RDS),* referred to by most as bronchopulmonary dysplasia (BPD).

BPD was originally defined as occurring when a premature newborn is treated with high oxygen concentration for more than 150 continuous hours under high pressure (CPAP, PEEP) by a respirator, resulting in injury to the lungs at the cellular level. After the initial destruction of the type I alveolar lining epithelium, with mucosal necrosis, peribronchial edema, and hem-

orrhage, the result over time is a clinical and radiographic picture of interstital edema, fibrosis, and emphysematous or atelectatic changes. By 4 weeks (28 days) of age, these changes are considered chronic and in the presence of oxygen dependency and respiratory symptoms, comprise the syndrome of BPD (see Fig. 2-23).

The radiographic appearance of BPD was classified into four stages, analogous to pathologic changes. The classification reflects the course of the insults caused by the treatment of immature lungs; however, it is of little practical use and is seldom used today:

- Stage I—represents the classic granularity described as ground glass at birth
- Stage II—develops at 4 to 10 days of age, producing a bilateral increased density caused by exudative necrosis
- Stage III—develops at 10 to 20 days of age, characterized by honeycomb appearance caused by overdistention of alveoli and terminal air sacs within dysplastic interstitium
- Stage IV—develops after 1 month of age, with fibrotic changes and scattered emphysematous, even cystic, changes; is associated with a mortality rate of 40% to 50%

If the infant survives, the appearance of the chest radiograph improves and may in fact be normal by 3 to 5 years of age in approximately 10% of patients. Pulmonary function studies, however, remain abnormal, and there is an increased incidence of lower respiratory tract infection.

Wilson-Mikity syndrome is rarely seen in premature infants and is characterized by respiratory symptoms at 2 to 4 weeks of age. Chest radiographs are normal at birth but reveal the typical changes indistinguishable

Table 2-2 Neonatal chest entities

	Hyaline membrane disease	Transient tachypnea of the newborn	Meconium aspiration	Neonatal pneumonia
Typical patient	Premature	Term Cesarean section	Postterm Meconium stained	Premature rupture of membranes
Time course	Within hours	24-48 hr	12-24 hr	Onset <6 hr
Lung volume	↓	±↑	±↑	↑
Imaging characteristics	Ground glass, granular	Interstitial "edema"	Coarse, nodular, asymmetric	Perihilar, "streaking"
Effusions	No	Yes	No	Maybe
Complications	Pulmonary interstitial emphysema or pneumothorax, Respiratory distress syndrome, patent ductus arteriosus	None	Persistent fetal circulation, extracorporeal membrane oxygenation (ECMO)	Sepsis, ECMO

Table 2-2 summarizes the causes of respiratory distress in neonates.

from RDS by 6 weeks. It is believed caused by injury of the air sacs by room air as opposed to high oxygen concentration or toxicity. Viral causes have also been suggested. Those that survive (50% to 70%) exhibit complete resolution of the radiographic findings by 1 year of age. Table 2-2 summarizes the causes of respiratory distress in neonates.

Retained fetal lung liquid (transient tachypnea of the newborn) The fetal lung is filled with fluid that contributes to the amniotic fluid. During delivery, part of this fluid is expressed into the airways, part is coughed or suctioned out, and part of it is resorbed by the lymphatics and the pulmonary veins. Delay of this process leads to difficulty breathing, clinically evident as respiratory distress in the newborn. This lung fluid clearing process can be quantified as cleared by the "birth canal squeeze" of the infant thorax during delivery (30%), resorbed by lymphatics (30%), and resorbed by capillaries (40%). Impairment of any of these mechanisms can result in a so–called "wet lung." Cesarean section, prolonged labor, maternal anesthesia or diabetes, and a precipitous delivery are all potential culprits. The infant is tachypnic during the first 6 hours of life, with a peak of symptoms at 1 day of age and a return to normal by 48 hours. Mild cyanosis, retraction, and grunting can occur. There is an equal gender distribution. Conventional chest radiographs may show a mildly enlarged cardiothymic silhouette, interstitial edema, fluid within the fissures, and small pleural effusions (Fig. 2-25). The lungs are hyperinflated and start to clear at 12 hours. This process should be complete and result in a normal chest radiograph by 48

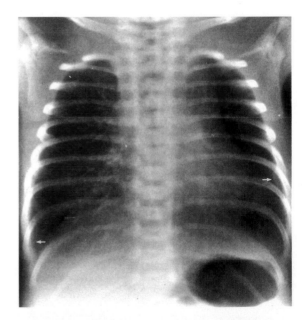

Fig. 2-25 Transient tachypnea of the newborn as evidence by hyperinflation, mild interstitial prominence, bilateral small effusions (*arrows*); all clearing by 48 hours after birth.

hours after birth. Differential diagnostic possibilities include CHD with congestive heart failure (CHF), pneumonia or aspiration, hypervolemia, or persistent fetal circulation (PFC).

Meconium aspiration Approximately 10% of all term deliveries are accompanied by meconium staining of the amniotic fluid. Aspiration of the meconium-containing fluid results in meconium's presence below the level of the vocal cords in approximately 1% of neonates. Meconium aspiration is related to perinatal stress (hypoxia, prolonged labor), with a vagal response postulated as the triggering factor for intrauterine evacuation of meconium by the fetus.

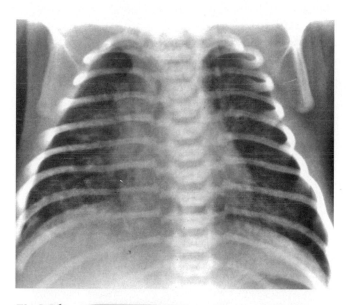

Fig.2-26 Meconium aspiration resulting in an asymmetric, somewhat nodular pattern in both lung fields in addition to areas of mild hyperaeration (*right apex*).

Concomitant fetal gasping caused by the intrauterine distress may facilitate the aspiration.

The aspirated meconium particles can produce bronchial obstruction, air trapping, and chemical pneumonitis. Conventional radiographs of the chest will reveal bilateral asymmetric areas of atelectasis and hyperaeration caused by a partial check-valve mechanism of the aspirate of meconium and by the irritative effect of meconium. The lungs are often hyperinflated, and there may be a concomitant pneumomediastinum or pneumothorax in approximately 25% of patients (Fig. 2-26).

Treatment is supportive and consists of antibiotics and oxygen. In severe cases when oxygenation cannot be maintained by the infant, ECMO is instituted to allow healing of the pneumonitis and to impove oxygenation. Meconium aspiration is often complicated by PFC.

Neonatal pneumonia Neonatal pneumonia can be acquired in utero or perinatally. Prolonged labor, premature rupture of membranes, placental infection, and ascending infection from the perineum are predisposing factors. Respiratory distress with tachypnea and metabolic acidosis (occasionally progressing to shock) is the most common clinical scenario. The most common caustive agent is group B β–hemolytic streptococcal infection acquired in the birth canal. Other causative agents are *Pseudomonas, Enterobacter, Staphylococcus, or Klebsiella.* The incidence of neonatal pneumonia is approximately one in 200 live births. Transplacentally acquired infections are rare.

The radiologic appearance is often identical to that of transient tachypnea of the newborn (TTN) or early HMD. A patchy, occasionally asymmetric, bilateral interstitial infiltrate is common (Fig. 2-27). A nodular pattern may predominate in hazy lungs, and an effusion is a common occurrence. Empyemas may develop and

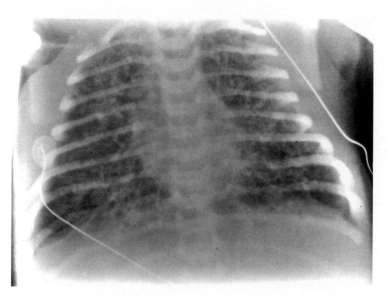

Fig. 2-27 **Neonatal pneumonia.** Bilateral, coarse interstitial infiltrate may occasionally be nodular.

suggest staphylococcal or *Klebsiella* infection. Untreated, the mortality and morbidity rates are high; thus early confirmation of the diagnosis to allow appropriate antibiotic therapy is critical.

Pulmonary lymphangiectasia   Pulmonary lymphangiectasia is characterized by dilated lymph channels. Lymph channels in utero regress to their expected neonatal caliber during 6 to 20 weeks gestation. This process may be interfered with by pulmonary venous obstruction or result from a developmental anomaly. Approximately one third of cases occur in association with congenital cardiac defects that cause pulmonary venous obstruction (e.g., total anomalous pulmonary venous return [TAPVR], hypoplastic left heart syndrome). Conventional radiographs mimic the changes of TTN and may have a more nodular pattern. The condition is often fatal early in life.

Persistent fetal circulation   PFC, a physiologic event of right-to-left shunting persisting after birth, has no clear cause. Increased sensitivity to intrauterine hypoxia, altered fetal pulmonary flow, and arterial muscle derangement have been implicated. It also may be a transition phenomenon similar to TTN in which time and maturation allow eventual return of the pulmonary circulation to normal as the high intrapulmonary pressure diminishes. Any of the neonatal pulmonary abnormalities discussed previously can be associated with PFC, likely secondary to increased pulmonary (interstitial) vascular resistance (pressure).

Inflammatory Lung Disease

Bacterial causes   Bacterial infection tends to cause alveolar exudates, lobar and segmental consolidations, and effusions. Most commonly caused by *Pneumococcus, Haemophilus influenzae* type b, and *Staphylococcus aureus*, these conditions clinically have little to distinguish them from each other.

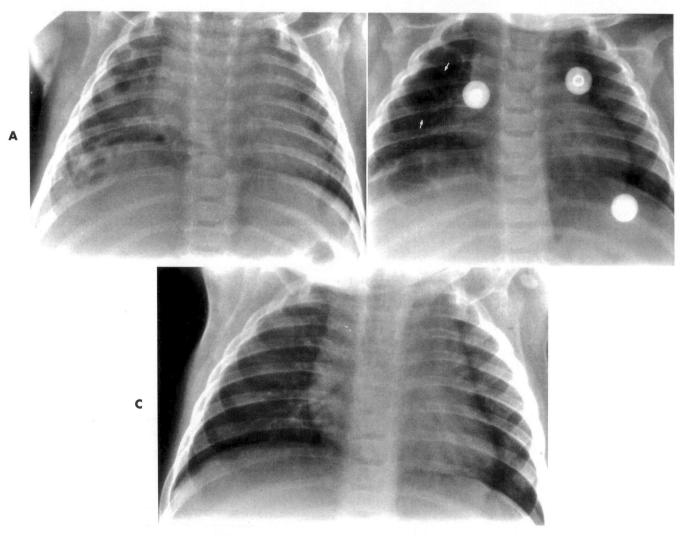

Fig. 2-28   Staphylococcal pneumonia shows progressive clearing of the consolidation with pneumatocele formation (*arrows*) (**A, B**) within 1 week, then clearing totally by 6 weeks (**C**).

Staphylococcal pneumonia occurs more commonly in early infancy, *H. influenzae* pneumonia most often between 6 and 12 months, and pneumococcal pneumonia more commonly from 1 to 3 years of age. Children with these pneumonias present with cough, chest pain, and often high fever, usually occurring after an upper respiratory infection. Staphylococcal pneumonia and *H. influenzae* pneumonia can also be complicated by the development of empyema. Pneumatoceles develop in 50% of patients with staphylococcal infection and are believed a form of PIE and local emphysema caused by airway obstruction and subsequent check-valve mechanism . They are often multiple but resolve completely in approximately 6 weeks (Fig. 2-28). Pneumatoceles are less likely to occur with streptococci.

Imaging is not usually helpful in determining the organism. Consolidation is usually lobar, may be accompanied by air bronchograms, and resolve in 2 or 3 weeks. Staphylococcal or pneumococcal pneumonia bacteria sometimes are spherical in children less than 8 years of age, with unsharp edges. This appearance can mimic that of a metastatic lesion and is called a "round pneumonia" (Fig. 2-29). It resolves completely after proper antimicrobial therapy. It probably results from centrifugal spread of the multiplying organisms through Kohn's pores and the channels of Lambert. Imaging may differentiate a complicating empyema from a sterile effusion in that an empyema will not change with position but free fluid should. CT may be able to demonstrate an enhancing ring around the empyema.

Chlamydia trachomatis pneumonia Pneumonia caused by *Chlamydia trachomatis* fits neither the bacterial nor the viral group. It is probably an obligate intracellular parasite and occurs as a neonatal infection acquired after passage of the fetus through the cervix and vagina. The infant at 3 to 6 weeks of age has respiratory symptoms and occasional associated pulmonary hemorrhage and often (30%) has developed chlamydial conjunctivitis. Clinical and radiologic findings are similar to viral bronchiolitis with diffuse perihilar interstitial involvement (Fig. 2-30). Effusions may occur; consolidations are rare.

Pertussis pneumonia Pneumonia resulting from pertussis is a contagious disease most common in children less than age 5 years. Latin for *severe cough* and

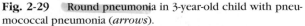

Fig. 2-29 Round pneumonia in 3-year-old child with pneumococcal pneumonia (*arrows*).

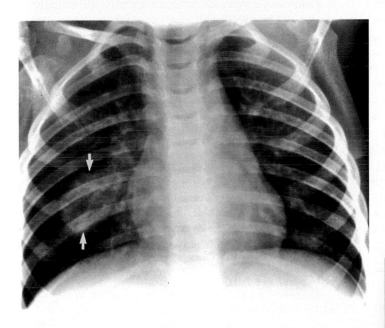

Fig. 2-30 Perihilar, diffuse interstitial infiltrates resulting in the "shaggy heart" sometimes seen in pertussis and *Chlamydia trachomatis* infection.

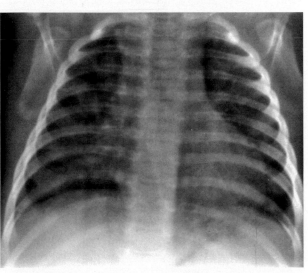

Chinese for *100 days*, it is caused by *Bordetella pertussis* and occurs more commonly in girls. Conventional radiographs reveal streaky perihilar infiltrates with (most often) unilateral hilar adenopathy, sometimes called the "shaggy" heart appearance.

Viral causes As noted, air space disease, either segmental or lobar, usually is bacterial in origin. Airway disease that manifests itself by peribronchial thickening, hyperinflation, and scattered atelectasis ("disordered aeration") more likely will be viral in origin.

In the age group less than 2 years, viral infection, most commonly with respiratory syncytial virus (RSV), parainfluenza types 1, 2, and 3, influenza, and adenovirus leads to inflammatory edema, surface cell necrosis, and increased mucus production. Radiographs of the chest show peribronchial cuffing and hyperinflation, a reflection of the airway involvement yet sparing of the air spaces. Often there are clear manifestations of disordered aeration—areas of atelectasis that, if sequential films were obtained, would be seen to clear within 24 to 48 hours and may reappear in other areas within the chest (see Fig. 2-2). The apices are spared; effusions and empyemas are rare. Resolution can take up to 2 weeks. After 2 years of age, this radiographic appearance is characteristic of reactive airway disease (asthma). Cystic fibrosis should be considered if repeated episodes of bronchiolitis occur in the appropriate patient population.

Mycoplasma pneumoniae Mycoplasma pneumoniae is a ubiquitous agent that causes epidemics of respiratory infection, primarily in older school-age children and adolescents. Of those infected, 50% get tracheobronchitis, 30% develop pneumonia, and in 10% each, pharyngitis and otitis media may occur. Clinically, symptoms are less severe but more common than with true bacterial pneumonias. Chest radiographs may reveal segmental, subsegmental, or reticulonodular insterstitial infiltrates. Lobar involvement is seen predominantly in the lower lobes. Effusions occur in approximately 20% of patients. Treatment is supportive and recovery slow.

Mycobacterial Infection

Tuberculosis Primary tuberculosis caused by *Mycobacterium tuberculosis* initially affects the lung but may spread throughout the body. Almost all cases, in infants and young children, begin in the lung parenchyma after exposure by inhalation. Initially, there is an exudate that, after 3 to 8 weeks as hypersensitivity develops, is followed by hilar and mediastinal nodal enlargement. Caseation and calcification, as well as parenchymal scarring, may ensue. Radiographically, this infiltrative process with local lymphatic and node involvement and parenchymal scarring is called the *primary complex of Ranke*. With the development of resistance, postprimary tuberculosis develops, with

consolidation of an entire segment or lobe, central lymph node enlargement, and pleural effusions and pulmonary cavitation. Seeding of organisms in the lungs through lymphatics and the venous system results in miliary (secondary) tuberculosis (2- to 3-mm nodules). The differential diagnosis of miliary nodular interstitial disease is listed in the box.

Other infections

Pulmonary mycosis Pulmonary mycotic infections are relatively rare in children except in endemic areas. Histoplasmosis is endemic in the midcentral United States, whereas coccidiomycosis is endemic in the southwestern United States. Radiographic findings are often lacking but clinically may be similar to those of primary tuberculosis, with characteristic hilar and mediastinal adenopathy and miliary granulomas in the pulmonary interstitium after 3 to 5 days. In children with histoplasmosis late calcification of the parenchyma and nodes is common. Effusions are rare.

Opportunistic infections In the patient with an altered immune response state (e.g., acquired immune deficiency syndrome [AIDS], or after chemotherapy for leukemia or lymphoma or transplant surgery), *Pneumocystis carinii* pneumonia, varicella, and fungal (mucormycosis, histoplasmosis) etiologies are more common.

P. carinii (a protozoa) *infection* occurs in debilitated or otherwise immunocompromised children and is seen most often in those treated for leukemia or lymphoma. The child clinically has a cough, tachypnea, and malaise, and the infection is often fatal. It is the most common opportunistic pulmonary infection in children with AIDS. Lung biopsy is necessary to confirm the diagnosis. Early chest radiographs may mimic those for a child with a respiratory viral infection, and then may progress from a reticulonodular interstitial process to a diffuse alveolar consolidation predominantly affecting the hila and bases. Lung volumes are normal to low. Pleural effusions may occur, but hilar adenopathy is uncommon (Fig. 2-32).

Differential Diagnosis of Miliary Nodular Interstitial Disease (Fig. 2-31)

Tuberculosis

Histoplasmosis, blastomycosis, cryptococcosis, and coccidiomycosis

Varicella (air space disease rare)

Lymphoid interstitial pneumontis (LIP), (human immunodeficiency virus[HIV]-positive mother)

Langerhans' cell histiocytosis (Hand-Schüller-Christian disease)

Metastatic thyroid carcinoma

Niemann-Pick disease or Gaucher disease (rare)

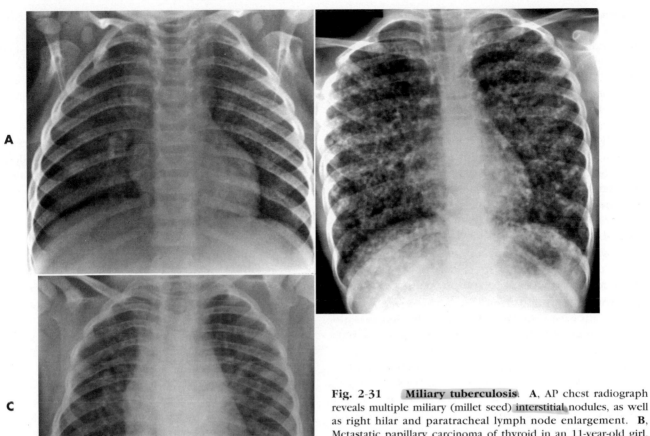

Fig. 2-31   Miliary tuberculosis. A, AP chest radiograph reveals multiple miliary (millet seed) interstitial nodules, as well as right hilar and paratracheal lymph node enlargement. **B,** Metastatic papillary carcinoma of thyroid in an 11-year-old girl. Note deviation of the trachea to the right. **C,** LIP: Lymphoid interstitial pneumonitis (biopsy proven).

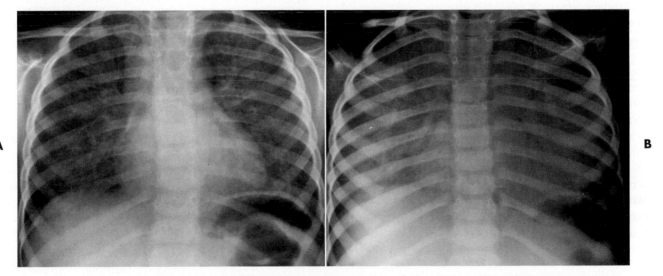

Fig. 2-32   A, *P. carinii* manifests as a diffuse reticular granular infiltrate bilaterally, progressing **(B)** to consolidation without hilar enlargement but with an effusion.

Varicella (chickenpox) is a highly contagious viral disease of childhood, with mortality highest in adults and the immunocompromised host. Clinically, cough, fever, and a vesicular rash are generally accompanied by mild constitutional symptoms. Air space disease (1%) associated with chickenpox in children occurs most often in the immunocompromised host. The younger the child, the less likely chickenpox complicated by air space disease will develop. Radiographs of the chest reveal initially nodular infiltrates that may progress to large segmental areas of patchy consolidation, predominantly in the bases and perihilar regions. Total clearing is virtually guaranteed, although punctate calcifications may occur within 2 years of the illness and persist through life.

Aspergillosis is one of the more common sporadic infections that frequently affect children with underlying conditions such as asthma, cystic fibrosis, or chronic granulomatous disease of childhood. It may be (1) a primary invasive process; (2) a suprainfection in a preexisting cavitary lesion; or (3) a hypersensitivity response.

Radiographs of the chest of the first two variants are characterized by air space disease consisting of mucus plugs with distal atelectasis, often involving several lobes. Cavitation may then occur. In such a cavity a "mycetoma" may form, consisting of aspergillosis spores. This condition is very rare in children. Hypersensitivity or allergic aspergillosis will mimic the imaging findings of bronchiolitis.

Aspiration pneumonia often mimics ordinary pneumonia, may lead to superimposed infection, may be acute or chronic, and may have either no respiratory effect at all or have fulminant pulmonary involvement. The effect depends to a large degree on what, how much, and how long the child aspirates. Aspiration is gravity dependent. If an infant (supine) aspirates, the right upper lobe and right lower lobe are common sites of involvement. If the (older) child is more vertical when aspiration occurs, the lower lobes will be predominantly affected. Chest radiographic findings range from normal to patchy air space consolidation, with or without confluent areas, to atelectasis or a mixture of both. Perihilar peribronchial involvement is also common, mimicking bronchiolitis. Effusions are rare.

In the diagnostic workup of a child with aspiration pneumonitis, it is important to search for an anatomic anomaly such as gastroesophageal reflux, an abnormal connection (e.g., tracheoesophageal fistula, cleft) between the trachea and esophagus or a swallowing dysfunction. To search for the anomalous connection between the esophagus and the trachea, the child should be evaluated in the prone position, using a nasogastric tube that is withdrawn at small increments while barium is injected. An upper gastrointestinal

examination (see Chapter 3) is useful to evaluate for the other two etiologies.

Populations at risk for aspiration pneumonia include anesthetized children, near-drowning victims, and those with convulsions (postictal). Hydrocarbon or lipid pneumonias can be the evidence that aspiration has occurred.

Asthma (reactive airway disease) is a common, diffuse, chronic lung disease characterized by hypersensitivity of the airways to a variety of stimuli (allergens, exercise, irritants such as smoke) that is IgE mediated. This results in recurrent bouts of wheezing, cough, and dyspnea, due to bronchospasm. Approximately 50% of children with asthma become symptomatic before 2 years of age, with 80% to 90% diagnosed by age 5 years. Chest imaging may reveal hyperaeration with peribronchial thickening or demonstrate complications, including atelectasis, effusions, pneumothorax, or pneumomediastinum. Most often the chest radiograph is normal (see Fig. 2-2).

Cystic Lung Disease

Cystic fibrosis   Cystic fibrosis (CF) is inherited as a single autosomal recessive trait. It is the most common semilethal genetic disease affecting Caucasians. This generalized dysfunction of the exocrine (mucous) glands affects approximately one out of 1500 Caucasian individuals. It is very uncommon in blacks (1:20,000) and Orientals (even less). Patients may have respiratory symptoms at all ages, although in a small group (approximately 5%) the earliest symptoms—meconium ileus, malabsorption, and failure to thrive—are related to the GI tract.

Pulmonary involvement, ranging from bronchiolitis in infants, chronic cough and recurrent respiratory infections in older children, and chronic pulmonary disease in adolescents, eventually occurs in almost all patients. Fatigue and weight loss from malabsorption and recurrent infections eventually develop. When respiratory insufficiency and progressive pulmonary arterial hypertension supervene, death usually occurs by the fourth decade, primarily because of pulmonary complications, including pulmonary hemorrhage.

Imaging findings on chest radiographs range initially from a completely normal radiograph to findings indistinguishable from those of bronchiolitis. Often there is hyperinflation, and when progressive mucus plugging with superimposed infection injures the pulmonary parenchyma, bronchial wall thickening, mucoid impaction, and resultant bronchiectatic cavities located predominantly in the upper lobes appear. Reactive nodal enlargement caused by recurrent bouts of infection are evidenced by prominent hilar regions (Fig. 2-33). The latter are due to reactive nodal hyperplasia

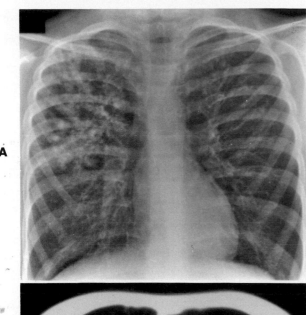

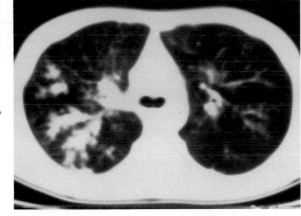

Fig. 2-33   CF. A, Chest radiograph with classic upper lobe bronchiectatic changes with a superimposed *P. aeruginosa* infection in the right upper lobe. **B,** CT examination confirms these changes.

caused by the recurrent infections (first due to *S. aureu,* later due to *Pseudomonas aeruginosa*) in the early stages of CF but eventually can also be attributed to large pulmonary arteries that are the result of developing pulmonary arterial hypertension.

Complications include pneumothorax, occasionally of the tension variety, that has only a 65% chance of being evacuated by chest tube. In addition, lobar atelectasis and pulmonary hypertension with cor pulmonale frequently occur. Bronchial artery hemorrhage is a grave complication, and the findings of cardiac silhouette enlargement in a patient with CF is ominous for the development of CHF.

In the evaluation of chest radiographs a number of scoring methods have been devised, with the method of Brassfield (0 = normal, 4 = severe changes) most often used. This scoring system correlates well with pulmonary function tests, clinical criteria, and morbidity and has a high degree of interobserver reproducibility.

Kartagener's syndrome   Kartagener's syndrome, an autosomal recessive entity, is characterized by thoracic and abdominal situs inversus and by the presence of immotile cilia that predispose to sinusitis, otitis media, and bronchiectasis. The ciliar immotility is due to a deficiency of the dynein arms of the cilia. Immotile cilia are also present in the inner ear and seminiferous tubules, leading to deafness and infertility. Imaging frequently suggests the diagnosis by matching two or more of these components. With a history of infertility or deafness, the diagnosis is confirmed.

Bronchiectasis   Localized bronchiectasis is most often caused by postinfectious causes such as tuberculosis (TB), viral or bacterial pneumonias, measles or is secondary to infections superimposed on immunodeficiency syndromes. It is less common than in the past because of improved medical therapy. Bronchography occasionally is useful, but thin-section high-resolution CT is preferred. It can reliably differentiate between cylindrical (tubular dilation), varicose (resembling varicose veins), or cystic or saccular (balloonlike dilation) types of bronchiectasis (see Fig. 2-33). An association of bronchiectasis with tracheal ectasia ("tracheobronchomegaly") and defective elastic tissue has been described (Mounier-Kuhn syndrome).

Swyer-James syndrome   Idiopathic unilateral hyperlucent lung (Swyer-James or Macleod's syndrome) is characterized by unilateral hyperlucency of the lung associated with a decrease in the number and size of the airways and pulmonary vessels. It is believed caused by a preceding viral pneumonitis that progresses to a necrotizing bronchiolitis. The resultant fibrosis produces bronchiolitis obliterans, manifested on chest radiographs by hyperlucency, diminished lung markings, and a lung often decreased in size (see Fig. 2-18).

The differential diagnosis of a unilateral hyperlucent lung includes endobronchial foreign body, pneumothorax, congenital lobar emphysema, hypoplasia of the lung or pulmonary artery and compensatory hyperinflation, and postradiation therapy shrinkage of the lungs.

Cysts

Solitary cysts   Solitary cysts include a pneumatocele (from staphylococci, tuberculosis, trauma), inflammatory (from staphylococci, Klebsiella), pulmonary foregut malformation, and bronchogenic or neurenteric cysts. Necrotic tumor is a rare occurrence, as are echinococcal cysts.

Multiple cysts   Multiple cysts often are caused by multiple occurrences of the above causes. A diaphragmatic hernia in neonates may be seen as multiple cysts once air replaces fluid after birth.

Bilateral cysts   Bilateral cystic lesions may be seen

with BPD (PIE, pneumatoceles), cystic fibrosis, septic emboli, and cavitary metastatic disease (papillomatosis, metastatic osteosarcoma, or rarely Wilms tumor). Very rare causes include Wegener granulomatosis and hyperimmunoglobulinemia E syndrome (Buckley syndrome), the latter characterized by skin lesions and abdominal abscesses.

Lung Neoplasms

Malignant neoplasms Metastatic disease to the lung is far more common than a primary lung tumor, with Wilms tumor the most common primary neoplasm during childhood. Osteosarcoma and Ewing sarcoma follow in incidence. Osteogenic sarcoma and rhabdomyosarcoma may be associated with pneumothorax or effusion. Primary malignant lung tumors are extremely rare and are often sarcomatous in origin.

Benign neoplasms Rare benign neoplastic lesions include pulmonary blastoma, bronchial adenoma, hamartoma, or a hemangioma. The carcinoid type of bronchial adenomas is more common then the salivary type. Approximately one half exhibit low-grade malignant characterization. The majority of them are located in the (right) mainstem bronchi and often present as a foreign body, with or without hemoptysis. Hamartomas or granulomas (e.g., TB, histoplasmosis) do occur, but postinflammatory pseudotumors (e.g., plasma cell granulomas) are rare. Arteriovenous malformations and hemangiomas are extremely rare in childhood. Bronchogenic cysts located in the parenchyma may appear as lung masses that seldom contain calcium and may be solid or air filled, depending on the degree of communication with the airways.

Miscellaneous Diffuse Interstitial Lung Diseases

Chronic granulomatous disease Chronic granulomatous disease of childhood is an X-linked recessive disorder that usually occurs before the age of 3 years, is rare, and presents with increased susceptibility to infection by normally nonpathogenic organisms, lymphadenopathy, hepatosplenomegaly, and pneumonia. The pathophysiology rests in an enzymatic defect that prohibits intracellular killing of bacteria and fungi. Granuloma formation in lung, liver, lymph nodes, and the wall of the GI tract can cause symptoms as well. Radiographs of the chest may reveal hilar enlargement, hepatomegaly, or antral or esophageal narrowing demonstrated after the administration of oral contrast.

Sarcoidosis Although relatively rare in children, sarcoidosis does occur between the ages of 5 and 15 years, predominantly in the black population without

Pulmonary Nodules

SOLITARY PULMONARY NODULES

Congenital
Bronchogenic cyst
Arteriovenous (AV) malformation or varix (lower lobes)
Sequestration

Inflammatory
Round pneumonia
Abscess
Granuloma (tuberculosis, fungal)
Plasma cell granuloma

Neoplastic
Bronchial adenoma
Metastasis (Wilms tumor, osteosarcoma)
Hamartoma, pulmonary blastoma

MULTIPLE PULMONARY NODULES

Inflammatory
Granuloma (TB, histoplasmosis, sarcoidosis)
Septic emboli

Neoplastic
Metastatic (Wilms tumor, osteosarcoma, thyroid cancer)
Laryngeal papillomatosis

Congenital
Multiple AV malformations (rare)

gender predominance. It presents as respiratory distress in 25%. Pulmonary function testing reveals restrictive change, which may be especially severe in the acute phase of disease. Rash, arthritis, and uveitis are much more frequent presenting symptoms.

Imaging findings always include bilateral hilar lymphadenopathy, almost always (80%) associated with bilateral paratracheal lymphadenopathy. This is in contradistinction to the one-third association of bilateral hilar adenopathy with paratracheal adenopathy in adults. The "1, 2, 3 sign" (adenopathy in both hilar [1, 2] and paratracheal [3] regions) as described in adults is unusual in childhood, occurring in only 10% to 15%. Reticulonodular, parenchymal involvement during childhood is seen in approximately two thirds of patients, about the same incidence as in adults (Fig. 2-34).

AIDS Approximately 2% of all AIDS cases occur in children, with nearly 80% diagnosed before 2 years of age. The major risk factors include maternal transmission and blood transfusions of the virus (HIV), leading to infection of the infant manifested by impaired helper T-cell function. The lung disease in pediatric patients

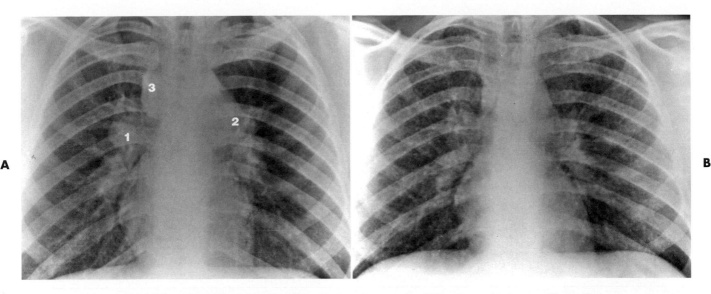

Fig. 2-34   Sarcoid. **A**, Bilateral hilar (*1, 2*) and paratracheal (*3*) adenopathy in sarcoidosis. **B**, Reticulonodular parenchymal involvement.

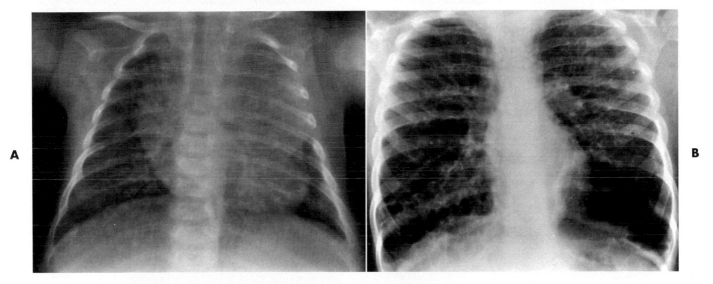

Fig. 2-35   A, Nodular interstitial changes of LCH. **B**, Chronic interstitial changes of eosinoplilic granuloma resembling those of BPD.

consists of acute pulmonary infections predominantly caused by P. *carinii* and cytomegalovirus (CMV), eventually leading to chronic lymphocytic infiltration or lymphatic interstitial pneumonia (LIP). Serious bacterial infections (*Streptococcus, H. influenzae*) may then supervene. The findings on radiographs of the chest in the early phases are predominantly a central parahilar interstitial infiltrate, which may become more diffuse and nodular in appearance, mimicking miliary TB. Lung biopsy is the diagnostic test of choice (Fig. 2-35, *A*).

Primary pulmonary histiocytosis X Langerhans cell histiocytosis (LCH) may affect the lung parenchyma in half of patients. Males are affected more often than females. Clinical signs include cough and dyspnea. Conventional chest radiographs reveal overaeration, peribronchial thickening resulting in perihilar infiltrates, and occasional nodular appearance of the interstitium (Fig. 2-35, *B*). Imaging findings rarely are confused with those of sarcoidosis in teenagers or RDS in infants and young children.

Mediastinal Masses

ANTERIOR MEDIASTINAL MASSES

Thymus: normal (rebound hypertrophy), thymoma
Teratoma (three layers),
Terrible **lymphoma**
Ectopic thyroid
Pericardial abnormalities
Bronchogenic cyst

MIDDLE MEDIASTINAL MASSES

Inflammatory lymph **nodes** or lympoma
Foregut abnormalities (esophageal duplication, bronchogenic cyst)
Prominant pulmonary **vessels**, aortic dilation or aneurysm

POSTERIOR MEDIASTINAL MASSES

Neural-based tumors: ganglioneuroma, ganglioneuroblastoma, neuroblastoma
Congenital pulmonary or pleural **lesions** (sequestration, bronchogenic or neurenteric cyst)

SUPERIOR MEDIASTINAL MASSES

Cystic hygroma
Bronchogenic cyst
Neural-based tumors
Rare vascular lesions

MEDIASTINUM

Anterior Mediastinum
  Thymus
  Neoplasms
    Hodgkin, Non-Hodgkin lymphoma
    Thymoma
    Germ cells tumors
Middle Mediastinum
  Foregut cysts
  Pericardial tumors
Posterior Mediastinum
  Neurogenic tumors
  Neurenteric cysts
  Extramedullary hematopoiesis

Mediastinal Masses

Mediastinal masses (see box) are the most common thoracic masses in children. The ones in bold in the box comprise 80% of these masses. Approximately 30% develop before age 12 years. Approximately 30% occur in the anterior, 30% in the middle, and 40% in the posterior compartment.

Compartmentalization of the mediastinum represents an arbitrary classification. Classically, the mediastinum has been divided into a superior and an inferior portion, with the inferior portion divided into anterior, middle, and posterior portions in slightly different ways by, among others, Felson and Hope. Although this division is slightly less easy to apply in infants and

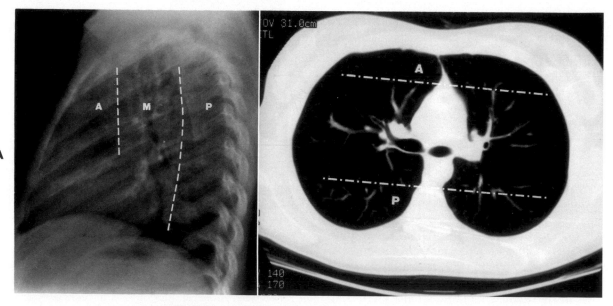

Fig. 2-36 Mediastinal compartmentalization on lateral radiograph (**A**) and CT (**B**).

children, for practical purposes the anterior mediastinum is delineated by a line drawn along the anterior edge of the vascular pedicle, whereas the posterior mediastinum consists of the structures posterior to a line drawn through the anterior edge of the vertebral bodies. The middle mediastinum is the resultant compartment between these two. These compartments are easily superimposed on transverse imaging modalities such as CT and MRI (Fig. 2-36). After identification of a mediastinal lesion on conventional chest radiographs, CT or MRI is the preferred modality for further evaluation of the middle and anterior mediastinum, whereas MRI is definitely the preferred modality for posterior mediastinal lesions.

Anterior Mediastinum

Thymus   The major occupant of the anterior mediastinum is the thymus, formed of two asymmetric lobes whose variability in size and shape is virtually limitless. The thymus shrinks dramatically under stress of systemic illness or steroid therapy. It regenerates with resolution of the stress or discontinuation of steroid therapy and may revert to the same shape or size. Twenty-five percent of those that rebound are larger than before the insult. Marked lobularity is never normal. The thymus also adapts to its surroundings and normally will not displace structures such as vessels or the trachea. On conventional radiographs, because of its location, the margins of the thymus may be indented by the anterior ribs (thymic wave) (Fig. 2-37); and the thymus changes shape during respiration (by elongating and narrowing during inspiration), which can be visualized better at fluoroscopy (see Fig. 2-1). Occasionally a

notch is seen along the left cardiothymic border, delineating the junction of heart and thymus. The right lobe can insinuate itself into the minor fissure (the "sail" sign) (Fig. 2-38). On conventional radiographs of the chest, thymic tissue is visible in a child up to 3 years of age. On a CT scan, thymic tissue may be distinct until the early teens. Hyperthyroidism or Addison disease can cause the thymus to enlarge abnormally, and infiltrative disorders such as lymphoma or leukemia and histiocytosis may also be implicated. On CT or MRI, the thymus is homogeneous throughout childhood,

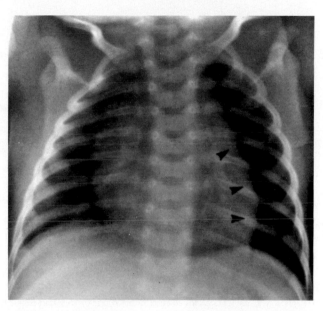

Fig. 2-37   Arrowheads mark the thymic "wave": anterior ribs indenting the thymic margin.

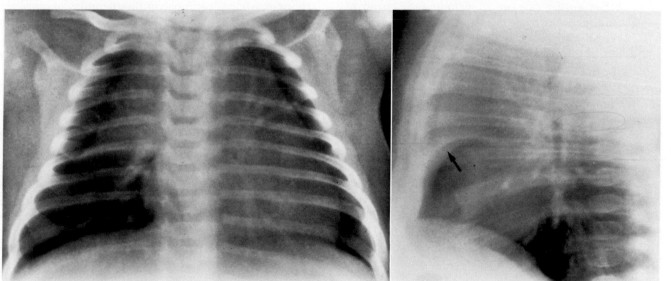

Fig. 2-38   A, The "sail" sign where the thymus insinuates itself into the minor fissure. B, Lateral radiograph illustrates same (*arrow*).

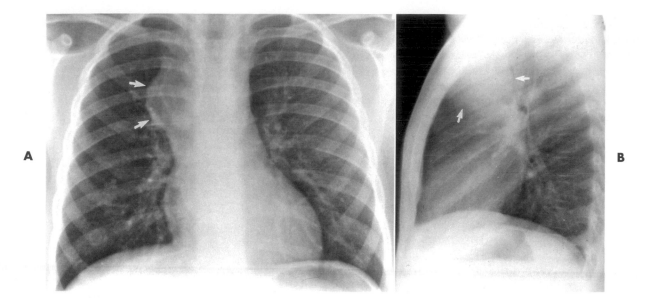

Fig. 2-39   **A**, Frontal and, **B**, lateral radiographs in a child with "lymphoma syndrome" demonstrating an anterior mediastinal mass posteriorly displacing the trachea.

with an attenuation similar or slightly greater than adjacent chest wall muscle on unenhanced studies. MRI characteristics include slightly hyperintense on T1 and slightly less intense than fat on T2 (see Fig. 2-22).

A hypoplastic thymus is often present in premature infants. In aplasia of the thymus (DiGeorge syndrome), infants are born with little or no thymic tissue or hypoparathyroid glands because of maldevelopment of the third and fourth pharyngeal pouches during the sixth to twelfth weeks of gestational life. Associated congenital anomalies may occur, including the tetrad of Fallot, truncus arteriosus, transposition of the great vessels, ventricular septal defect, or absent pulmonary valve.

Neoplasms   Approximately 30% of all mediastinal masses occur in the anterior mediastinum.

After leukemia and central nervous system (CNS) tumors, lymphoma is the third most common neoplasm of childhood. It is the most common anterior mediastinal mass, accounting for a quarter of all mediastinal masses. Approximately 30% of patients have (bilateral) mediastinal lymphadenopathy. Approximately 15% of children with acute lymphocytic leukemia (ALL) have "lymphoma syndrome," associated with a mediastinal mass in nearly 60% of patients (Fig. 2-39).

Non-Hodgkin lymphoma   Non-Hodgkin lymphoma (NHL) usually appears in an insidious fashion with few specific symptoms. Approximately 60% of lymphoma in children is NHL, which represent 6% of all childhood cancers, and it has marked similarities to ALL; thus in

Types of Lymphoma

I   Lymphoblastic (30%), supradiaphragmatic, T cell
II   Undifferentiated non-Burkitt (30%), abdomen, B cell
III Undifferentiated Burkitt (25%), abdomen, B cell
IV   Large cell (histiocytic) (15%), various locations, cells

the pediatric age group lymphoma and leukemia are often referred to as a single entity. The peak age of presentation is 9 years, and males outnumber females 3:1. More than 70% of patients have disseminated disease at the time of presentation.

There are four major types of NHL (see box). Type I is usually supradiaphragmatic; types II and III are subdiaphragmatic; and group IV can occur anywhere but is rare in the mediastinum. Of note is that abdominal NHL is often B cell in origin, whereas mediastinal NHL is often T cell in origin. In addition, the disease presents primarily *extranodal*; the most frequent primary site is the ileocecal region, followed by the mediastinum. It spreads hematogenously and has a mediastinal mass in approximately 50% of patients. Tracheobronchial compression occurs in 85%. A pleural effusion often is seen.

CT and MRI are the modalities of choice for staging.

Treatment revolves around chemotherapy, and the critical prognostic factor is bone marrow involvement.

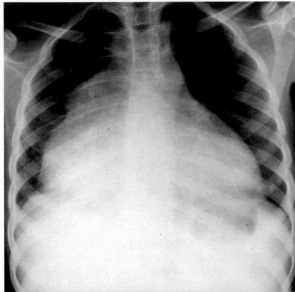

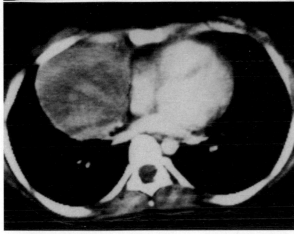

Fig. 2-40   Hodgkin lymphoma. A, Chest radiograph demonstrating an anterior mediastinal mass with ipsilateral hilar adenopathy. **B,** Contrast enhanced CT scan confirms the extent of the mediastinal lesion.

cervical adenopathy w/ concomitant mediastinal involvement

Hodgkin lymphoma   Hodgkin lymphoma occurs in the pediatric age group in approximately 10% of all cases. Its incidence is slightly less than NHL in children (40%). There is no difference from the adult disease in its mode of presentation, imaging appearance, histologic features, treatment, and prognosis except for a male predominance. The diagnosis is made on biopsy, with the Reed-Sternberg cell the classic marker. The nodular sclerotic type occurs in 60%, mixed cellularity in 25%, lymphocyte prominent in 10%, and lymphocyte depleted in 5%.

The site of origin is almost invariably *nodal* and spreads by direct continuity (Fig. 2-40). Most (85%) initially have a mediastinal mass, and 30% have hilar adenopathy. The most common primary configuration is cervical lymphadenopathy with concomitant mediastinal involvement (90%). Paraaortic and celiac nodes are much more commonly involved than mesenteric lymph nodes. In contradistinction to NHL, the initial presentation of Hodgkin lymphoma is anything but insidious. Significant tracheobronchial compression occurs in more than 50% of patients.

Staging is extremely important in determining therapy. CT and MRI are the modalities of choice. Emergency radiation therapy may be needed for tracheobronchial compression, which occurs in up to half of the patients at presentation with Hodgkin lymphoma. Scintigraphy (gallium 67 citrate) is useful for determining response to therapy in the mediastinum.

Thymoma   (Unilocular) thymic cysts, thymolipomas, and thymomas are rare in the pediatric age group. Approximately 15% of thymomas are aggressive. Associated paraneoplastic syndromes include myasthenia gravis most commonly and red cell aplasia. Half of patients with thymoma have myasthenia, and 10% to 15% of all patients with myasthenia have a thymoma. Calcifications occur in 25%. MRI and CT complement conventional radiography.

Germ cell tumors   Germ cell tumors include teratoma, dermoid, or endodermal sinus (yolk sac) tumor that can be distinguished from other masses on CT scanning when calcium and fat are present. Teratoma is the most common germ cell tumor. It is derived from multipotential cells in the third pharyngeal pouch that have descended into the mediastinum with the thymus. Most benign teratomas are cystic, containing a thick wall as well as fat. Calcification is often present and best demonstrated on CT, which also can be used to evaluate for local invasion. Malignant teratoma is much less common than its benign counterpart and occurs in (male) adolescents. It more commonly occurs in the sacrococcygeal region (10% in the mediastinum).

Middle Mediastinum

Lesions in the middle mediastinum also comprise approximately 30% of all mediastinal masses. The differential diagnosis of middle mediastinal lesions includes *nodes*, esophagus-related abnormalities such as a duplication cyst, hiatus hernia, or *bronchopulmonary foregut* abnormalities, including a bronchogenic cyst or sequestration. Common entities included in lymphadenopathy are from either neoplastic (e.g., in lymphoma or leukemia) or infectious (primarily granulomatous ones such as TB, histoplasmosis, or sarcoidosis) causes. Common *vascular* lesions include rings, slings, and aortic arch abnormalities.

Foregut cysts   Foregut cysts are usually single and round. Depending on their communication with the

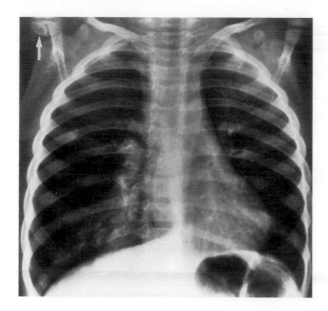

Fig. 2-41   AP radiograph reveals hyperinflation of right lung, right middle lobe atelectasis, and well circumscribed right humeral proximal epiphyseal lesion (*arrows*) in a patient with tuberculosis.

Fig. 2-42   Neuroblastoma.   A, Frontal radiograph reveals a large posterior mediastinal mass containing calcification (*arrowhead*) and causing rib erosion (*arrows*) and displacement of the mediastinum to the right. **B,** CT image confirms radiographic findings and demonstrates an effusion (*arrow*). MR images define the axial extent with "dumbbell" extension (*arrow*) of lesion into the neural foramen (**C**) and the coronal spinal canal extent (**D**).

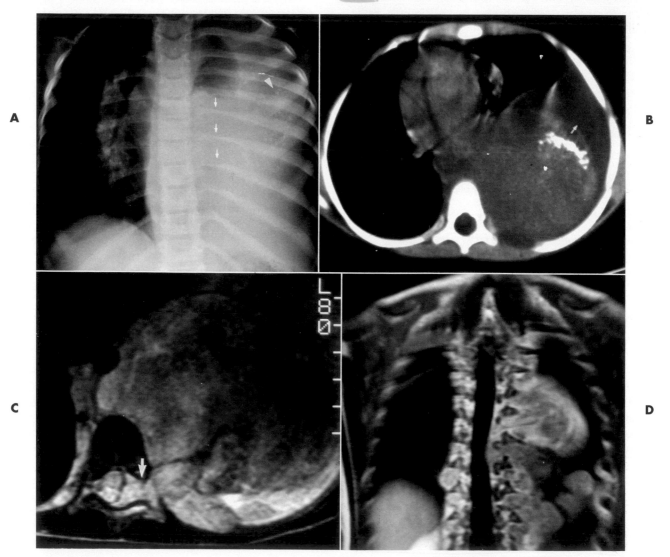

GI tract (enteric), the airways (bronchogenic), or the spinal canal (neurenteric), they may be solid, contain an air-fluid level, or be air filled (enteric cysts are discussed in Chapter 3). All foregut-related cystic lesions are more common on the right than on the left side and are often related to the carina.

CT or increasingly MRI is the imaging modality of choice after initial demonstration of the mass on conventional (contrast) studies (Fig. 2-41; see Fig. 2-22).

Pericardial tumors   Tumors of the (peri)cardium are extremely rare in childhood.

Posterior Mediastinum

Posterior mediastinal masses comprise approximately 40% of all pediatric mediastinal masses.

Neurogenic tumors   Neurogenic tumors comprise 90% of the posterior mediastinal masses in the pediatric age group. Neuroblastoma, ganglioneuroblastoma, and ganglioneuroma represent a group of neurogenic tumors with an increasingly higher benign cell composition. Neuroblastoma is by far the most common (15% of all neuroblastomas occur here), followed by ganglioneuroblastoma (more highly differentiated than neuroblastoma) and ganglioneuroma (a benign lesion occurring in older children with an excellent prognosis). Schwannomas, neurofibromas (seldom solitary), and paragangliomas occur rarely as compared to adults. Mediastinal neuroblastoma is also associated with a more favorable prognosis when diagnosed in a child before 1 year of age, and the lesion usually occurs in children less than 2 years of age.

Neurenteric cysts   Neurenteric cysts are identical to foregut cysts except for the association with vertebral anomalies. The latter can vary from hemivertebrae to spina bifida to blocked vertebrae and clefts.

MRI is the imaging modality of choice, especially with its multiplanar capabilities (Fig. 2-42). CT primarily is useful to evaluate for calcifications and bony erosion (rib, neural foramen). The classic dumbbell appearance of thoracic neuroblastoma is also exquisitely demonstrated on MRI; MRI also has a definite advantage in the postoperative, postirradiation therapy follow-up.

Extramedullary hematopoiesis   Extramedullary hematopoiesis is usually unilateral, can result from severe hereditary anemias (e.g., thalassemia, hereditary spherocytosis), and usually is located between T8 and T12. CT and MRI delineate the extent optimally.

HEART

Developmental Anomalies
Increased pulmonary vascularity without cyanosis
Ventricular septal defect
Atrial septal defect
Atrioventricular canal defect
Patent ductus arteriosus
Increased pulmonary vascularity with cyanosis
Transposition of great arteries
Corrected transposition
Persistent truncus arteriosus
Total anomalous pulmonary venous return
Partial anomalous pulmonary venous return
Double outlet right ventricle
Single ventricle
Decreased pulmonary vascularity with cyanosis
Tetrad of Fallot
Tricuspid atresia
Ebstein anomaly
Obstructive lesions
Coarctation of the aorta
Congenital aortic stenosis
Pulmonary stenosis
Miscellaneous conditions
Hypoplastic left heart syndrome
Cor triatriatum
Heterotaxy
Cardiac malposition
Dextrocardia
Levocardia
AV concordance
AV discordance
Cardiosplenic syndromes
Heterotaxy syndrome
Asplenia
Polysplenia
Acquired Cardiac Anomalies
Pericardial disease
Congenital absence of pericardium
Pericarditis
Myocardial Disease
Kawasaki disease
Rheumatic heart disease
Endocardial anomalies
Endocardial fibroelastosis
Endocarditis
Vignettes
Conventional radiographic findings in CHD
Congested pulmonary vasculature
Persistent fetal circulation
Pulmonary artery segment
Common surgical procedures
Right aortic arch

Table 2-3 Correlation of imaging findings with hemodynamics in left-to-right shunts

	Atrial septal defect	Ventricular septal defect	Patent ductus arteriosus (AP window)	Atrioventricular canal defect
ENLARGEMENT	RV, RA	RV, LV, LA	LV, LA	All chambers
CARDIAC CONTOUR	Enlarged right side	Biventricular enlargement	Enlarged left side	Both sides enlarged
AORTIC SEGMENT	(Rotationally) smaller	Normal	Larger (theoretically), usually normal	Normal
PULMONARY TRUNK	Enlarged	Enlarged	Enlarged	Enlarged
PULMONARY VASCULAR OBSTRUCTIVE DISEASE	Most common	Rare	Rare	Often in Down syndrome
CONGESTIVE HEART FAILURE	Rare	Often if large	Often if large	Common

RV, Right ventricle; *RA,* right atrium; *LV,* left ventricle; *LA,* left atrium.

Developmental Anomalies

Congenital heart disease (CHD) occurs in approximately 1% of all live births. Approximately 25% of these babies become symptomatic in the first year of life, approximately 25% of patients with CHD eventually die of their disease, and approximately 25% of these deaths occur in the first month of life. However, earlier detection and intervention have made increasing survivability possible by using palliative intervention, physiologic revisions, and true anatomic correction of the lesions.

The more common radiographic patterns of CHD are discussed below.

Increased pulmonary vascularity without cyanosis Acyanotic communications between the systemic and pulmonary circuits include intracardiac left-to-right shunts and large systemic arteriovenus (AV) connections. Common examples of the former include ventricular septal defect (VSD), atrial septal defect (ASD), atrioventricular canal (AVC) defect, and patent ductus arteriosus (PDA) (Table 2-3). Less common are aorticopulmonary window and coronary artery fistula. The hemodynamic effect of these lesions varies with the size and location of the communication between the pulmonary and systemic circuits. Longstanding shunts with eventual development of pulmonary vascular obstructive disease (formerly known as *Eisenmenger physiology*) may be evident as increased central pulmonary arterial size and tapering of peripheral vessels.

Large systemic AV connections are rare in children but include vein of Galen aneurysm and hepatic, GI, or cutaneous AV malformations.

Classification of VSDs

TYPE I
Conal (outlet) defect (5%); supracristal (subpulmonic) in location*

TYPE II
(Peri)membranous defect (80%); located just below the crista supraventricularis

TYPE III
Inlet or AV canal type (5%), posterior septum

TYPE IV
Muscular defects (often multiple) (10%)

*Types II and IV often close spontaneously; type I never does.

Ventricular septal defect Approximately 20% of patients with CHD have an isolated VSD. In addition, VSD is the most common congenital intracardiac lesion in children (25%). Many small VSDs close spontaneously; thus anatomic classification of VSDs is important in planning whether surgical treatment is necessary. The most common classification of VSDs is shown in the box.

Clinically, patients classicially are seen with a prominent blowing pansystolic murmur at the lower sternal border. These patients can have CHF, repeated respiratory infections, or failure to thrive, usually after 1 month of life because the pulmonary vascular resistance gradually falls during this period. In an older child, if pulmonary vascular resistance remains high, a large VSD may lead to pulmonary hypertension. Rarely the development of pulmonary vascular obstructive disease causes reversal of blood flow, creating a right-to-left shunt across the septal defect. This may lead to cyanosis (formerly known as *Eisenmenger physiology*). Most patients, however, will have undergone surgery to correct the defect before pulmonary flow reversal occurs.

Conventional chest film findings usually are evident only in patients with a medium- to large-sized defect (i.e., when the ratio of pulmonary to systemic blood flow is greater than 2:1). The pulmonary vascularity is increased with biventricular enlargement and dilation of the central pulmonary trunk (Fig. 2-43). Left atrial enlargement and resultant posterior displacement and elevation of the left mainstem bronchus are also often present. Radiographic signs of CHF may appear after the first month of life as the pulmonary vascular resistance decreases.

Therapy is surgical closure of the defect(s); up to half of VSDs close spontaneously. Detachable catheter devices for closure of VSD are under development.

Atrial septal defect   The second most common cardiac anomaly in children, ASD, accounts for 10% of all CHD. An ASD is the most common shunt that persists into adulthood. It is classified according to its location in the atrial septum.

- An ostium secundum (II) ASD is most common (60%) and is located in the midseptum in the area of fossa ovalis. It is usually an isolated anomaly.
- An ostium primum (I) ASD (30%) is situated low in the atrial septum (foramen ovale) and is synonymous with a partial AV canal defect (large opening in the inferior septum always associated with a cleft mitral valve).
- A sinus venosus ASD (5%) is a defect in the posterior septum, usually near the entrance of the superior vena cava. It is often associated with partial anomalous pulmonary venous drainage, usually (85%) from the right upper lobe pulmonary vein into the superior vena cava (SVC).
- A patent foramen ovale represents a defect in apposition of the septum secundum to the septum primus, functional only in right-to-left shunts.

ASDs are six to eight times more common in females than in males. The association of an ASD with mitral stenosis in a child with rheumatic disease (rare today) is known as Lutembacher's syndrome. An ostium secundum defect associated with conduction defects and skeletal abnormalities of the upper extremities (absent or froglike thumb) is known as the Holt-Oram syndrome, an autosomal dominant entity.

Clinically the patients are most often asymptomatic. When entering adolescence or young adulthood, the patient may have mild dyspnea or an asymptomatic heart murmur with a harsh systolic murmur along the high left sternal border. There is fixed splitting of a loud S2. A patient with an ostium primum ASD often has a blowing pansystolic murmur of mitral regurgitation.

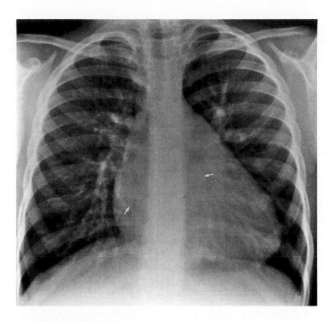

Fig. 2-43 VSD. Increased pulmonary vascularity, enlarged left atrium (*arrows*), and mildly enlarged cardiac silhouette in a 3-month-old with failure to thrive.

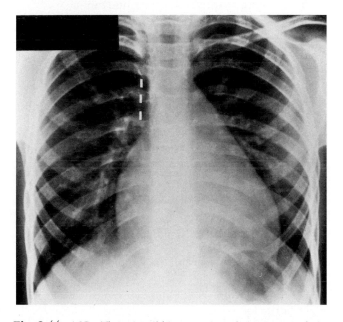

Fig. 2-44 ASD. There is mild increase in pulmonary vascularity and "rotation" of mediastinal contour. Note the "absent" SVC contour and prominent ipsilateral pulmonary trunk.

Conventional chest radiographs are normal in infancy. Later in childhood, increased pulmonary vascularity may appear, with mild leftward rotation of the heart and the great vessels. This position may make the aorta appear disproportionally small, whereas the pulmonary trunk becomes disproportionally large (Fig. 2-44). In addition, the superior vena cava's contour is often "absent" because it is rotated over the spine and no longer forms a border. Right ventricular dilation is present. Left atrial enlargement is absent because of immediate decrompression of the increased volume of blood to the right atrium during both systole and diastole.

Treatment consists of elective surgical closure, although percutaneous closure with a "clam shell" device is being done experimentally.

Atrioventricular canal defect   AVC defect (endocardial cushion defect) is the result of abnormal development of the endocardial cushion tissue. It can include any or all of the following: common AV valves, a low ostium primum ASD; a cleft anterior mitral leaflet; a posterior (inlet) VSD; and a cleft septal tricuspid leaflet. The extreme result is a complete AV canal; most commonly, a partial defect includes a primum ASD and cleft mitral valve. Partial AV canal defects occur more commonly, with the entire range of defects comprising 4% of congenital heart disease:

- Complete canal defects: ASD[1], VSD, common AV valves
- Partial canal defects: ASD[1], cleft mitral septal leaflet

Clinically, mild-to-moderate shunting at the atrial level may lead to pulmonary hypertension (more common with Down syndrome); more commonly encountered are failure to thrive, dyspnea, and fatigue.

Patients with trisomy 21 (Down symdrome) comprise 40% to 50% of patients with an AV canal defect (partial or complete forms). Complete AV canal defects are often seen in patients with asplenia or polysplenia (heterotaxy syndrome).

Conventional chest radiographs of a partial AV canal are often indistinguishable from those of an ASD. When there is a complete defect, the radiographic findings reflect enlargement of the right side (right atrium and ventricle) and large blood volumes in the lungs. Surgery with low mortality is possible for both the partial and complete AV canal variants.

Patent ductus arteriosus   PDA, the persistence of (normal) fetal circulation after birth, constitutes 8% to 10% of CHD (one in 3000 term infants) and is more common in girls and premature infants (50% of those less than 1500 g). The ductus connects the left pulmonary artery to the descending aorta just distal to the origin of the left subclavian artery (sixth aortic arch). It functionally closes by 48 hours after birth; it is anatomically closed by 1 month of life. Closure begins at the pulmonic end, and the ligamentum calcifies in some children.

PDA is usually asymptomatic, but if it is large, symptoms can range from a (machinery-like) murmur in a newborn to CHF in infancy (caused by left ventricular failure). It can be aggravated by hyaline membrane disease (HMD) in premature infants in whom it occurs in 25% of patients, and it may then require surgical (clip) or medical (indomethacin) therapy. The ductus thus closes (or stays open) for chemical—not pressure—reasons.

Conventional chest radiographs in the neonate with PDA may reveal increased pulmonary vascularity, pulmonary edema, or left atrial enlargement. These findings may be difficult to evaluate if changes of HMD or RDS are present. In the older child an enlarged aortic knob is theoretically possible but seldom noted; increased pulmonary vascularity may be noted. In a child less than age 3 years, the thymic shadow makes it even more difficult to evaluate the aortic knob; in fact, it often is impossible. In reality, there is no way to differentiate VSD and PDA on conventional chest films in children. Color-flow Doppler evaluation of the left atrial to aortic root ratio (normal, <1) is also important in evaluating PDA.

Radiographic evidence of a closed duct may be evident as ligamentum calcification or as a surgical device (clip or "clam shell") (Fig. 2-45).

Increased pulmonary vascularity with cyanosis Common anomalies in this category include transposition of the great arteries (TGA), corrected transposition, persistent truncus arteriosus (PTA), and total anomalous pulmonary venous return (TAPVR), whereas less common anomalies include partial anomalous pulmonary venous return (PAPVR), double outlet right ventricle (DORV), occasionally tricuspid atresia, and a single ventricle.

Transposition of great arteries   TGA, the most common form of cyanotic CHD, comprises approximately 5% of CHD. The origin of both the aorta and the pulmonary artery are from the "wrong" (discordant) ventricle; the aorta originates from the right ventricle, whereas the pulmonary artery arises from the left ventricle. The aorta lies mostly anterior to the pulmonary artery and somewhat to the right (dextro-TGA).

This anomaly results in delivery of deoxygenated blood to the body and then its return to the right ventricle, whereas oxygenated blood is circulated from the heart to the lungs and back again. This condition is incompatible with life unless there is a communication at the atrial, ventricular (40%), or ductus arteriosus level. Approximately 70% of infants have an intact ventricular septum. The incidence of dextro-TGA is one in 4000 live births and is higher in infants of diabetic mothers; boys outnumber girls 2.5:1. It is the most common CHD presenting with cyanosis in the first 24 hours of life.

Clinically these newborns are intensely cyanotic at birth and are unresponsive to 100% oxygen if they do not have a VSD. Bidirectional flow of blood at the atrial and/or ventricular level leads to an admixture of oxygenated and nonoxygenated blood. Large pulmonary blood flow results in CHF with less cyanosis, whereas diminished pulmonary flow (pulmonic stenosis) results in more intense cyanosis, with normal or slightly increased pulmonary vasculature.

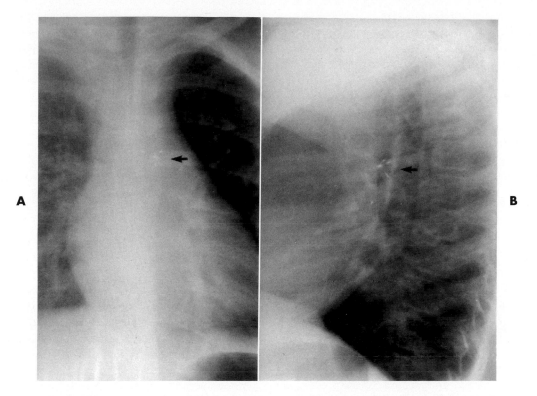

Fig. 2-45   PDA. **A,** Frontal and **(B)** lateral radiographs demonstrate a "clam shell" device used to close the patent ductus arteriosus (*arrows*).

Conventional chest radiographs may reveal mild cardiomegaly, although a normal-size cardiac silhouette is the rule immediately after birth. There is increased, occasionally asymmetric, pulmonary vascularity as soon as the physiologic neonatal pulmonary hypertension resolves. There are hyperinflation and lack of a normal thymic contour (stress). Descriptions of this appearance include "egg-on-side" and "apple-on-a-string" configurations (Fig. 2-46).

Palliative therapy centers around creation of a large ASD to improve bidirectional flow by catheter balloon septostomy (Rashkind's procedure).

Corrective surgery is achieved through an arterial switch procedure (sometimes called the *Jatene procedure*). Radiographically the appearance of the heart often reverts to normal. The survival rate is 70% to 80% to age 2 years.

Corrected transposition   A congenitally corrected, or "levo," TGA represents inversion of the ventricles in a patient with a normal atrial relationship (situs solitus). The morphologic right ventricle is located on the left, with blood reaching it from the left atrium through a tricuspid valve and the blood leaving it through the aorta. The morphologic left ventricle is on the right side, receiving blood through a mitral valve from the

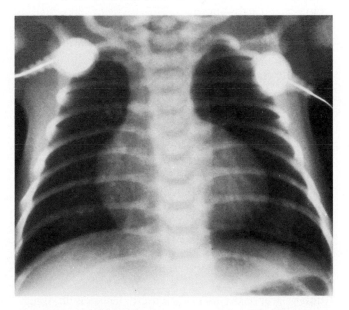

Fig. 2-46 Transposition of the great arteries is suggested in 1-day-old infant by "egg-on-side" appearance of a mildly enlarged cardiac silhouette and loss of thymic contour in the superior mediastinum. There is asymmetric slight "shunt" vascularity.

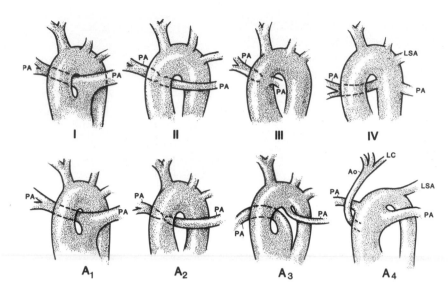

Fig. 2-47   Classification of truncus arteriosus. Top row: Collett-Edwards types 1-4, bottom row: van Praagh types A1-A4 (*LSA*, left subclavian artery, *LC*, left carotid artery). (Courtesy S. W. Miller, M.D.)

right atrium and giving rise to the pulmonary artery. Only 1% of children with the defect are without significant other cardiac defects. VSD (50%), single ventricle (35%), and pulmonary stenosis (PS) (50%) commonly coexist. Tricuspid valve regurgitation occurs in 30%.

Clincally, the findings relate to severity of the intracardiac lesions. These patients may be entirely normal and live a normal life span or may die early as a result of cyanosis and arrhythmias.

Conventional chest radiographs are often normal but may show an abnormal fullness in the left upper heart border and mediastinum caused by the ascending aorta and right ventricle being border-forming on the left. Pulmonary vascularity varies according to the presence and type of associated intracardiac lesions, but it is usually normal or decreased because most levo-TGA have PS or VSD.

Persistent truncus arteriosus   PTA represents a developmental failure of the septation of the primitive truncus arteriosus into the aorta and pulmonary artery. This single trunk arises from a single semilunar valve possessing anywhere from two to six cusps. It comprises less than 2% of CHD and occurs in one in 10,000 live births. It classically has been classified on the basis of the origin of the pulmonary artery. The pulmonary arteries may have a common origin from the trunk or arm of the ascending arch. There is an obligatory shunt at the ventricular level. The former type IV truncus (Collette-Edwards) has been reclassified as a *pseudotruncus arteriosus*, type I, in which the atretic pulmonary artery is supplied by a branch of the

descending aorta. A pseudotruncus, type II (the most severe form of the tetrad of Fallot) can then be visualized as the PDA supplying the atretic pulmonary artery. A variant of this classification is by van Praagh (Fig. 2-47).

The patients present early in infancy with cyanosis, failure to thrive, dyspnea, and CHF.

Chest radiographs reveal mild "oval" bilateral cardiomegaly and increased, occasionally asymmetric pulmonary vascularity. An aortic arch on the right side is present in 35% of patients, and the pulmonary waist is often quite prominent (thymic stress atrophy). Therapeutically, in infancy a valved conduit is placed between the right ventricle and the pulmonary artery, and the VSD is closed. It may be necessary to revise this conduit as somatic growth demands.

Total anomalous pulmonary venous return Occurring twice as often in males as in females, TAPVR accounts for 1% of CHD. There are four types of anomalous pulmonary venous drainage: supracardiac (50%), cardiac (30%), infracardiac (15%), and mixed (5%).

In each of these types, obstruction of venous flow occurs in 50% to 60% except for the intracardiac type, in which it occurs 100% of the time. Clinically, if there is high pulmonary flow and good admixture, cyanosis is mild. With pulmonary venous obstruction, cyanosis is severe, and intervention is mandatory to prevent death. These infants normally present in the first 2 weeks of life.

Chest radiographs of patients with TAPVR *with* obstruction reveal a normal cardiac silhouette with

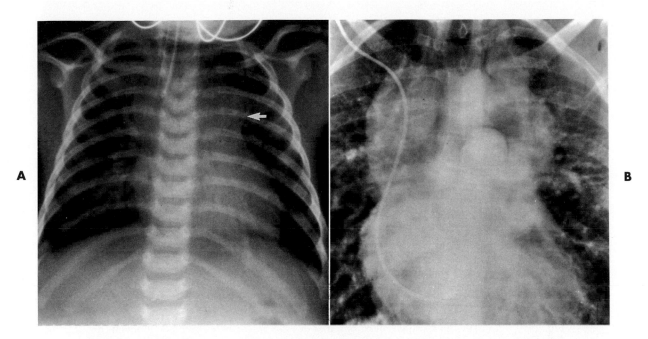

Fig. 2-48   A, "Figure-eight" cardiomediastinal silouette in a child with a left sided SVC (*arrow*) and PAPVR. B, Angiographic demonstration of supracardiac TAPVR without obstruction in a teenager.

severely congested pulmonary vessels and interstitial pulmonary edema; in patients with TAPVR *without* obstruction there is cardiomegaly (dilated right ventricule and atrium), an enlarged pulmonary artery segment, and increased pulmonary flow. The classic "snowman" or "figure-eight" cardiac silhouette occurs in older children with nonobstructive TAPVR but not in infants (Fig. 2-48).

Cardiac US and MRI are very useful in identifying the anomalous venous drainage types as well.

Treatment involves surgical connection of the common pulmonary vein to the left atrium and closure of the ASD.

Partial anomalous pulmonary venous return PAPVR is usually associated with a sinus venosus ASD. The chest radiographs are similar to those for an ASD because most PAPVR is to the SVC or a SVC on the left side. The anomalous venous return may be identified on US but demonstrated better by angiocardiography.

Double outlet right ventricle DORV is characterized by both the aorta and the pulmonary trunk originating from the right ventricle, the presence of a VSD, and a normal-size left ventricle. Because the aorta and pulmonic valve are side by side, the cardiac silhouette becomes somewhat oval in configuration, although normal in size, especially early in life. Pulmonary flow is often normal. Cineangiography is the imaging modality of choice.

Single ventricle An infant with a single ventricle is seen with early cyanosis and CHF. The aorta and pulmonary trunk are often transposed (dextro-TGA), and the condition is invariably associated with the asplenia syndrome.

Decreased pulmonary vascularity with cyanosis The congenital lesions included in this group have a common denominator: pulmonary stenosis of varying severity with a shunt that causes cyanosis. These lesions include the tetrad of Fallot (PS and VSD), tricuspid atresia, and Ebstein anomaly (dysplastic right ventric and ASD), all resulting in right-to-left shunt.

Tetrad of Fallot Tetrad of Fallot is the most common cyanotic CHD of children and adults. It comprises 8% to 10% of all CHD and consists of infundibular pulmonary stenosis, resultant right vetricular hypertrophy, a VSD, and an overriding aorta. The probable cause of this lesion is aberrant development of the infundibulum. If the pulmonary valvular obstruction is mild (one third of cases) and the VSD large (invariably), there is sufficient pulmonary flow to allow for a "pink tet." At the other end of the spectrum is pseudotruncus arteriosus (pulmonary atresia and a VSD). Many infants, however, are desaturated but not clinically cyanotic for the first 3 to 6 months of life. In babies in whom cyanosis appears after 1 month of age, the tetrad of Fallot is the most common congenital heart lesion. Exertional dyspnea and hypoxemic spells occasionally relieved by

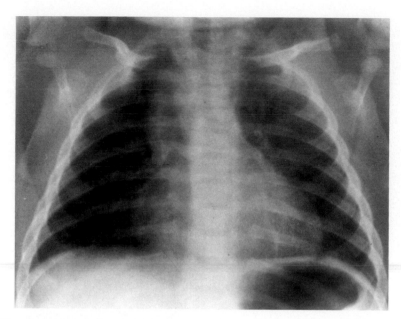

Fig. 2-49 A classic "boot-shaped" heart of tetrad of Fallot in a cynotic 2-month-old infant. An absent left pulmonary artery segment, decreased pulmonary blood flow, right aortic arch, and right ventricular hypertrophy result in an upturned cardiac apex.

squatting, which increases systemic venous return, are common clinical vignettes. The right ventricular hypertrophy is evident on electrocardiogram (ECG). There is a high association with trisomy 21, tracheoesophageal fistula (TEF), and the VATER complex.

Radiographic findings in the chest are characterized by (1) decreased pulmonary flow, although it is normal or increased in patients with a pink tet; (2) a cardiac waist that is notably narrow because of the absence of the pulmonary artery segment and thymic atrophy (stress); (3) the presence of a collateral flow with a reticular pattern (with pseudotruncus) (this occasionally is seen on conventional radiographs in the upper medial lung fields and may be verified on MRI); and (4) right ventricular hypertrophy, resulting in an upturned and prominent cardiac apex. This results in the classic appearance of the "coeur-en-sabot" or "boot-shaped" heart (Fig. 2-49). This contour can be enhanced by an aortic arch on the right side, present in 25% of patients.

Treatment consists of surgical correction. In the past palliative procedures included the Potts procedure, in which an anastomosis was created between the left pulmonary artery and the descending aorta; the Waterston procedure, which created an anastomosis between the ascending aorta and the right pulmonary artery; and the Blalock-Taussig operation, which involved a graft (previously the subclavian artery) to the ipsilateral pulmonary artery. These procedures were aimed at palliation of the oligemic lung. The current treatment in most surgical centers is complete correction in infancy, with closure of the VSD and a patch on the right ventricular outflow tract.

Tricuspid artesia   Absence of the tricuspid valve comprises 1% of all congenital heart lesions. Infants with this condition are cyanotic at birth and have an obligatory ASD, a VSD, and (rarely) a PDA coexisting. Tricuspid atresia has varible features that have in common absence of any direct communication between the right and left ventricles. In 30% of cases there is transposition (right or left) of the great vessels. Absence of the tricuspid valve is accompanied by PS (or rarely pulmonary atresia) in 50% of cases, rarely by TAPVR. An obligatory right-to-left shunt at the arterial level causes left ventricular enlargement.

Radiographs of the chest reveal normal or decreased pulmonary flow and a "rounded" cardiac apex caused by the left ventricular hypertrophy or enlargement. A concave pulmonary artery segment may be present (Fig. 2-50). The aorta is on the right side in 5% of these patients. Palliation consists of maintaining pulmonary flow by either keeping the PDA open with prostaglandins or surgically creating a modified Blalock-Taussig shunt. Further surgical correction consists of a Fontan procedure. The survival rate is approximately 70% at 5 years.

Ebstein anomaly   Ebstein anomaly is an uncommon (<1%) congenital cardiac anomaly consisting of displacement of the tricuspid valve tissue into the right ventricle accompanied by severe insufficiency of the valve. It is due to failure of undermining of the tricuspid valve, and there is a resultant enlarged right atrial cavity with a partially atrialized right ventricle. An ASD is always present. The larger the atrialized right ventricle, the smaller is the normally functioning portion of

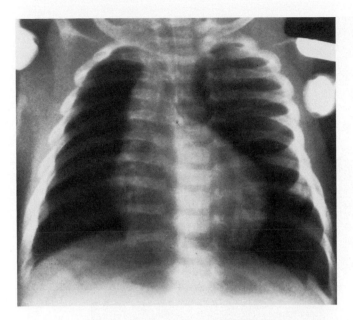

Fig. 2-50 Tricuspid atresia in 1-month-old infant reveals a rounded cardiac apex and a somewhat rounded right atrial contour. There is markedly decreased pulmonary vasculature.

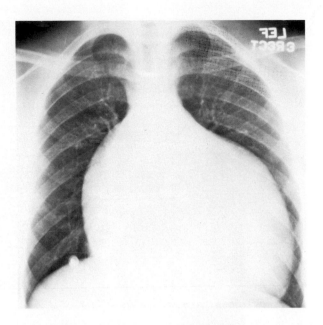

Fig. 2-51 Ebstein malformation in this teenager is demonstrated by massively enlarged boxlike cardiac configuration with diminished pulmonary vasculature.

the right side of the heart, resulting in increasing cyanosis because of right-to-left shunting through the ASD (a poorly functioning right ventricle). However, the severity of the right-to-left shunt depends more on the severity of the tricuspid regurgitation and pulmonary artery resistance than the contractibility of the right ventricle. Most infants present in the first month of life; some survive to adolescence or even childhood with severe pulmonary hypertension. Palpitations caused by arrhythmias are a common clinical problem.

The chest radiograph findings depend on the degree of dilation of the right side of the heart. The cardiothymic silhouette may resemble that of a pericardial effusion and be quite enlarged ("box-shaped" heart). There is often diminished pulmonary vascularity because of the right-to-left shunting at the atrial level. As the child reaches the teens and young adulthood, there may be normal vascularity, a large (massive) right atrium with increased rounding of the SVC-right atrial junction and a large right ventricle (Fig. 2-51). MRI also readily demonstrates the morphology.

Treatment in the newborn is palliative and includes the use of ECMO while the pulmonary vascular resistance is allowed to drop. The prognosis is variable, with a 50% mortality rate in the neonate by the first month for severe forms.

The differential diagnosis of the imaging findings in patients with Ebstein anomaly also includes tricuspid insufficiency and Uhl anomaly. The latter consists of focal or complete absence of right ventricular

myocardium, which results in a poorly functioning right ventricle with tricuspid insufficiency.

Obstructive lesions Common obstructive lesions with normal pulmonary flow can occur anywhere along the left ventricular outflow tract. They include coarctation of the aorta and aortic stenosis. The most common obstructive lesion on the right side is pulmonary stenosis (PS).

Coarctation of the aorta Coarctation of the aorta occurs just distal to the origin of the left subclavian artery and comprises 5% of all congenital heart lesions. Males are affected twice as often as females. The narrowing may be diffuse, occurring preductally and in infants, or localized, usually occurring postductally and in adults. This coarctation is associated most often (80%) with a bicuspid aortic valve but may also be associated with PDA (60%), VSD (30%), tracheoesophageal fistula, and circle of Willis aneurysms. Some of these patients present with CHF, which occurs either in infancy or after the third decade, but the rest of the patients usually are asymptomatic. Frequently these patients come to clinical attention with lower extremity hypotension relative to upper extremity hypertension as a result of the aortic narrowing. The collateral blood flow to a great extent determines the classic imaging findings.

The chest radiograph may reveal left ventricular enlargement, especially on the lateral view. The descending aorta is often dilated *poststenotically*, and the ascending aorta usually is dilated as a result of tur-

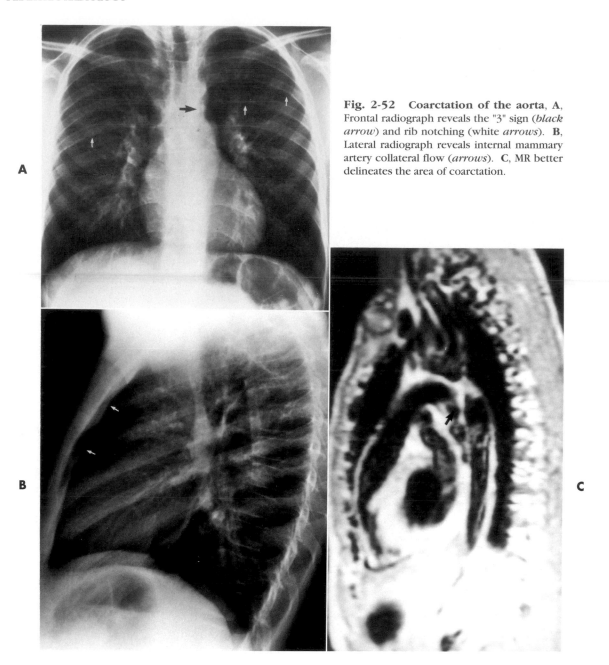

Fig. 2-52   Coarctation of the aorta, **A**, Frontal radiograph reveals the "3" sign (*black arrow*) and rib notching (white *arrows*). **B**, Lateral radiograph reveals internal mammary artery collateral flow (*arrows*). **C**, MR better delineates the area of coarctation.

bulence caused by the bicuspid aortic valve. This combination explains the "figure 3 sign" on the chest radiograph, which is made up of the dilated aortic arch projected above the poststenotic dilated segment of the descending aorta. The "reverse 3" or E sign may be noted on an esophageal contrast study. Rib notching is rare in a child before 8 to 12 years of age, typically is located along the inferior aspects of ribs three through eight, and represents pressure erosion of hypertrophied intercostal arteries serving as collaterals. The first and second ribs are spared because their intercostal arteries originate from the intercostal trunks rather than the descending aorta. Rib notching is seen bilaterally unless an aberrant right subclavian artery is present; notching then is absent on the right side. MRI

has replaced angiography and illustrates the exact site and length of the coarctation (Fig. 2-52).

Treatment consists of surgical excision of the narrowed segment, with or without patch augmentation of the aorta.

Congenital aortic stenosis   Congenital aortic stenosis occurs most commonly in boys (4:1). It is usually of the valvular type, with a deformed, frequently bicuspid aortic valve (50%), but subvalvular (fixed or dynamic) or supravalvular stenosis may also occur. The lesion eventually results in pressure overload of the left ventricle that, if severe, leads to clinical symptoms, often by the teen years. Subvalvular stenosis caused by a fibromuscular ring is considered fixed, whereas idiopathic hypertrophic subaortic stenosis (IHSS) is the cause for

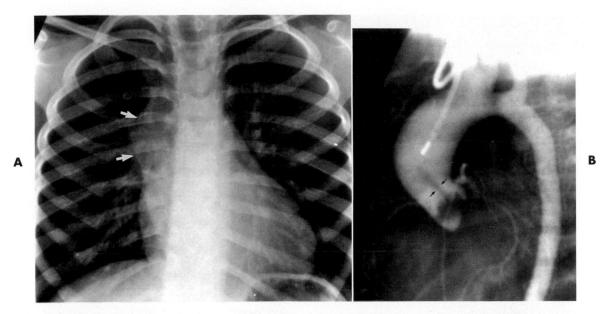

Fig. 2-53 Congenital aortic stenosis (CAS). A, Frontal radiograph reveals a dilated poststenotic segment of the ascending aorta (*arrows*). **B,** An aortic root injection illustrates the jet effect of the unopacified blood through the stenotic aortic valve (*arrow*).

dynamic subvalvular stenosis. This entity is familial in 35% of patients and has an equal gender incidence. The age at presentation of congenital aortic stenosis is inversely related to the severity of the obstruction, and the spectrum ranges from critical stenosis with CHF in the newborn to mild stenosis and an asymptomatic murmur in children and adolescents. Congenital aortic stenosis usually is progressive with age and is characterized by a harsh stenotic murmur at the upper right sternal border. Supravalvular stenosis is frequently (30%) associated with Williams syndrome (elfin faces, mental retardation, and neonatal hypercalcemia). Conventional chest radiographs reveal, in the absence of CHF, a normal heart size. The ascending aorta is seen as a border forming on the right side of the mediastinum as a result of poststenotic dilation (Fig. 2-53). It is abnormal for the ascending aorta to be border forming on the right side of the mediastinum before the age of 10 years. Cardiac catheterization and MRI may delineate the degree of obstruction further.

Initial treatment of valvular aortic stenosis consists of balloon dilation. If it is unsuccessful, aortic valve commissurotomy is performed. Subvalvular and supravalvular aortic stenoses are treated by resection of the obstructing segment.

Pulmonary stenosis   PS is the most common of acyanotic lesions found either isolated or in combination with other cardiac lesions. Commonly (95%) the lesion is characterized by commissural fusion with a central small orifice. Dysplastic valves occur in the remaining 5%, associated with Noonan syndrome. Chest radiographs show poststenotic dilation of the

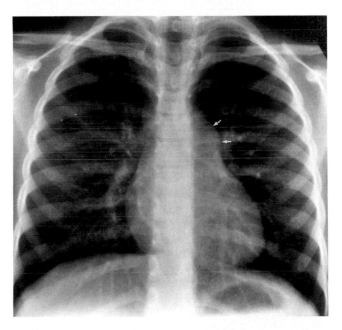

Fig. 2-54 Pulmonic stenosis (PS). Frontal radiograph demonstrates poststenotic dilation of the left pulmonary artery segment (arrows).

main pulmonary artery segment and the left main pulmonary artery as a result of the "jet" effect of the ejecting blood. Right ventricular hypertrophy may lead to an upturned cardiac apex (Fig. 2-54). Most patients are asymptomatic until adolescence. Treatment consists of balloon valvuloplasty. A few patients will need surgical relief of the destruction.

Table 2-4 Cardiosplenic syndromes

Lesions	Asplenia	Polysplenia
Heart	Complex CHD: corrected TgA, AV canal TPVR with obstruction, pulmonary stenosis/atresia, single ventricle	ASD, VSD, AV canal, single ventricle Azygous continuation of IVC
Lungs	Trilobed Eparterial bronchi Right pulmonary arteries	Bilobed Hyparterial Left pulmonary arteries
Abdomen	Heterotaxy Midline gallbladder Midline liver and stomach Malrotation	Heterotaxy Absent gallbladder, biliary atresia Malpositioned liver and stomach Rare anomalies

Miscellaneous Conditions

Hypoplastic left heart syndrome   HLHS is the most common cause of CHF in the neonate and presents at birth. The major components of HLHS are hypoplasia or atresia of the aortic and mitral valves; the ascending aortic arch, left atrium, and left ventricle also are hypoplastic. There is an obligatory left-to-right shunt, most often at the atrial level. The infant often appears septic because peripheral circulation is poor, and the infant may be in shock.

Chest radiographs reveal globular cardiomegaly with congested pulmonary flow within 24 hours of life. US is the definitive imaging modality to delineate the lesion.

Treatment consists of a two-step Norwood procedure. The lesion is usually fatal (80%) within the first week without surgery.

Cor triatriatum   Cor triatriatum reflects the failure of the left atrium to incorporate the common pulmonary veins. This failure results in a perforated membrane dissecting the left atrium and impeding blood return from the lungs as in mitral stenosis. Clinically this is seen as CHF. US may be diagnostic.

Heterotaxy

Cardiac malposition   Cardiac malpositions are complex and are best left to specialty texts. A few terms and definitions follow.

Dextrocardia implies that the cardiac silhouette is predominantly "pointed" to the right side of the spine, and there is associated inversion of the cardiac chamber (mirror image).

Levocardia refers to the cardiac silhouette "pointing" to the left, with normal chamber orientation.

In addition to the direction of the cardiac apex, the position of the gastric air bubble and the configuration and position of the liver will determine situs solitus (totalis). This is the normal appearance. The mirror image, situs inversus (totalis), is associated with only a slight increase in CHD.

Ambiguous viscera (visceral heterotaxy) exists when there is a midline stomach and a horizontal liver. There are multiple associated cardiac anomalies (Table 2-4).

AV concordance indicates that the right atrium is appropriately aligned with the right ventricle like the left atrium is with the left ventricle. There then is a much smaller chance of CHD.

AV discordance includes the abnormal right atrium to left ventricle and left atrium to right ventricle anatomic relation. Angiography and MRI can shed further light on whether the ventricles are inverted, whether there is levo- or dextro-loop bending, or whether there is transposition of the great vessels. It is often associated with CHD.

Cardiosplenic syndromes   Heterotaxy syndrome includes developmental complexes characterized by a tendency for symmetric development of normally asymmetric organs or organ systems (see Table 2-4). Thus these abnormalities should be considered whenever there is a discordance between the cardiac apex and abdominal site. Although rare, they are accompanied by severe CHD. Most infants die in the early postnatal period.

Asplenia, a teratogenic insult at 4 weeks gestation, is characterized by bilateral trilobed (right sidedness) lungs with eparterial bronchi, constantly severe CHD, an asymmetric liver, and GI tract malformations (microgastria biliary atresia).

Polysplenia is characterized by bilateral bilobed (left sidedness) lungs with hyparterial bronchi, variably severe associated CHD, and renal anomalies.

Both conditions have bilateral superior venae cavae,

Acquired Cardiac Anomalies

Pericardial disease Congential *absence of the pericardium* happens most often on the left side (70%) and is associated with PDA, ASD, and tetrad of Fallot. Absence on the right side is rare. Chest radiographs of children with small defects often demonstrate a protuberance in the region of the left atrial appendage that may involve the entire heart if there is total absence of the pericardium.

Pericarditis (pericardial effusion) most often is caused by *H. influenzae* in children and is initially seen with fever and dyspnea. There is usually an enlarged cardiac silhouette; US demonstrates the effusion best.

Myocardial disease Kawasaki disease is a mucocutaneous lymph node syndrome characterized by fever, rash, conjunctivits, and cervical adenopathy. Its peak incidence occurs between 1 and 3 years of age. The symptoms are due to a generalized vasculitis, but eventually, after approximately 1 month, the disease involves the myocardium. The vasculitis of the coronary arteries may progress to aneurysms and stenosis of the proximal portions of both left and right coronary arteries. These conditions may result in myocardial infarction, which is silent in one third of patients. Conventional chest radiographs most often reveal a normal chest except for cardiac enlargement in severe cases of myocardial involvement. Cardiac US is the imaging modality of choice to detect the coronary artery aneurysm. Treatment is medical and consists of gamma globulin.

Rheumatic heart disease is uncommon in children less than age 5 years and is rare in the Western world as compared to 40 years ago. It is the most common reason for acquired valvular insufficiency and/or stenosis and is caused by group A β-hemolytic streptococcus. In approximately 50% of patients, acute rheumatic fever results in myocarditis, with involvement of the mitral (85%) and aortic valves (55%) most commonly. If left ventricular failure or mitral regurgitation occurs, chest radiographs often show left atrial enlargement or enlargement of the left atrial appendage. If pulmonary venous hypertension occurs, there may be signs of congestive failure, with Kerley "B" lines and interstitial edema. In children treatment with appropriate antibiotics is often sufficient, with complete resolution of valvular disease common.

Endocardial anomalies *Endocardial fibroelastosis*, an endocardial thickening often associated with myocardial necrosis, possibly the result of myocardial fibrosis, can cause congestive failure in the neonate in the absence of murmurs. These changes can happen *secondarily* in aortic stenosis, coarctation of the aorta, PDA, and other causes of left ventricular overload.

Viral infection or inheritance has been implicated but not proved. Between 1 and 3 months of life marked cardiac enlargement on the left side becomes evident on chest radiographs, and the heart may develop a globular configuration. There is often compression of the left lower lobe bronchus in association, resulting in atelectasis of the left lower lobe. A cardiac transplant is the definitive treatment of choice.

Endocarditis, although rare, can be acute, subacute, or chronic. Usually it affects children with underlying CHD who are older than age 2 years. It can occur in children less than age 2 years and affect a normal valve. Offending agents include streptococci and staphylococci; the condition manifests in the child as fever and CHF. The valvular disease is best identified on US.

Pearls

Conventional radiographic findings in CHD

- If the cardiac apex reaches the lateral chest wall on the AP view or if the cardiac silhouette accounts for more than 50% of the chest diameter on the lateral view (trachea displaced posteriorly), chamber enlargement (CHD) is suggested.
- An increase in cardiac size is due to dilation secondary to increased blood flow, regurgitant valves, or failure.
- Cardiothoracic ration (<0.6 is normal in newborns) is of little value in evaluating children.
- The lateral chest radiograph is most useful for determining left atrial and left ventricular enlargement.
- Premature sternal fusion is associated with cyanotic CHD, a hypersegmental sternum with trisomy 21.
- CHD can be associated with thin ribs (trisomy 13, 18, or 21), 11 pairs of ribs (Down syndrome), and rib notching (coarctation of the aorta).
- Vertebral body anomalies are seen more often in VATER, tetrad of Fallot, and truncus arteriosus.
- Pulmonary artery calcification may be seen in patients with pulmonary hypertension.
- A ductus arteriosus "bump" with or without a calcified thrombus, although mostly a radiographic myth, can be noted.

Congested pulmonary vasculature The pulmonary artery normally is equal or slightly smaller in diameter as compared to the accompanying bronchus. The descending right pulmonary artery normally has the same diameters as the trachea. If the vessel diameter is increased:

- At 1 week
  Persistent fetal circulation
  Hypoplastic left heart syndrome
  TAPVR (with obstruction)
  Volume overload
  Transposition
  Severe coarctation
  Critical aortic stenosis

- At 2 to 4 weeks
    TAPVR (unobstructed)
    Large left-to-right shunts
    Truncus arteriosus
- Later
    Cardiomyopathy
    TAPVR (no obstruction)

Persistent fetal circulation
- Right-to-left shunting through the PDA occurs in the first few days of life when persistent pulmonary hypertension is present.
- Predisposing lesions include a diaphragmatic hernia, meconium aspiration, or neonatal infection.
- ECMO is the treatment of choice until the pulmonary pressure decreases.

Pulmonary artery segment
- Prominent
    Valvular PS
    Left-to-right shunts (VSD, ASD, PDA)
    TAPVR
- Concave
    Tetrad of Fallot
    Pulmonary atresia
    TGA (rotated)

Common surgical procedures
- Blalock-Taussig shunt: Gortex graft from subclavian artery to pulmonary artery
- Fontan procedure: SVC or IVC to pulmonary artery connection with ASD closure (for single ventricle hearts)
- Mustard procedure: dextro-TGA repair (atrial shunt)
- Senning procedure: dextro-TGA repair (atrial baffle)
- Jatene procedure: dextro-TGA repair (atrial switch)
- Waterston procedure: ascending aortic window to right pulmonary artery
- Potts procedure: descending aortic window to left pulmonary artery (rarely done)
- Blalock-Hanlon operation: removal of atrial septum in dextro-TGA (no longer done)

Right aortic arch
- Tetrad of Fallot
- Truncus arteriosus
- Dextro-TGA
- Tricuspid atresia (rarely)

Suggested Readings
Texts

Elliot LP, editor: Cardiac Imaging in Infants, Children and Adults, 1991, Lippincott, Pa.

Freedom RM, Culham JAG, Moes CAF: Angiocardiography of congenital heart disease, 1984, MacMillian, NY.

Kirks DR, editor: Practical Pediatric Imaging, 1992, Little Brown and Co., Boston, pp 516-702 (chest), pp 418-508 (cardiac).

Moss' Heart Disease in Infants, Children and Adolescents, ed 4, Baltimore, 1989, Williams & Wilkins.

Poznansky AK, Kirkpatrick JA, editors: Syllabus for the Categorical Course in Pediatric Radiology, Oakwood, Ill, 1989.

Silverman FM, Kuhn JP, editors: Caffey's Pediatric X-Ray Diagnosis, ed 9, vol 1, St Louis, 1991, Mosby-Year Book, pp 355-696 (chest), pp 697-892 (cardiac).

Silverman FM, Kuhn JP, editors: Caffey's pediatric X-ray Diagnosis, ed 9, vol 2, St. Louis, 1992, Mosby-Year Book, pp 1969-2028.

Sty JR, Wells RG, Starshak RJ et al: Diagnostic Imaging of Infants and Children, vol 3, 1992, Aspen Publishers, pp 1-232.

Swischuk LE: Imaging of the Newborn, Infant and Young Child, ed 3, Baltimore, 1989, Wiliams & Wilkins, pp 1-245 (chest), pp 246-354 (cardiac)

Van Praagh R, Vlad P: Dextrocardia, mesocardia and levocardia: the segmental approach to the diagnosis in congenital heart disease. Keith JD, Rowe RD, Vlad P, editors: Heart Disease in Infancy and Childhood, MacMillan, NY, ed 3, 1978, p. 638.

Articles

Ambrozino MM, Genieser NB, Krasinski K et al: Opportunistic infections and tumors in immunocompromised children, Radiol Clin North Am 30:639, 1992.

Berdon WE, Baker DH: Vascular anomalies and the infant lung: rings, slings and other things, Semin Roentgenol 7:39, 1972.

Ellis K: Developmental abnormalities in the systemic blood supply to the lungs, AJR 156:669, 1991.

Griscom NT: Pneumonia in children and some of its variants, Radiology 167:297, 1988.

Griscom, NT, Wohl ME, Kirkpatrick JA: Lower respiratory infections: how infants differ from adults, Radiol Clin North Am 16:367, 1978.

Heithoff KB, Sane SM, Williams GH et al: Bronchopulmonary foregut malformations: a unifying etiological concept, AJR 126:46, 1975.

Kirkpatrick JA: Pneumonia in children as it differs from adult pneumonia, Semin Roentgenol 15:96, 1980.

Lowe GM, Donaldson JS, Backer CL: Vascular rings: 10 year review of imaging, Radiographics 11:637, 1991.

Merten DF: Diagnostic imaging of mediastinal masses in children, AJR 158:825, 1992.

Northway WH Jr, Rosan RC: Radiographic features of pulmonary oxygen toxicity in the newborn: brochopulmonary dysplasia, Radiology 91:49, 1968.

Panicek DM, Heitzman ER, Randall PA et al: The continuum of pulmonary developmental anomalies, Radiographics 7:747, 1987.

Reid L: The lung: its growth and remodeling in health and disease, AJR 129:777, 1977.

Siegel MJ, Glazer HS, Wiener JI et al: Normal and abnormal thymus in childhood: MR imaging, Radiology 172:367, 1989.

Sivit CJ, Taylor GA, Eichelberger MR: Chest injury in children with blunt abdominal trauma: evaluation with CT, Radiology 171:815, 1989.

Strife JL: Upper airway and tracheal obstruction in infants and children, Radiol Clin North Am 26:2, 1988.

Strife JL et al: The position of the trachea in infants and children with right aortic arch, Peditr Radiol 19:226, 1989.

Swischuk LE, Hayden CK: Viral versus bacterial pulmonary infections in children (is roentgenographic differentiation possible?), Pediatri Radiol 16:278, 1986.

Winer-Muram HT, Tonkin IL: The spectrum of heterotaxy syndromes, Radiol Clin North Am 27:1147, 1989

CHAPTER 3

Gastrointestinal Tract

Imaging Techniques

Conventional Radiographs
  Abnormal gas patterns
    Adynamic ileus
    Dynamic ileus
    Ascites
    Calcifications
Contrast Examinations
  Barium sulfate suspension
  Water-soluble contrast agents
    Hyperosmolar agents
    Isotonic agents
    Low-osmolar agents
  Air
Ultrasound
Computerized Tomography
Magnetic Resonance Imaging
Nulear Medicine

Conventional Radiographs

In a child with abdominal symptoms, conventional radiographs of the abdomen comprise the usual initial imaging evaluation requested by the clinician. Familiarity with the proper age at presentation, the symptomatology of pediatric gastrointestinal (GI) diseases, and the great variability in radiographic patterns in the abdomen is very important. To arrive at a proper differential diagnosis in the abdomen, an abdominal radiograph must be exposed with the child in both the upright and supine positions. This positioning allows appropriate evaluation of the entire large and small bowel and assists greatly in pinpointing sites of pathology. In the neonatal age group a lateral decubitus

view, preferably the left, is easier to obtain than the erect radiograph that is preferred in the child that can cooperate. This applies even more because on a cross-table lateral view, it may be difficult to differentiate intraluminal from extraluminal air.

Pertinent points of difference from an adult abdominal radiograph are that the liver takes up a relatively larger space in the peritoneal cavity of children; the spleen should not be visible or at least should not displace the gastric contour; and the retroperitoneal fat stripes (psoas shadows) frequently are not seen because of the relative paucity of fat in the infant's and small child's retroperitoneum. In contrast, the properitoneal fat stripes are visible from infancy. Soft tissue pseudomasses in the abdomen may include the urinary bladder, the fluid-filled stomach or intestine, an umbilical hernia, or rarely a myelocele.

In the newborn there should be air in the stomach at birth. At 6 hours, the stomach and greater portion of the small bowel should be filled with air, and by 24 hours of life, air should be present in the rectum. A variation in this sequence (e.g., the absence of air in the stomach at 1 hour) should raise the possibility of an esophageal atresia. Clinically, absence of meconium passage by 24 hours should cause concern (Hirschsprung disease, a meconium plug or ileus), whereas abdominal distention or marked dilation of any viscus in the first 12 to 24 hours of life should lead to further imaging evaluation, most often by contrast enema.

Abnormal gas patterns Abnormal gas patterns can be distinctive in the neonate. Duodenal and proximal jejunal atresia may have a suggestive radiographic appearance, as may distal ileal atresia (Fig. 3-1). In the infant and young child pyloric stenosis and intussusception occasionally are suggested on the conventional abdominal radiograph: the former by an "hourglass" or

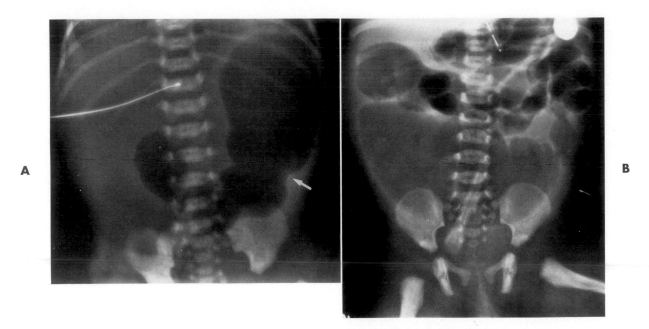

Fig. 3-1 **A**, Abdominal radiograph revealing air in the stomach and duodenal bulb with visualized peristaltic wave in the stomach (*arrow*) with no air distally. Duodenal atresia. **B**, Markedly dilated loops of bowel with a transverse orientation in a 1-day-old child. Ileal atresia.

"caterpillar-shaped" dilated stomach, the latter by revealing the soft tissue mass density of the intussusceptum (Fig. 3-2). Abnormal collections of air such as in a scrotal hernial sac or within the bladder (anorectal malformations) or in the bowel wall (neonatal necrotizing enterocolitis) may also support a definite diagnosis based on the conventional abdominal radiographs. Unfortunately, in neonates it is often impossible to differentiate small from large bowel, especially if the viscus is dilated. It is therefore often useful to speak of high- or low-bowel obstruction.

Although it is difficult if not impossible to differentiate large from small bowel in the presence of bowel dilation, determining the location or orientation of the distended loops often helps. Valvulae conniventes and haustral markings may distinguish small from large bowel, respectively, while the distended colon is more peripheral in location than the centrally located distended small bowel.

In infants and older children an *adynamic ileus* occurs after surgery, sepsis, or gastroenteritis or can be associated with electrolyte disturbances such as dehydration and hypokalemia and with drugs such as meperidine (Demerol), morphine-containing substances, and anti-cholinergics.

A *dynamic (mechanical) ileus* usually has an anatomic or congenital cause. The differential diagnosis in ascending order of likelihood includes (appen-

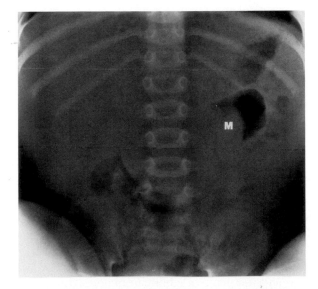

Fig. 3-2 Abdominal radiograph in a 2-year-old child with abdominal pain suggests the intussusceptum (*M*) invaginating the intussuscipiens.

diceal) inflammation, intussusception, malrotation, hernia, or adhesions.

The differential diagnosis of a gasless abdomen includes vomiting, use of medication that decreases peristalsis (e.g., pancuronium [Pavulon]), and obstruction of a fluid-filled viscus. Peritoneal irritation (peritonitis) or ascites can also displace ultraluminal air.

Ascites has many causes. In the neonate ascites may be urinary in origin (25% to 30%) secondary to obstruction and subsequent forniceal rupture, or chylous, caused by rupture of the lymphatic ducts. Other causes include peritonitis resulting from bowel perforation (meconium peritonitis) or appendicitis, congestive heart disease or erythroblastosis fetalis.

Conventional abdominal imaging classically illustrates centralization of bowel loops (air rises), blurring of the inferior hepatic edge, and obliteration of the properitoneal fat planes caused by fluid in the paracolic gutters. Ultrasound (US) is much more sensitive, as is computerized tomography (CT), with which small amounts of ascites can be detected in Morrison's pouch or the pouch of Douglas.

Calcifications Structures that may contain calcifications include the peritoneal wall (meconium peritonitis), viscera (appendicolith, torsed ovary), tumors (dermoid), and the retroperitoneal organs (adrenal hemorrhage, neuroblastoma, Wilms' tumor). The differential diagnosis of calcified structures in the pediatric abdomen may also include mesenteric or duplication cysts, calcified thrombi resulting from arterial or venous line placement, and renal or gallbladder calculi. Rare liver and spleen calcifications may occur in entities such as chronic granulomatous disease of childhood, hemangiomas, hamartomas, and hepatoblastoma.

Contrast Examinations

Barium sulfate suspension Indications for barium examinations of the GI tract are discussed in the subsequent sections.

There are two relative contraindications to using barium as a contrast agent: suspected bowel *perforation* or a predisposition for pulmonary *aspiration* of barium. Neither one is an absolute contraindication because barium in the retroperitoneum, mediastinum, or the peritoneal cavity that is removed shortly after entering these spaces will only hold minimal risk for sequelae such as granuloma formation, adhesions, or peritonitis. The same reasoning holds for aspirated barium, for it provokes a cough reflex. Thus when routine care is taken, barium constitutes a useful and safe contrast agent in the pediatric age group.

Water-soluble contrast agents The most commonly used water-soluble contrast agents are Gastrografin and Hypaque. Conray or Cysto-Conray also is used.

These agents are *hyperosmolar water-soluble media* and should not be used routinely in the upper GI tract. There is a serious risk of pulmonary edema or death when these agents are aspirated, caused by release of histamine or histamine-like substances in the lung. In addition, they can be toxic to the bowel mucosa, and their hydrophilic nature can result in massive fluid shifts in neonates. These contrast agents also cause a fluid shift into the lumen of the GI tract, resulting in their marked dilution, as early as the third portion of the duodenum, thus limiting their diagnostic use. In the large bowel, on the other hand, these agents can be used to exploit this hyperosmolar quality (e.g., to facilitate meconium plug evacuation by absorbing fluid into the bowel lumen, the "lubricating" effect of Tween•80, an additive of Gastrografin).

By appropriately diluting the above agents, near isotonicity can be achieved.

Isotonic contrast agents are useful when perforation is suspected or when the anatomic integrity must be evaluated in the sick neonate. Indications include necrotizing enterocolitis (NEC) and bowel anastomoses after surgery.

In recent years *low-osmolar water-soluble contrast agents* (e.g., metrizamide, Isovue, Omnipaque) have become available. They have the advantage of not being diluted during passage through the GI tract, of having virtually no effect on lungs or peritoneum, and of not being systematically absorbed. Their major disadvantage is their cost, a factor 10 times more expensive when compared to the conventional hyperosmolar agents.

When obtaining a pyelogram using low-osmolar contrast agents for GI investigatory purposes, visceral perforation is present, even if its location is not identified.

Air Air has been a useful contrast agent for as long as x-ray examinations have been performed. In pediatric imaging air (or CO_2) has been used by some in the reduction of intussusception. Reluctance to use it has been attributed to its being more cumbersome to use: the air pressure must be regulated and monitoring the air column may be difficult. Also, the perforation rate is higher compared to barium reduction (2.8% vs. 0.7%). In a patient with suspected esophageal atresia, however, air is very useful as a contrast agent. Only a little need be administered through a nasogastric (NG) tube to outline the atretic pouch without the risk for aspiration that would be present if a positive contrast agent were used.

Contrast studies of the small and large bowels do differ significantly from those of the adult in that clinical circumstances to a large degree dictate which study will be performed and in what fashion. Congenital abnormalities of the bowel such as malrotation occur more frequently, whereas in children less than 10 years of age inflammatory bowel disease (IBD) rarely occurs. Thus, it is doubly important that the pediatric imager be aware of the potential yield of an examination, its risks, and the effect on subsequent therapeutic regimens.

In pediatric upper gastrointestinal (UGI) studies the imager assesses the swallowing mechanism, the presence or absence of nasopharyngeal reflux, the contours and motility pattern of the esophagus and gastroesophageal junction, and the anatomic and functional integrity of the stomach, duodenum, and proximal jejunum, especially the ligament of Treitz. Air-filled and barium-filled views of the stomach and duodenum are worthwhile for mucosal evaluation but are not as mandatory as in the adult population. The evaluation of gatroesophageal reflux (GER) is controversial. There are some who, while intermittently fluoroscoping, assess the presence or absence of GER over 5 minutes, whereas others rely on a combination of incidental observation of GER during the UGI study and the pH probe study or nuclear medicine evaluation (milk scan) to fully demonstrate and evaluate GER. Imaging thus tends to objectify the subjective, because therapy should be guided more by the clinical spectrum of findings.

The contrast enema (or barium enema [BE]) examination in children is done primarily for anatomic evaluation of meconium-related obstruction, for determination of a transition zone in children with Hirschsprung's disease, and in the evaluation of lower GI bleeding. Routine rigorous preparatory cleansing of the colon as is done in adults is not usually necessary since intraluminal lesions (carcinoma, polyps) are less common. To evaluate the colonic mucosa in patients suspected of IBD or polyps, adequate preparation is mandatory. In the evaluation of meconium-related obstruction or Hirschsprung disease there need be no preparation of the colon in the latter instance because it could preclude determination of a transition zone, especially if located in the rectum. Therefore, in evaluating for Hirschsprung, a straight-tipped nonbulbous catheter is used to minimize disturbing the anorectal anatomy. The use of a balloontype enema tip is contraindicated in virtually all lower GI tract examinations in children. Proper taping in position of a soft, malleable bulbous enema tip is sufficient in all others and virtually atraumatic. Whether fluoroscopy should be performed with the patient in a prone or supine position is a personal preference; however, at the outset of the study the patient should be in the lateral position so that the retrorectal space and puborectalis sling can be evaluated adequately. The 'spot' films of the splenic and hepatic flexures and of the sigmoid colon are necessary only in specific instances in which overhead views have not properly elucidated these areas.

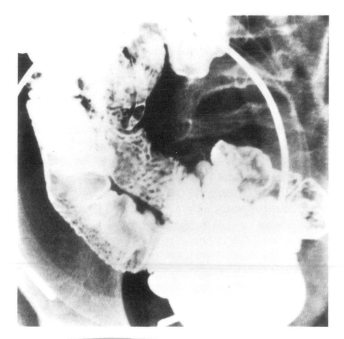

Fig. 3-3 Prominent lymphoid follicles in the terminal ileum.

Obtaining a postevacuation film is mandatory, especially after intussusception reduction and after all other single-contrast enema examinations to evaluate for mucosal detail, but it can be omitted after double-contrast examinations. A 24-hour postevacuation film is useful in suspected aganglionosis or megacolon cases to assess for diminished peristaltic evacuation activity.

Finally, throughout the entire small and large bowel, prominent lymphoid follicles, a normal finding particularly well seen in the terminal ileum, should not be confused with pathology. This holds true for all children through the teen years (Fig. 3-3).

Ultrasound

US is the screening modality of choice in the child suspected of intraabdominal pathology. Ionizing radiation is not used, and US is easy and quick to perform, with minimal if any patient preparation. There is no known risk associated with the procedure, and the lack of fat in infants and children allows better visualization of intraabdominal and retroperitoneal structures than in the adult. It is seldom necessary to use sedation, and manually immobilizing the child is often sufficient. When minimal restraint is necessary the use of sandbags or a papooseboard may be useful.

In general, a directed approach (e.g., right upper quadrant [RUQ] pain) leads to a higher yield than if vague symptomology (e.g., abdominal pain) is allowed to be the indication. Systematic evaluation of the abdominal or pelvic organs can best be accomplished by using a 3.5 or 5 MHz (sometimes 7.5 MHz) mechanical sector or, for the right lower quadrant (RLQ) a 5- or 7.5- MHz linear transducer. Color-flow Doppler evaluation of all major vessels should be routine.

Computerized Tomography

CT is an extremely accurate and fast-imaging modality, especially for retroperitoneal anatomy. As a rule, children less than 4 months and more than 4 years of age do not require sedation. The different regimens used for sedation reflect personal preferences and are influenced by the availability of pediatric anesthesia monitoring. An abdominal CT scan should be performed using both oral and intravenous (IV) contrast. Requirements and suggestions for the pediatric age group are listed in the box.

The advantages in the use of CT is its superior tissue plane resolution as compared to that with conventional radiographs. Disadvantages are relative. An average abdominal CT scan exposes the patient to approximately 2 rad, an amount that compares favorably to that of abdominal angiography (28 rad) and excretory urography (1 rad), especially when the amount of information is compared.

Indications include the evaluation of intraabdominal solid masses, abscesses, trauma, and hepatobiliary abnormalities and tumor staging. It is also useful in the guidance of drainage catheter placement and in establishing radiation therapy portals.

Spiral scanning further decreases scan time, limits exposure, and allows the use of improved three dimensional reconstruction algorithms, especially in trauma settings and in (facial, skull) reconstructive surgery planning.

Magnetic Resonance Imaging (MRI)

Advantages of MRI include superior multiplanar capabilities, absence of ionizing radiation, and excellent tissue and vascular resolution.

A disadvantage is that patients less than 6 years of age usually require sedation. Older patients need sedation only on a case-by-case basis. The total scan time for MRI is usually considerably longer than for CT, with claustrophobia a real issue for pediatric patients. MRI frequently is more expensive than CT or US.

Avoidance of motion artifacts Techniques used to minimize artifacts secondary to physiologic motion are as useful in children as they are in adults. They include respiratory ordered-phase encoding ("Resp Comp"), cardiac gating, gradient moment nulling ("Flow Comp"), and presaturation. The bellows used as a detector for respiratory motion to reduce artifacts is usually too big for use in children. Thus it is helpful to

---

CT Contrast Agents

ORAL CONTRAST

The contrast material commonly suggested to opacify the GI tract is meglumine diatrizoate (Gastrografin), 5 ml in 180 ml (6 oz) of, preferably, orange juice because Gastrogafin's taste in water is not pleasant.

- Neonates: one 6-oz cup of the prepared contrast agent, administered with the infant on the CT table (after entering the CT suite)
- Young children (1-6 yrs): two 6-oz cups (350 ml) of prepared contrast agent—one 2 hr before the examination and one while on the CT table
- Older children (>6 yr): four 6-oz cups (approximately 700 ml)—two 4 hr before, one 2 hr before the examination, and one while on the CT table

INTRAVENOUS CONTRAST

(Informed consent varies from institution to institution). It is strongly suggested to use low-osmolar water-soluble (physician administered or supervised) because contrast reactions and discomfort in case of extravasation are much less than with hyperosmolar water-soluble contrast agents.

SUGGESTED DOSAGE:

Child's Weight (lb)	Dosage
Up to 12	2 ml/lb
13-25	25 ml
26-50	1 ml/lb
51-100	50ml

---

wrap the bellows twice around the child's waist or to isolate part of the bellows with a plastic paper clip to fit the bellows to the patient's waist. If cardiac gating is being used, it is important to place the electrodes before the child falls asleep; otherwise, the sedation may fail during placement of the electrodes.

MRI protocols

The imaging protocols for MRI are, for the most part, identical to the protocols used for imaging adult patients. Some specific considerations in pediatric patients follow:

- *Use of coils.* For infants and newborns, the head coil can be used as a body coil. For this age group, the 3-inch surface coil provides excellent imaging of joints, with the exception of hips, which can be imaged with the head "body" coil or the 5-inch coil, and knees, which can be imaged with the extremity coil or the 5 inch coil.
- *Field of view (FOV).* Measurement of abdominal or thoracic girth provides a good indication of the FOV. As a rule of thumb, thoracoabdominal imaging in newborns and infants can be done, with FOV ranging from 24 to 32 cm.

Table 3-1 Common pediatric nuclear medicine procedures

Procedure	Radioisotope	Dosage
Meckel scan	$^{99m}TcO_4$ *Pertechnetate*	1-5 mCi IV
Liver or spleen scan	^{99m}Tc-sulfur colloid	0.5-5 mCi IV
Biliary scan	^{99m}Tc diSIDA	1 mC IV
Milk scan	^{99m}Tc-sulfur colloid	1 mCi by mouth (PO) or per nasogastric (NG) tube
Gastric emptying studies	^{99m}Tc-sulfur colloid Indium-111-DTPA	Less than 1 mCi PO or per NG tube

Table 3-2 Schematic representation of intestinal rotation in the fetus (Fig. 3-4, C)

Stage	Failure result	Duodenum (degrees)	Large bowel (degrees)	Embryology (wk)
I	Nonrotation	90	90	<6
II	"Reversed" rotation	90	0	6-10 (midgut into yolk sac)
III	Short mesentery	90	180	>10
	TOTAL	270	270	

Contrast

Oral To opacify the bowel, newborns and infants undergoing abdominal or pelvic examinations may be given a bottle of formula with a high iron content 2 hours before imaging. If patients are to undergo general anesthesia, the stomach should be evacuated before induction. If oral contrast is administered, glucagon (0.2 ml IV) should be given before imaging to minimize motion artifacts.

Intravenous Use of Gd-DTPA (0.1 mmol/kg is the usual pediatric dose) currently requires written consent from the parents.

Nuclear Medicine

Radioisotopes   The pediatric radioisotope examinations of the abdomen include studies for GER (milk scan) and gastric emptying, liver and spleen scans, and ectopic gastric mucosa (Meckel diverticulum) studies. They are reviewed in depth in the volume *Nuclear Medicine* in this series. Table 3-1 reviews the common pediatric procedures and dosages.

Developmental Anatomy

In the first 4 weeks cephalocaudal growth of the embryo with lateral "folding" results in the formation of the primitive gut. There is free communication between the foregut and amniotic sac at this stage, and by 28 days the tracheobronchial diverticulum and the liver bud have started to develop. Thus the foregut (from the oral cavity just distal to the pancreatic ductal buds), the midgut (from the primitive pancreas to the distal transverse colon), and the hindgut (from distal transverse colon to anus) are recognizable by 6 weeks gestation. The bowel is then formed in three steps: after forming the primitive tube, the lumen solidifies and then recanalizes, a process known as canalization. Anomalies of this process result in atresias or duplications.

Normal positioning of the intestinal tract results after a process of fetal rotation of the midgut and subsequent fixation of the mesenteric structures to the posterior abdominal wall (Table 3-2). In the fifth week of gestation the foregut (supplied by the celiac axis), hindgut (supplied by the inferior mesenteric artery [IMA]), and midgut (supplied by the superior mesenteric artery [SMA]) are suspended from the posterior peritoneal wall. By the eighth week, the midgut has rotated 90 degrees counterclockwise. The next 90-degree rotation allows the stomach and proximal (prearterial) portion of the duodenum to be anterior to the SMA and the third and fourth (postarterial) portion of the duodenum and rest of the small and large bowel to be posterior to the SMA.

These 90-degree rotations occurs with the entire GI tract outside of the peritoneal cavity (extracoelomic). By the tenth week of gestation, the midgut begins to return to the peritoneal cavity, a process that is complete by the eleventh week, all the while undergoing an additional 90 degrees of counterclockwise rotation. The total rotation thus totals 270 degrees counterclockwise around the SMA (Fig. 3-4). The cecum then gradually descends into the right lower quadrant by 4 to 5 months gestational age. This fixation process may not be complete until after birth and is the reason neonates and young children often have a "high-riding" or loose

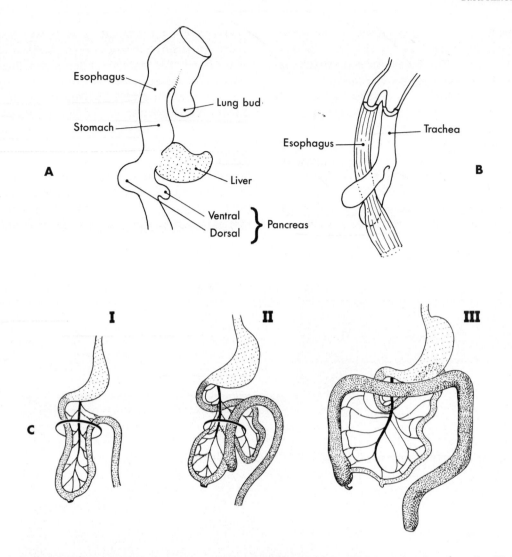

Fig. 3-4 Diagramatic representation of the embryology at 22 days (**A**) and at 5 to 6 weeks (**B**) and intestinal rotation (**C**) of the GI tract.

cecum. This "looseness" of the bowel mesentery may lead to internal hernias.

Internal hernias occur when a normal viscus protrudes through a hole in the mesentery or other apertures in the peritoneal cavity. Paraduodenal (on the left side more often than the right) hernias are most common. They account for approximately 2% of all intestinal obstructions.

"ACUTE" GASTROINTESTINAL CONDITIONS

Necrotizing Enterocolitis
Midgut volvulus
Hypertrophic Pyloric Stenosis
Intussusception
Pneumoperitoneum
Gastrointestinal Bleeding

Necrotizing Enterocolitis

NEC occurs most commonly (85%) in premature neonates who weigh less than 2500 g and are of less than 37 weeks gestation. The clinical presentation, with bloody diarrhea (25%) or abdominal distention, possibly signs of sepsis, and vomiting, apnea, or lethargy, is often at 3 to 4 days of life. The occurrence of NEC has been associated with hypoxia, stress, low blood pressure, and infection.

The cause of NEC is probably multifactorial, with premature rupture of the membranes, preeclampsia, diabetes mellitus, multiparity, early feeding with (high osmolar) formula, and placement of umbilical artery and venous catheters all implicated as placing the infant at a higher risk for NEC.

The pathophysiology implicates bowel ischemia as a result of low blood flow. Subsequent breakdown of the mucosal barrier allows bacteria and/or air to enter the bowel wall. This may be caused or facilitated by necrosis or autolysis of intestinal flora. A viral role in this process is controversial. The interstitial bowel wall air can then enter the portal venous circulation, often accompanied by the development of metabolic acidosis and disseminated intravascular coagulation (DIC).

The most common site of occurrence in infants with NEC is the distal ileum or the ascending colon, although the entire bowel can be involved. Strictures are more common in the colon (80%) and can occur in up to one third of all patients with NEC.

Perforation occurs most often within the first 36 hours, and most commonly in the ileocecal region.

Treatment for NEC involves bowel rest and antibiotics. If perforation does occur, surgical exploration is mandatory. The value of abdominal radiographs in predicting perforation is controversial. Some centers believe that an acute change in orientation of the bowel loops heralds impending perforation, whereas others believe that perforation has occurred if a loop or loops remain in a fixed configuration over a period of time.

Abdominal radiographs obtained at the time of clinical presentation of NEC reflect the friable and edematous quality of the bowel wall, which is manifested by a jumbled pattern secondary to bowel wall edema that

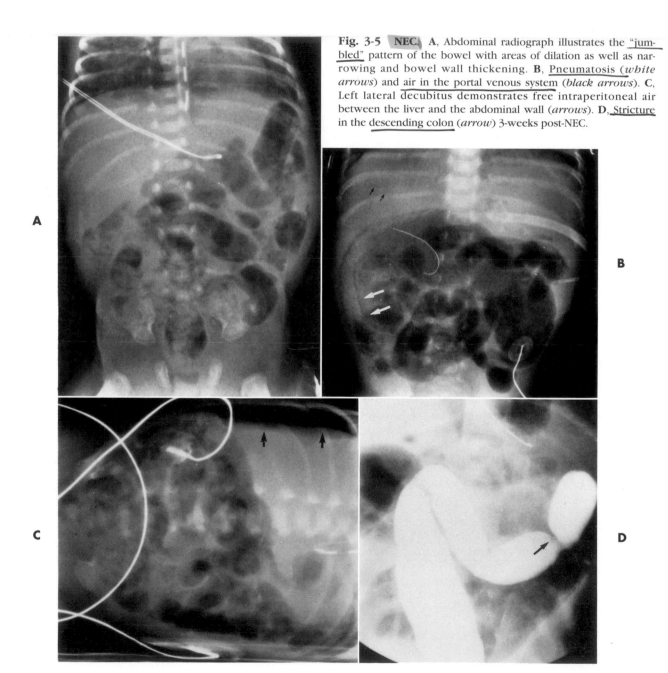

Fig. 3-5 NEC. **A,** Abdominal radiograph illustrates the "jumbled" pattern of the bowel with areas of dilation as well as narrowing and bowel wall thickening. **B,** Pneumatosis (*white arrows*) and air in the portal venous system (*black arrows*). **C,** Left lateral decubitus demonstrates free intraperitoneal air between the liver and the abdominal wall (*arrows*). **D,** Stricture in the descending colon (*arrow*) 3-weeks post-NEC.

either compresses the lumen in some areas or causes an ileus to appear in other areas. Frequently both coexist with or without pneumatosis.

The air in the bowel wall may present as either linear or bubbly pneumatosis. The air is located in either the submucosal or subserosal layer and is of a fleeting nature. It either resorbs or enters the portal venous system.

Air in the portal venous system distributes itself from the porta hepatis to the hepatic periphery, and used to be thought of as being associated with increased mortality. It currently is considered part of the overall NEC imaging spectrum and does not appear to alter the morbidity or mortality (Fig. 3-5).

If perforation is suspected either on clinical grounds or after a physical examination, a left lateral decubitus film is preferred over the supine cross-table examination. Approximately two thirds of perforations are heralded by free air; approximately one third will develop ascites. Free air is identified on conventional radiographs by air outlining the falciform ligament ("football" sign) or both sides of the bowel wall (Rigler's sign) (Fig. 3-6).

Bowel wall thickening and ascites of NEC are shown in reproducible fashion with US. Air can be identified within the portal vein. Recently, attempts have been made to use color-flow or duplex US to better demonstrate air bubbles flowing through the portal vein and

its tributaries. The predictive value of this finding is not yet clear.

The use of contrast studies is rarely if ever indicated in the acute phase of NEC. Nonionic contrast agents would be preferred in such a setting. Evaluation for the presence of strictures, which are most frequently seen 6 to 12 months after the acute stage, necessitates performing a contrast enema. Balloon dilation of the strictures has been attempted but without consistent success.

Midgut Volvulus

Midgut volvulus can occur at any age but is more common in the term infant. It represents a true emergency condition that can lead to necrosis of the twisted portion of intestine. The twisted portion rotates around the SMA as its fulcrum. It can happen in utero but is most commonly diagnosed (80%) in the first few weeks of life. Bilious vomiting, usually at 2 to 3 days of life, is the classic presenting symptom. Abdominal distention is not common.

The condition occurs because there is malfixation of bowel and a resultant short mesentery, allowing the small bowel to twist around the SMA. It is an absolute emergency, making imaging imperative so that surgical intervention can prevent vascular compromise to the bowel. It has been shown that three and one-half turns

Fig. 3-6 Abdominal radiograph in a patient with NEC demonstrates free air outlining the falciform ligaments (*large arrow*) as well as Rigler's sign (*double arrows*).

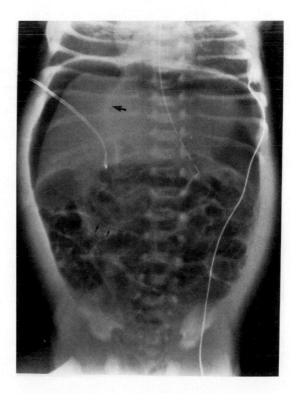

around the SMA is the critical point that leads to high mortality secondary to bowel necrosis; fewer turns may only compromise venous and lymphatic drainage.

Conventional radiographs are suggestive in the majority of cases by demonstrating mild dilation of duodenal loops proximal to the volvulus and edema of the bowel wall involved. Relatively little distal intestinal air is present. This results in a "high" obstruction with or without air-fluid levels. Static air-fluid levels often indicate bowel necrosis (Fig. 3-7).

Contrast studies A peroral contrast examination is the initial examination of choice to demonstrate the volvulus if there is no obstruction. Barium is a safe contrast agent; a nonionic agent may also be used. A classic corkscrew appearance of the second and third portion of duodenum is seen in case of midgut volvulus. There is, by definition, an abnormal position of the ligament of Treitz, the anatomic landmark of the duodenojejunal junction. Use of contrast enema to diagnose malrotation is unreliable because a high-riding cecum is seen in 15% to 20% of healthy neonates and infants. (Cecal position is thus not as reliable as the position of the ligament of Treitz to rule out malrotation).

US may demonstrate dilated and fluid-filled small bowel loops, as well as reversal of the orientation of the superior mesenteric vein (SMV) with regard to the SMA. This finding is helpful but not diagnostic for midgut volvulus.

Hypertrophic Pyloric Stenosis

Hypertrophic pyloric stenosis (HPS) is characterized by acquired hypertrophy of the circular pyloric muscle in the neonate, but the longitudinal muscle is unaffected. Immature coordination between antral contractility and emptying may explain this condition. Genetic (firstborn male, familial incidence) or gastric humoral (high gastrin levels) factors also have been implicated. HPS usually is seen 2 to 6 weeks after birth, although 20% of these infants have symptoms from birth. The symptoms include vomiting, projectile in 10% to 15%, in association with dehydration, hypochloremic alkalosis, or jaundice. HPS is rare after 12 weeks of age.

The incidence of HPS is variable: one in 500 live births in the United States, one in 2000 in African-Americans, and one in 25 live births in Sweden.

Boys outnumer girls 4:1. In addition, there is a seasonal variation in incidence. On physical examinations 10% of patients have either hyperperistaltic waves or a palpable pyloric olive. In that instance, imaging usually is not indicated.

A *conventional radiograph* of the abdomen may show a distended stomach with or without an air-fluid level and relatively little gas distally in approximately 15% to 20% of cases. The gastric hyperperistalsis may be evident in a "caterpillar" configuration of the stomach.

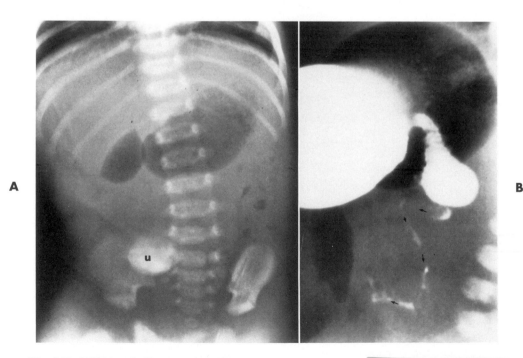

Fig. 3-7   Midgut volvulus. A, Abdominal radiograph demonstrates air in the distended stomach and duodenal bulb with a few pockets of air distally. These findings remained unchanged over 6 hours. Note the umbilical hernia (*u*). **B**, Contrast study illustrates the "cork screw" appearance of a midgut volvulus (*arrows*).

Table 3-3 Diagnosis and treatment of suspected pyloric stenosis (Fig. 3-8)

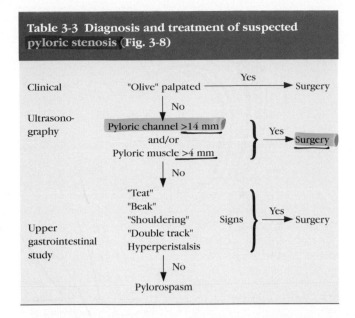

Clinical — "Olive" palpated — Yes → Surgery

↓ No

Ultrasonography — Pyloric channel >14 mm and/or Pyloric muscle >4 mm — Yes → Surgery

↓ No

Upper gastrointestinal study — "Teat" "Beak" "Shouldering" "Double track" Hyperperistalsis — Signs — Yes → Surgery

↓ No

Pylorospasm

The role and imaging characteristics of US and an upper GI evaluation are summarized and illustrated in Table 3-4. Using US, a 5-MHz or 7.5-MHz linear transducer is most useful. True HPS presents no difficulty for the operator. A donut, or bullseye, should be readily apparent with the infant slightly turned on its right side to take advantage of gastric contents in the antrum as an acoustic "window" (Fig. 3-8).

A UGI examination is performed with only a relatively small amount of contrast swallowed, or inserted through an NG tube as preferred by some. After an examination with the positive results, the contrast agent should be removed from the stomach before the infant leaves the imaging suite.

Pylorospasm, the main differential diagnostic entity, is a controversial entity and can best be regarded as delayed gastric emptying. After a variable time period (days to weeks), symptoms disappear in these children. Whether or not this represents a "forme fruste" of

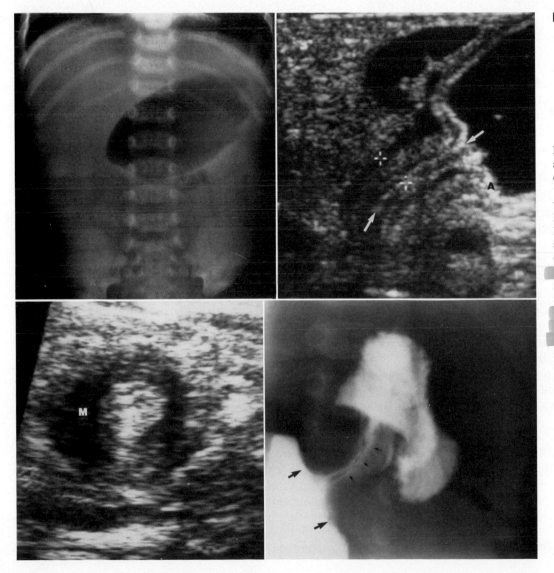

Fig. 3-8 HPS. **A**, Supine abdominal radiograph demonstrates a dilated "contracting" stomach with little air distally. **B**, Longitudinal US depicts hypertrophied muscle (*X*) and an elongated canal (*arrows*). "Shouldering" of the antrum (*A*) is also noted. **C**, Transverse US reveals the thickened muscle (*M*) surrounding the echogenic pyloric channel (bull's eye). **D**, UGI demonstrates the "shouldering" (*large arrows*) and the elongated and narrowed pyloric channel with a "double-track" (*small arrows*).

pyloric stenosis is not certain since adrenogenital syndrome, dehydration, and sepsis have also been implicated as causes. Finally, gastroenteritis, pyloric channel (stress) ulcer, and congenital abnormalities such as an antral web or gastric duplication can lead to a symptom complex similar to that of HPS.

Intussusception

Intussusception is the invagination of a portion of proximal bowel (intussusceptum) into a contiguous segment of distal bowel (intussuscipiens). It occurs in patients ranging in age from newborn to 18 years; the peak incidence (40%) occurs between 5 and 9 months of age, and 60% occurs before the first and 90% before the second birthday. Boys outnumber girls 3:2. The incidence varies according to season and geographic location, occurring most commonly in winter and spring and in Australia and Europe.

Because a discernable lead point causing intussusception occurs infrequently, the cause is most often deemed idiopathic.

Idiopathic intussusception is believed triggered by hypertrophy of lymphoid tissue (Peyer's patches) in the terminal ileum that may be related to an antecedent (7 to 10 days) viral infection. Adenovirus has been isolated frequently from children with intussusception and has been thought to play a role in some cases by increasing motility of the bowel or producing hyperplasia of the lymphoid tissue.

Lead points that may cause intussusception include duplication cysts, Meckel diverticulum, lymphoma, polyps, hemorrhage into the wall of the bowel such as with Henoch-Schönlein purpura, appendiceal inflammation, and inspissated stool in patients with cystic fibrosis. Lead points most often are present in neonates in the first month of life or in children more than 5 years of age. The most common lead point in patients more than 5 years of age is lymphoma; in infants it is a Meckel diverticulum.

With regard to location, approximately 90% of all intussusception are ileocolic, with the remaining 10% ileoilea or colocolic. Ileoileal intussusceptions most commonly are seen in postoperative patients, with the mechanism thought abnormal peristalsis during resolution of an ileus. Colocolic intussusceptions are very rare (Fig. 3-9).

The most frequent clinical symptoms include abdominal pain and vomiting (each >90%), blood per rectum and a palpable abdominal mass (each in approximately 60%). Approximately 20% of afflicted children have an upper respiratory tract infection at presentation, and 10% have had diarrhea before the onset of symptoms. Fever is common. The typical "currant jelly" stools, consisting of blood and mucus mixed with

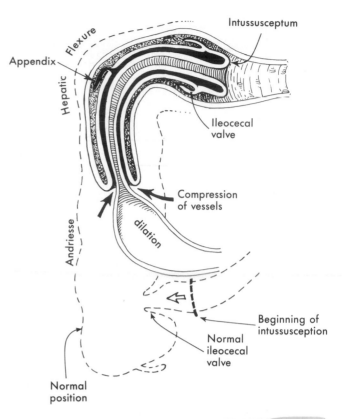

Fig. 3-9 Schematic representation of an ileocolic intussusception.

stool, occur in 15% to 20% and usually appear within 24 hours, although they may not appear until 2 days after the onset of symptoms. Differential diagnostic considerations include viral gastroenteritis, peritonitis caused by a ruptured viscus (appendix), or sepsis.

Conventional abdominal radiographs of the abdomen never rule out an intussusception but may confirm this suspicion by showing a mass a colon devoid of its contents (see Fig. 3-2). This emptying of the distal colon occurs because intussuscepted bowel leads to hyperperistalsis of the distal colonic segment that is related either to the event itself or to the cathartic properties of intraluminal blood.

Reduction of an intussusception can be achieved by surgical or nonsurgical means. The mortality rate associated with surgical reduction is currently estimated at approximately 0.1%; with imaging reductions, no mortality has been reported. The advantage of imaging or pressure reduction lies in the avoidance of generalized anesthesia and laparotomy.

Current imaging in patients suspected of having an intussusception consists of a preliminary radiographic examination of the abdomen followed by a diagnostic examination using a contrast-agent enema. (US and CT may identify intussusception, but their use in the therapeutic phase of this entity is limited.) If results of the diagnostic examination are positive, a *therapeutic*

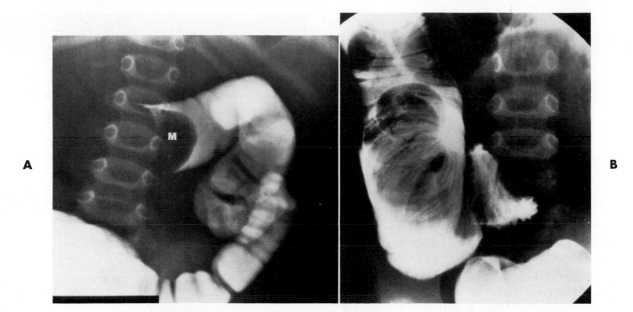

Fig. 3-10 **Intussusception.** **A,** A diagnostic enema encounters the intussusceptum in the mid-transverse colon (*M*). **B,** The "coiled spring" appearance of an ileocolic intussusception: the contrast has interdigitated between the intussusceptum and the intussuscipiens.

enema is administered in sequence. Definitive therapy has occurred when the intussusception is reduced as shown radiographically when the contrast agent refluxes freely into the terminal ileum.

The only absolute *contraindications* to performing a diagnostic enema examination when intussusception is suspected are intestinal perforation and peritonitis. The duration of symptoms (>24 hours) need not be a contraindication, although a lower success rate of reduction has been noted in the presence of obstruction.

The patient should be in satisfactory clinical condition before any form of treatment for intussusception is undertaken. The operating room should be ready and the surgical team notified and in the hospital if not in the imaging suite. (Mild sedation and immobilization of the patient before the enema is administered have been advocated by some.)

The choice of contrast agent for "imaging reduction" is controversial. Air, water, barium, and a water-soluble agent have all been used successfully. The height of the contrast column traditionally is placed 3 feet above the table. Further elevation of the reservoir does not significantly alter the intraluminal pressure, but the "bag at eye level" is a convenient height. After insertion of the enema tip (a balloon is not used), the intussusception is sought. Monitoring is done most easily by fluoroscopy; as noted, US is also suggested by some. Reducing an intussusception should be attempted three times. The end point of a successful reduction procedure consists of *free* flow of the contrast agent into the

terminal ileum (TI). Care should be taken to determine the presence of residual ileoileal intussusception and to allow identification of a possible lead point (Fig. 3-10).

A postevacuation film is of paramount importance, for recurrence may occur during evacuation. A recurrence is revealed by complete evacuation of the colon on the postevacuation film. Significant residual contrast in the colon is the rule after successful reduction.

In addition, after successful reduction the ileocecal valve may remain enlarged up to 24 hours, but this is not deemed pathologically significant. Perforation does occur in 2.8% of patients reduced with air and in 0.7% of those reduced with barium. This is a surgical emergency, and its major sequelae are peritonitis caused by fecal contamination of the peritoneum, adhesions, and granuloma formation.

The recurrence rate for intussusception varies from 1% to 8% following hydrostatic or surgical reduction, with most instances occurring within 48 hours after the reduction procedure.

Pneumoperitoneum

Free air within the peritoneal cavity may represent an emergency, depending on the clinical history (see box on p. 70). Air present in the peritoneum after surgery usually will have disappeared by 3 days but may last as long as 1 or 2 weeks. If it is diminishing in amount, it can be clinically followed; however, if it is increasing in amount, a patent connection between the peritoneum and an air-containing structure must be excluded. Pneumoperitoneum after insertion of a rectal thermometer or an enema tip or secondary to other iatrogenic procedures also can be a cause.

Supine abdominal radiographs often can be diagnostic. Rigler's sign (visualization of both sides of the bowel) and the football sign (air outlining the falciform ligament) are indicative of free air. Horizontal beam radiography is most useful and often diagnostic in determining intraperitoneal free air before exploratory laparotomy (see Fig. 3-6).

Gastrointestinal Bleeding

It is less useful in the pediatric age group to differentiate between upper and lower GI hemorrhage than in adults. The most common cause of GI bleeding is an anal fissure, followed by a Meckel diverticulum, polyps, or intussusception (see box). By age group, infections and stress are seen most often in neonates and infants. In infants and young children less than 5 years old, a Meckel diverticulum, juvenile polyp, or intussusception must be considered. Clinically, in those presenting with brisk bleeding, a Meckel diverticulum or stress ulcer should be considered and in those presenting with melena or trace blood, a juvenile polyp, intussusception, or anal fissure.

The yield of a conventional *abdominal radiograph*, US, or CT is unpredictable and often low. Contrast studies using barium may be useful to delineate underlying pathology.

Radionuclide studies using ^{99m}Tc-labeled red blood cells can localize the bleeding site. This study sometimes helps visualize a Meckel diverticulum because the ectopic gastric mucosa cells of the diverticulum secrete ^{99m}Tc pertechnetate. Endoscopy in skilled hands is extremely accurate.

Esophagus

Anatomy and Development Anomalies
  Pharynx and esophagus: embryogenesis
  Esophageal atresia and tracheoesophageal fistula
  Cystic foregut malformations
  Vascular impressions
    Concomitant posterior esophageal and anterior
      tracheal impressions
    Anterior tracheal impressions
    Posterior esophageal impression
    Lesion between esophagus and trachea
Acquired Conditions
  Strictures
  Esophagitis
  Foreign bodies
  Achalasia
  Neoplasms

Differential Diagnosis of Free Air

Gastric perforation in the newborn
Necrotizing enterocolitis
Visceral obstructions such as with Hirschsprung
  disease and meconium-related ileus
Dissection of air from a pneumomediastinum
Perforated ulcers, Meckel diverticulum, or appendix

GI Hemorrhage

NEONATES
  NEC, infectious colitis
INFANT
  Stress ulcer, Meckel diverticulum, intussusception
CHILD
  Polyp, inflammatory bowel disease

Anatomic and Developmental Anomalies

Pharynx and esophagus   During the fourth and fifth weeks of gestation, lateral ridges appear in the foregut that fuse medially, separating the trachea and esophagus. The esophagus then elongates and resembles the adult esophagus (see Fig. 3-4, *A* and *B*). However, in children the normal impression of the aortic arch, left mainstem bronchus, and left atrium is not seen as consistently, but the stripping wave is usually quite prominent.

Intermittent sucking and swallowing of amniotic fluid and mandibular movements have been observed as early as 24 weeks by US. The swallowing mechanism matures rapidly after birth. Nasopharyngeal regurgitation is abnormal after 2 to 3 days of life. Aspirating small amounts usually is followed by a clearing cough in struggling or crying infants. Repeated aspiration of contrast during UGI study is a reason to terminate the UGI study immediately. Video evaluation may be of diagnostic assistance in these disorders.

Swallowing mechanism failure caused by poor relaxation of the upper esophageal sphincter (cricopharyngeal spasm), neuromuscular disorders such as cerebral palsy, familial dysautonomia (i.e., Riley-Day syndrome in Ashkenazi Jews), and other rare conditions affecting the esophagus (e.g., cranial nerve palsies, scleroderma, dermatomyositis) may all occur in children but are rare.

Esophageal atresia and tracheoesophageal fistula Failure of differentiation, ridge formation, and elongation of the primitive foregut can result in various combinations of esophageal atresia (EA) and tracheoesophageal fistula (TEF) (Fig. 3-11).

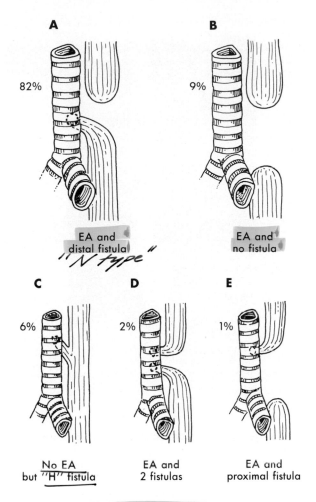

A 82% EA and distal fistula "N type"

B 9% EA and no fistula

C 6% No EA but "H" fistula

D 2% EA and 2 fistulas

E 1% EA and proximal fistula

Fig. 3-11 The common (**A, B**) and less comon (**C, D, E**) combinations of EA and TEF.

The incidence of these abnormalities varies from one in 2000 to one in 5000 live births, with a sporadic familial occurrence.

In one third of these patients prenatal US as early as 24 weeks gestation can suggest the presence of these abnormalities if polyhydramnios is present. Clinically, approximately 30% of infants with EA and TEF are born prematurely, and inability to introduce an NG tube should suggest that EA is present. Coughing, choking, or cyanosis associated with the first feeding is the most common clinical presenting symptom on the first day of life. There is an increased incidence of TEF in infants with Down syndrome.

Imaging of EA and TEF with conventional radiographs (1) may reveal the air-distended esophageal atretic pouch; (2) may show the NG tube curled up in this pouch; or (3) may show excessive dilation of stomach and/or small bowel as a result of a distal fistula communicating between the lungs and the esophagus (Fig. 3-12). A gasless abdomen usually indicates there is no coexisting distal fistula. In addition, conventional radiographs are useful to evaluate for associated abnormalities, most commonly the vascular and (cardiac) vertebral defects, anorectal malformation, TE fistula, and radial and renal dysplasia comprising the (VATER) association. Associated anomalies occur in approximately one third of patients with EA and TEF (see box on p. 72). Contrast evaluation is usually not necessary, but if it is requested, it should be performed with less than 1 ml of contrast agent. Treatment consists of primary anastomosis of the proximal and distal esophagus.

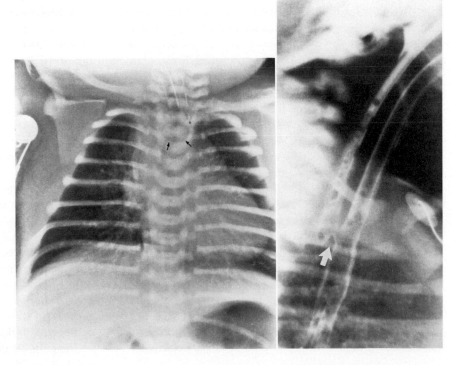

Fig. 3-12 EA/TEF. A, Inability to pass NG tube and air-distended proximal esophageal pouch (*arrows*) illustrated on admission chest radiograph. Note stomach bubble. **B,** Contrast study illustrates the proximal TEF (*arrow*).

A   B

Anomolies Associated With EA and TEF

CARDIAC
Patent ductus arteriosus, ventricular septal defect, right sided arch

GASTROINTESTINAL
Duodenal atresia, imperforate anus

GENITOURINARY
Renal agenesis (unilateral)

SKELETAL
Vertebral anomalies

DOWN SYNDROME
30%

Colonic interposition or gastric tube surgery may be needed if primary repair proves impossible. Nonionic (barium) contrast evaluation may then be used to exclude postoperative leaks.

Furthermore, the distal esophageal segment exhibits disordered motility in more than 90% of the infants after surgical repair of EA. The upper esophagus exhibits dysmotility in less than 10% of patients.

Rare anomalies of tracheal and esophageal separation include laryngotracheoesophageal cleft, tracheal agenesis (with or without a fistula), and esophageal bronchus. The clinical presentation of these anomalies is not different from that of EA or TEF.

Cystic foregut malformations Foregut malformations consist of a spectrum that can range from webs to duplication, with considerable overlap. In the chest, foregut malformations may appear on chest radiographs as a middle or posterior mediastinal mass. There may be associated malformations of the vertebral bodies, whereas the cysts themselves may contain respiratory (bronchogenic), or GI mucosa or both. The secretory properties of these lesions in the respiratory epithelium may cause the lesions to enlarge and cause symptoms. They can then be divided into three broad categories: bronchogenic cysts, neurenteric cysts, and esophageal duplications.

Neurenteric cysts usually are located more posterior than bronchogenic cysts; the latter are discussed in Chapter 2. Neurenteric cysts may hemorrhage or enlarge as a result of epithelial secretions and may be associated with neurologic symptoms (paraplegia) secondary to cord compression. They are virtually always associated with vertebral body anomalies. Esophageal duplications are half as common as ileal duplications. Stomach and duodenal duplications rank next in incidence. Gender incidence is equal, and symptoms usually are related to obstruction. There is seldom communication between the duplication and the true lumen of the GI tract unless repeated inflammation has occurred.

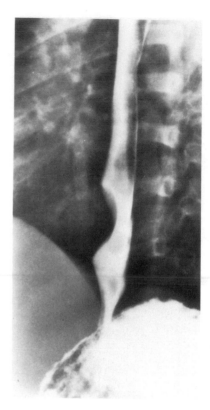

Fig. 3-13 Esophageal duplication. Smooth submucosal lesion narrowing the distal esophageal lumen.

Conventional radiographs may demonstrate a middle mediastinal soft tissue density or, on contrast examination, a smooth submucosal lesion narrowing the esophageal lumen (Fig. 3-13).

CT displays the anatomic relationships to a better extent. MRI proves the presence of a cystic component on T2-weighted images.

Vascular impressions In infants presenting with feeding disorders, spitting, or dyspnea, congenital vascular anomalies of the esophagus are high on the list of differential diagnostic possibilities. "Rings and slings" may appear in the neonate with symptoms or constitute an incidental finding in infants and children. Their embryogenesis springs from six paired ascending branchial arches present during fetal life that pass on either side of the developing foregut. The first two arches disappear. The third arch gives rise to the carotid vessels. The fourth arch gives rise to the aortic arch and the sixth arch to the pulmonary artery and the ductus arteriosis. The fifth arch fails to develop. All congenital vascular rings and resultant impressions on foregut derivatives ultimately are determined by which portion of these paired ascending arches has persisted or degenerated during this developmental period.

Imaging by conventional radiographs, with or with-

Trachea   Esophagus

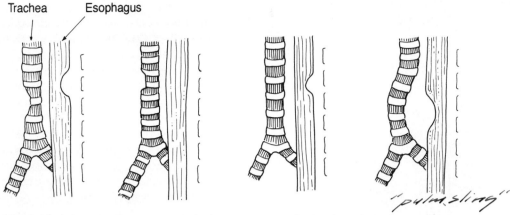

"pulm sling"

Fig. 3-14   Schematic diagram reveals the four common tracheal and esophageal impressions.

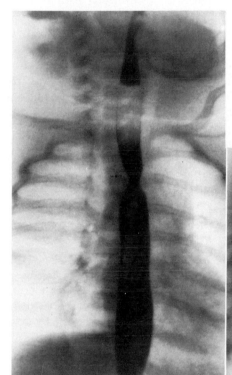

Fig. 3-15   **Double aortic arch.** **A,** Frontal view reveals an indentation on both sides of the contrast-filled esophagus, the right being slightly more cephalad (*arrow*). **B,** Lateral view reveals the posterior esophageal impression and a subtle anterior tracheal narrowing (*arrow*).

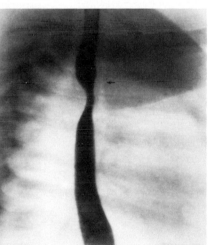

A   **B**

out the use of contrast to outline the esophagus, then reveals one of the following four common patterns (Fig. 3-14).

Concomitant posterior esophageal and anterior tracheal impressions   Concomitant posterior esophageal and anterior tracheal impressions result from a true vascular ring. The most common entity is a double aortic arch or a right aortic arch combined with an aberrant left subclavian artery. The ring in this instance is completed by the ductus remnant. If the ring is tight enough and causes tracheal compression, surgical treatment may be necessary. In 75% of cases of double aortic arch, the descending aorta is on the left with the posterior arch more cephalad. The descending aorta is on the right in the remaining 25%, with the posterior arch more caudad. The posterior arch is the larger arch in the majority of cases. On conventional radiographs the frontal projection reveals an indentation of the contrast-filled esophagus on both sides, usually with the right side impression slightly cephalad to left. The lateral view may illustrate both the esophageal and tracheal impression (Fig. 3-15). The surgical treatment is the same for both of these possibilities and consists of dividing the smaller arch.

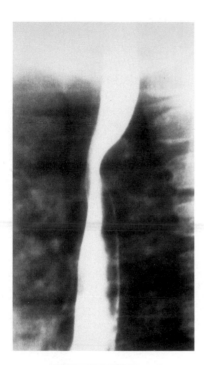

Fig. 3-16 Aberrant right subclavian artery causing a posterior impression on the esophagus.

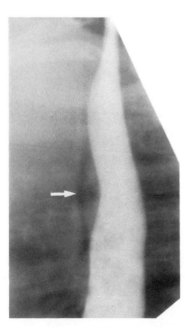

Fig. 3-17 Lateral view with contrast in the esophagus illustrates the aberrant left pulmonary artery between it and the trachea (*arrow*).

Anterior tracheal impression An anterior tracheal impression is caused by the innominate artery arising to the left of the trachea and ascending anteriorly. It is also considered a normal finding unless accompanied by symptoms. Its presence can be proven on endoscopy or MRI. Symptoms of respiratory compromise may necessitate aortopexy (see Fig. 2-9).

Posterior esophageal impression The appearance of a posterior esophageal impression is fairly common as a result of an aberrant right subclavian artery in cases of a *left* aortic arch. It is caused less commonly by an aberrant left subclavian artery with a *right* aortic arch. It is caused by disappearance of the fourth branchial arch. If it is not accompanied by symptoms, it is normal and does not require treatment. Dysphagia has been reported rarely. The trachea is normal (Fig. 3-16).

Lesion between esophagus and trachea Even though lymph nodes and the very rare bronchogenic cyst can be considered in a differential diagnosis, they are usually more lateral in location than a lesion between the esophagus and trachea. A rounded soft tissue density between the esophagus and trachea represents the pathognomonic appearance of an aberrant left pulmonary artery. The left pulmonary artery arises from the right pulmonary artery and slings to the left, a variant of the sixth branchial arch. Tracheomalacia frequently is present. Tracheal compromise may be present at birth, with severe respiratory distress, and correction of this abnormality is necessary to avoid continued respiratory problems. Conventional lateral radiographs (with barium) are usually diagnostic (Fig. 3-17).

Acquired Conditions

Strictures Although symptomatic narrowing of the esophagus can be congenital, it is usually acquired. In infants with rare congenital stenosis there are two types, with the most common form consisting of a stenosis at the junction of the middle and distal thirds of the esophagus. Symptoms usually do not occur until solid foods become part of the diet. The less common form has a long segment of narrowing anywhere along the esophagus. The cause for the congenital stenosis is unknown, although intramural tracheobronchial remnants and gastric or pancreatic tissue rests have been reported.

Acquired esophageal stenosis is usually the sequela of GER, ingestion of caustic substances (lye), and candidal or viral esophagitis (see box).

GER can occur with or without a hiatus hernia but is most commonly seen in association with immaturity of the gastroesophageal junction. GER can be considered a normal finding in infants up to 1 year, but longer standing GER may cause inflammation of the mucosa. Inflammatory changes and subsequent strictures are

Differential Diagnosis of Esophageal Strictures

Esophagitis due to GER, caustic substances, or
   chronic infection (Candida)
After tracheoesophageal fistula repair, more than
   4 months after radiation therapy
Barrett's esophagus, epidermolysis bullosa
Chronic granulomatous disease of childhood
   (see Fig. 3-23), eosinophilic gastroenterities

best documented by contrast studies or endoscopy.
Barrett's esophagus (replacement of squamous eiptheli-
um by columnar epithelium as a result of GER) is rarely
seen in children but, if present, can result in strictures
over time.

Lye (alkali) ingestion is the most common cause of a
stricture and leads to mucosal necrosis in 3 to 5 days
and to fibrous contraction by 3 to 5 weeks, with strictures occurring in one third of patients as early as 3
weeks after the insult. Boys less than age 3 years represent the majority of patients. Long- or short-segment
strictures occur most often in the middle and lower
third of the esophagus. They may be amenable to balloon dilation (Fig. 3-18).

Esophagitis Infectious causes of esophagitis most
commonly include Candida (in patients receiving
chemotherapy), herpes simplex virus (HSV-1), and
cytomegalovirus (common in patients with AIDS).
Rarer types of esophagitis are probably secondary to
mucosal trauma and can occur in Crohn disease or epidermolysis bullosa. The latter is a congenital blistering
disorder of the skin and mucous membranes. It is autosomal recessive. These bullae can ulcerate and
progress to strictures. Eosinophilic gastroenteritis
rarely affects the esophagus but can produce dilation,
dysmotility, and strictures, as can Crohn disease and
graft-versus-host disease (GVHD). Iatrogenic causes
such as medications (eg., antibiotics, antiinflammatory
drugs), prolonged intubation, and radiation must be
considered but are usually evident from the clinical
history.

Esophagitis can be suggested on *conventional radiographs* of the chest by a dilated, air-filled atonic
esophagus. This appearance is rare as are accompanying air-space changes in the lungs, suggesting aspiration. Esophagoscopy with biopsy usually is used to
confirm the diagnosis of esophagitis. The extent of
esophagitis can be evaluated best by using isosmolar
contrast medium to prevent extravasation from developing into mediastinitis or aspiration resulting in pulmonary edema. Fine mucosal ulceration, loss of peristalsis (spasm), and eventually stricture formation are
the most common imaging findings.

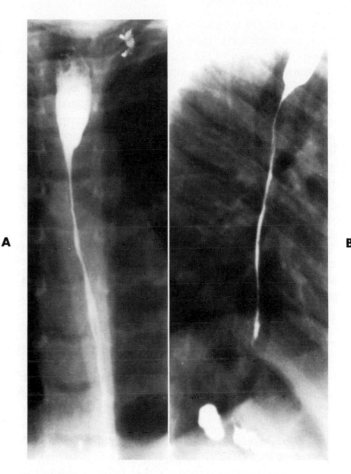

A   **B**

Fig. 3-18   AP (**A**) and lateral (**B**) views demonstrate an
esophageal stricture caused by accidental lye ingestion.

Foreign bodies Because infants and young children
can and do swallow many types of foreign bodies, these
objects occasionally become impacted at any of the
four normal sites of relative narrowing in the esophagus. These sites include the thoracic inlet or at the
level of the cricopharyngeus muscle (75%), at the levels
where the aortic arch or the left mainstem bronchus
crosses the esophagus (20%), and at the level of the gastroesophageal junction (5%). The patients are often
acutely symptomatic. The risk of aspirating the foreign
bodies compels the clinician to decide to remove them.
If the foreign object can be propelled to the stomach,
nature frequently will eliminate them. Remember that
25% of objects larger than a quarter cannot pass the
ileocecal valve because it is the narrowest part of the
GI tract. If the foreign body remains stuck in the
esophagus, its removal can be performed easily through
a flexible endoscope. Foley catheter removal under fluoroscopic guidance is somewhat controversial because
of the risk for aspiration, but it has the advantage of
avoiding sedation. In experienced hands, it has a high
success rate.

Imaging should include an AP radiograph of the chest and abdomen (mouth to anus) and a lateral soft tissue examination of the neck (Fig. 3-19).

Coin-shaped foreign bodies have a distinctive plain film appearance in the upper esophagus. They will be oriented en-face on AP radiographs when lodged in the esophagus but en-face on the lateral radiograph when located in the trachea. If a foreign body is suspected but is not radiopaque, fluoroscopy is needed to evaluate for mediastinal shift or to assess for symmetric hemidiaphragmatic motion. Contrast studies with barium or nonionic agents may be useful in the diagnosis of non-opaque foreign bodies, but the contrast medium may obscure small or minimally opaque foreign bodies. The presence of edema of the esophageal wall around the object suggests that the foreign body has been present more than 24 hours. Perforation or fistula formation then becomes more likely, and catheter removal probably should be avoided.

Achalasia Achalasia is rare in children, with 3% of all cases occurring in children less than 10 years of age. There is no gender predilection. Achalasia is caused by failure of relaxation of the lower esophageal sphincter in response to swallowing as a result of the absence or destruction of the myenteric plexus. Radiographs of the chest may demonstrate pulmonary changes secondary to aspiration, an air-fluid level in a dilated esophagus, or a gasless stomach (in 70% of patients). A contrast study will demonstrate the classic beaking and disordered peristalsis of the esophagus.

Neoplasms Benign esophageal tumors are uncommon in children but may include leiomyomas, hamartomas (Peutz-Jeghers syndrome), and polyps.

Malignant esophageal tumors are exceedingly rare in children. Lymphoma (extrinsic pressure) and very rarely esophageal carcinomas secondary to esophagitis (lye) occur.

As in adults, these lesions most often are detected on a contrast (barium) study. They are characterized by a filling defect with acute angles to the wall, occasionally with ulceration. CT or MRI is then used to better characterize the extent of these lesions.

Stomach and Diaphragm

Anatomy and Developmental Anomalies
  Embryogenesis and variants
  Gastroesophageal reflux
  Diaphragmatic hernia
Acquired Conditions
  Air distention
  Inflammation
  Ulceration
  Bezoars
Neoplasms
  Benign
  Malignant
  Imaging

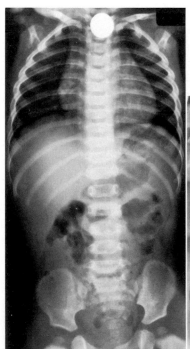
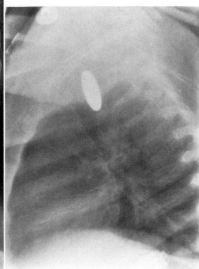

Fig. 3-19 **A**, AP "mouth to anus" radiograph demonstrates a coin en face and therefore stuck in the esophagus. **B**, Lateral view confirms this position and suggests mild edema surrounding the coin.

A

B

Anatomic and Developmental Anomalies

Embryogenesis and variants The embryogenesis of the diaphragm involves a ventral portion formed from the septum transversum, which is located between the pericardial cavity and the coelomic cavity, as well as the posterior portion, formed by the pleuroperitoneal membrane that will develop striated muscle to form the muscular diaphragm. Defective development of either portion may result in hernias.

The stomach first appears as a fusiform dilation of the foregut in the fifth gestational week. A ninety-degree rotation around the longitudinal axis results in a relatively larger greater curvature that will "sink" to its adult position. This explains the stomach's being predominantly transverse in orientation during the first year of life ("cascade" stomach). After gradual change in shape during the subsequent years (differential growth of opposite sides of the stomach), it attains the adult shape by the early teen years.

Microgastria (small stomach) and agastria (absent stomach) are extremely rare conditions that present in patients with massive GER and usually are associated with a normal remainder of the GI tract.

Gastric duplication is the rarest (5%) form of GI tract duplication. These cystic lesions are located on the (antral) greater curvature and do not communicate with the lumen. They enlarge as a result of secretions and hemorrhage and are more common in girls. The imaging (US) appearance of duplications is characteristic because of the echogenic appearance of the GI mucosa (Fig. 3-20).

Both diverticula and webs are uncommon. The former are located posterolaterally in the fundus, the latter in the antrum. Diverticula usually occur in adults. If the web totally occludes the antral lumen, it may be associated with gastric or pyloric atresia, probably as an ischemic event rather than a failure of recanalization since it may be associated with jejunal or ileal atresias (Fig. 3-21).

The stomach is fixed by ligaments connecting the stomach to the liver, diaphragm, spleen, and colon. Rarely, laxity of these ligaments or deficient fixation can lead to volvulus of the stomach. There are two types described: organoaxial and mesenteroaxial (Fig. 3-22). In organoaxial rotation the axis of rotation is

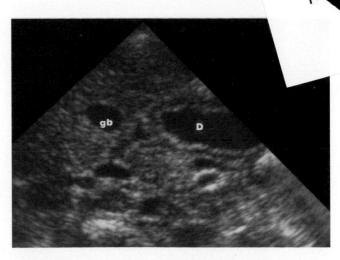

Fig. 3-20 Coronal US image demonstrates the characteristic US appearance of gastrointestinal duplications (*D*): an echogenic mucosa bordered by a relatively hypoechogenic rim representing muscle. Gallbladder (*gb*).

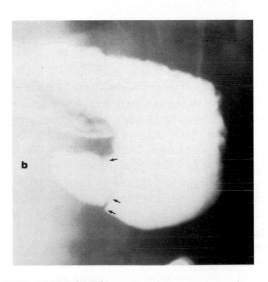

Fig. 3-21 Antral web. A linear structure in the antrum (*arrows*) on UGI examination (*b*, Duodenal bulb) in a vomiting child.

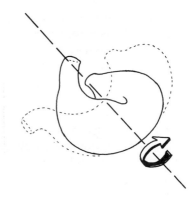

Fig. 3-22 Schematic representation of an organoaxial (A) and a mesenteroaxial (B) volvulus.

A

B

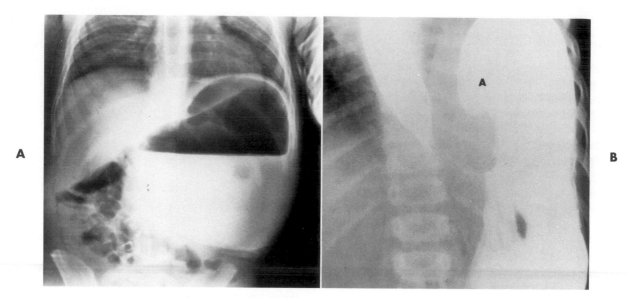

Fig. 3-23 Mesenteroaxial gastric volvulus. **A**, Conventional radiograph reveals a markedly dilated gastric contour with an air-fluid level. **B**, Contrast examination reveals the antrum (*A*) in the region of the fundus and a GE junction that is in a lower than normal position.

parallel to the long axis of the stomach, a condition rare in children. It is often associated with aerophagia. In mesenteroaxial rotation, the axis of rotation is at right angles to the stomach parallel to the mesentery. Mesenteroaxial rotation, the more common of the two types, often is seen acutely, is usually posttraumatic in origin, and is associated with a higher risk of vascular compromise and diaphragmatic herniation as a result of trauma to the diaphragm. The antrum is located in the region usually occupied by the fundus (Fig. 3-23).

Gastroesophageal reflux GER most often is an incidental abnormality in an otherwise healthy infant. It is defined as regurgitation of gastric contents into the esophagus. Lack of competency of the gastroesophageal (GE) junction is implicated, with or without a hiatus hernia. GER often improves with age as the angle of the esophagus to the fundus matures, i.e., becomes more acute and thus competent.

The GE junction consists of the lower esophageal sphincter (LES), which is in the process of maturation up to 6 months after birth. The LES prevents GER from occurring because the LES normally relaxes only during swallowing. Its anatomic location is at the junction of columnar and squamous epithelium—below the diaphragm (about 4 cm long) in adults and at the diaphragm (about 1 cm long) in infants. This sphincter creates a 15 to 30 mm Hg barrier to regurgitation. In addition, the incident angle of the esophagus in relation to the cardia is less acute in infants than in the adult. During infancy this combination may allow gastric contents to reflux into the esophagus. This can be considered physiologic and should cease by 9 to 12 months of age. GER can become clinically significant if

aspiration occurs, esophagitis results, or the child fails to thrive. GER is less likely to resolve when present after 1 year of age. It may be associated with a hiatus hernia and predominates in males (3:1). There is also an increased incidence in children with Down syndrome, cystic fibrosis, and neurologically impaired states.

Conventional radiographs of the chest or abdomen do not detect GER itself but can suggest aspiration secondary to GER with air space disease in infants, particularly in the upper lobes. In a supine patient aspiration preferentially will enter the dependent (upper lobe) region. The radiograph of the chest may also reveal the presence of a hiatus hernia with or without an air-fluid level.

US has shown reasonable correlation with the upper GI evaluation of GER with contrast medium (barium). For both these studies, sensitivity does not necessarily correlate with specificity. Because GER is an intermittent phenomenon and therefore may not be detected during intermittent imaging observation, a false negative result from the examination is common. Some observe the GE junction with fluoroscopy for 5 minutes; others use a variety of GER-provoking maneuvers. Neither way is definitive. Grading of GER is used at some institutions but is of limited clinical use. If the contrast agent reaches the level of the hila or clavicles, GER is considered significant. In short, the main use of the UGI examination is to verify normal anatomy and function.

Studies using ^{99m}Tc-sulfur colloid in milk or food are easy and sensitive evaluations that allow better quantification of GER but resolve little anatomic detail.

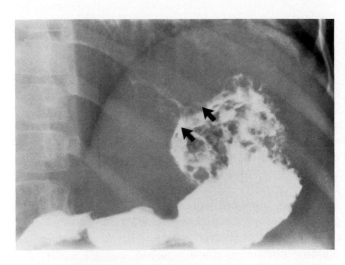

Fig. 3-24 Status-post Nissen fundoplication resulting in a gastric cardia pseudotumor (*arrows*).

However, these studies correlate well with the 24-hour pH probe test, an invasive test that requires hospitalization but nonetheless is considered the gold standard. Treatment of GER is medical in infants, but if recurrent aspiration, esophagitis, or failure to thrive occur, surgery is considered. The Nissen fundoplication (esophageal wrap using the gastric fundus) is the operative procedure often performed in children older than 18 months. This may be evident on UGI as a "pseudotumor" (Fig. 3-24).

Diaphragmatic hernia The most common congenital diaphragmatic hernia is a herniation of peritoneal contents through the foramen of Bochdalek. It occurs in approximately one in 2000 live births and occurs much more frequently on the left side (5:1). Left-sided preference may be either because the pleuroperitoneal canal on the right closes earlier or because the liver "protects" against herniation on the right side. Clinically, if the defect is large, the patient usually has severe respiratory distress, cyanosis, and a scaphoid abdomen at birth. Some infants are seen slightly later in the neonatal period with respiratory distress; in such an instance, the hernia is often smaller.

In the neonate conventional radiographic examination of the abdomen and chest ("babygram") initially may demonstrate an opaque hemithorax with a paucity of bowel loops under the diaphragm. Once swallowed, air enters the viscus, and chest radiographs are classically diagnostic (see Fig. 2-17). Multiple radiolucencies in the affected hemithorax consistent with the presence of air-filled bowel loops are often seen. Some loops of bowel remain fluid filled, but most become at least partially air filled. There may be mediastinal shift

to the contralateral side and a persistent paucity of bowel gas in the abdomen. Occasionally, a hydrothorax is present. Because of the volume effect of the herniated bowel, pulmonary hypoplasia results, the severity of which largely determines morbidity and mortality. Malrotation is invariably present. A rare form of diaphragmatic herniation occurs a few weeks after birth and for unknown reasons (diaphragmatic motion?) becomes evident after a (often streptococcal) pneumonia.

The differential diagnosis of this conventional radiographic finding includes cystic adenomatoid malformation, pneumatoceles, and an elevated right hemidiaphragm secondary to pulmonary hypoplasia (scimitar syndrome) or eventration.

Contrast evaluation through a NG tube often is diagnostic if conventional radiographs have not been. Prenatal US often detects the herniation in utero, facilitating immediate postnatal intervention.

Treatment is usually surgical, assisted by extracorporeal membrane oxygenation (ECMO), depending on the degree of pulmonary hypoplasia. Intrauterine intervention currently is being developed.

Acquired Conditions

Air distention A stomach distended by air may be caused by anxiety or crying (air swallowing), attempted intubation (NG or endotracheal), or gastric outlet obstruction (hypertrophy of the circular pylorus muscle [HPS]). The clinical history usually contains sufficient explanation in these instances. However, it may be necessary to rule out congenital lesions if there is too much air (antral web or EA with a distal fistula) or too little or no air (EA), depending on age of presentation.

Causes of outlet obstruction include HPS, pylorospasm, and antropyloric ulcers. Benign ulceration in infants and children is usually stress related and medically treated.

Inflammation Gastritis can be of a primary or secondary nature. Rare primary causes include eosinophilic gastroenteritis, chronic granulomatous disease of childhood (CGDC), Crohn disease (predominantly involving the antrum), and Ménétrier disease (giant hypertrophic gastritis). Secondary causes include stress, medications, infection (in particular, *helicobacter* sp. or candidiasis in immunosuppressed children), and the ingestion of caustic substances (i.e., acid). Imaging (barium) may reveal thickening of the rugae (except the antral narrowing seen in children with Crohn disease), mucosal nodularity, and decreased peristalsis. Increased secretions also are often noted.

Ulceration Gastric ulcers rarely are seen in children but present with GI bleeding and pain. They are very unlikely in children less than 10 years of age except for neonatal ulcers that are considered stress or hypoxemic insults. Gastric and duodenal ulcers in older children mimic the symptoms and causes of those in adults. They may be associated with chronic pancreatitis, Zollinger-Ellison syndrome, cystic fibrosis, and multiple endocrine adenomatosis (MEA) syndrome. Antiinflammatory agent (e.g., aspirin)–induced ulcers may also occur.

Bezoars   Indigestible organic material can form a collection in the stomach called a *bezoar*. It can be composed of hair (trichobezoar), vegetable matter (phytobezoar), or milk curd (lactobezoar) and is seen as a solid, mobile mass that fails to exit the stomach on conventional or barium evaluation. The former two types are seen in children and adolescents with bad breath and frequently are associated with anorexia and weight loss. The lactobezoar is seen in infants, probably as a result of improper mixing of formula with sufficient water. Vomiting and the resultant dehydration constitute the clinical picture.

Conventional radiographs of the abdomen are often characteristic and may be diagnostically sufficient, with a rim of air outlining an intragastric, often mottled mass. Contrast (barium) also can be of use to outline the (mobile) bezoar (Fig. 3-25). The treatment of choice is surgical removal.

Neoplasms

Neoplasms in the pediatric stomach are rare.

Benign lesions   Benign lesions constituting secondary gastric involvement in children with Gardner syndrome, Peutz-Jegher syndrome, and familial polyposis can manifest as polyps in the stomach, most often of the regenerative type. Benign lymphoid hyperplasia can be seen but often is associated with immunoglobulin deficiency. Most primary benign gastric tumors are mesenchymal in origin. They include leiomyomas, teratomas, and lipomas. All are rare. Aberrant (ectopic) pancreatic tissue most often is located along the greater curvature (antrum) and pylorus. It often contains a draining duct seen as a dimple on contrast studies in 50% of these children, and it may grow to obstructive size.

Primary malignant tumors   Primary malignant tumors are exceptionally rare but may include leiomyosarcomas or lymphomas. A rare locally aggressive lesion with a benign course has also been described, termed an *inflammatory pseudotumor*, which initially presents as an epigastric mass.

Although conventional radiographs can suggest masses or rarely calcifications (teratoma) of the stomach, most often a contrast agent (barium) is needed to

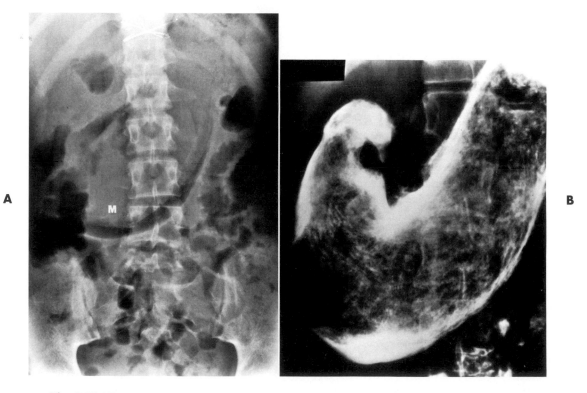

Fig. 3-25   Bezoar. A, Conventional radiograph reveals a mass (M) within the stomach outlined by gastric air. **B,** Contrast study confirms the trichobezoar.

delineate the mucosa and the anatomy better. The extent of the tumor can be evaluated with US but is better assessed with CT, using both peroral and IV contrast. Endoscopy also is used frequently for diagnostic purposes.

Intestinal Tract

Anatomy and Developmental Anomalies
Malrotation
Omphalocele
Gastroschisis
Atresia and stenosis
Duplication anomalies
Meckel diverticulum
Meconium
Meconium peritonitis
Meconium ileus
Meconium-ileus equivalent
Meconium plug
Hirschsprung disease
Anorectal malformations
Acquired Anomalies
Gastroenteritis
Crohn disease
Ulcerative colitis
Other colitides
Pseudomembranous colitis
Typhlitis
Appendicitis
Neoplasms
Polyposis syndromes

Anatomic and Developmental Anomalies

Malrotation Interference with the orderly sequence of rotation and fixation of the GI tract between 6 and 10 weeks gestation can result in malposition and/or malrotation of the bowel. Malrotation may be totally asymptomatic for life, or the neonate may present acutely with obstruction (midgut volvulus). This "twisting" of bowel is facilitated by a shortened mesenteric attachment to the posterior peritoneal wall. The duodenum and midportion of the transverse colon are the only segments properly attached so that rotation with the SMA as its fulcrum can occur.

The entire process of bowel rotation during embryology does not always go smoothly. During the bowel's return to the peritoneal cavity during the process of extracoelomic rotation, there may be interference with cecal descent if normal bowel rotation is not complete. This results in malpositioning of the bowel, with the mesentery attempting to "fix" the colon to the posterior peritoneal wall. This attempt is evident in fibrous peritoneal (Ladd) bands oriented diagonally across the abdomen that can obstruct the bowel lumen, most often the duodenum (Fig. 3-26). To assess for proper anatomic location of the small bowel, the most reliable indicator is the normal position of the ligament of Treitz (duodenal-jejunal junction), which is best demonstrated on UGI examination (Fig. 3-27).

Imaging by conventional radiographs of the abdomen will show a high obstruction or abnormal position of bowel loops in most instances. Partial duodenal obstruction is the most important finding. A horizontal beam radiograph is useful, and absence of small bowel air in the presence of peritoneal signs is an omi-

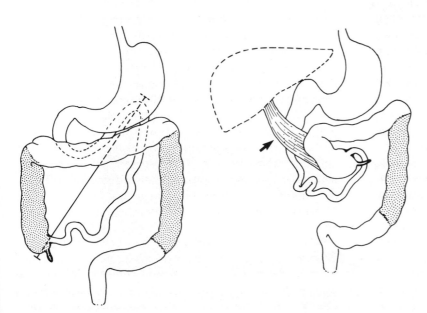

Fig. 3-26 Schematic representation of normal fixation (*stippled*) (**A**) and malpositioned intestinal tract (**B**). Note Ladd bands (*arrow*).

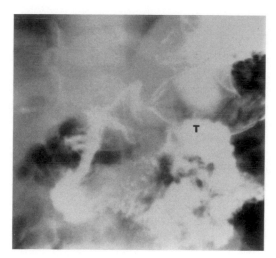

Fig. 3-27 Normal location of the ligament of Treitz (*T*) (duodenal jejunal junction).

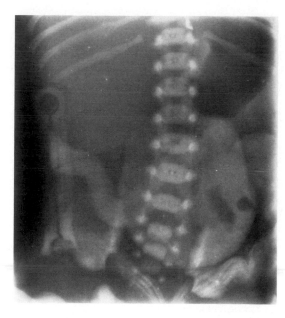

Fig. 3-28 Omphalocele. The umbilicus comes off the dome of the soft tissue mass projecting anteriorly from the abdomen.

nous finding. A UGI study using barium or nonionic agents will reveal the site of obstruction or an abnormal course of the second and third portion of the duodenum (see Fig. 3-7). Use of contrast enema is not as reliable in excluding malrotation because a "floppy" cecum occurs in 10% to 15% of patients with a normally positioned bowel. US has been used to screen for malrotation by assessing the normal location of the SMA to the left and lateral to the SMV. In children with malrotation this relationship has been observed as reversed, but this observation currently is not considered clinically reliable.

Omphalocele   Failure of the midgut to return completely to the peritoneal cavity during the tenth week of intrauterine life creates an exomphalos, or an omphalocele. By definition, the interrupted rotation of the bowel results in malrotation. The liver and spleen may also be malpositioned. Thus the omphalocele's contents can vary from a single loop of bowel to the entire GI tract. Rarely, only the liver is contained in the omphalocele. The herniated sac is covered by peritoneum and amnion, and the umbilical cord inserts at its apex. There is a slight male predominance for this condition. Approximately 30% of patients are premature, and the incidence is one in 5000 live births. Associated cardiac anomalies may be present. The kidneys may "over ascend" and thus be located just under the diaphragm. Beckwith-Wiedemann syndrome may also be present.

US imaging may be diagnostic prenatally. Conventional radiographs of the abdomen after birth may reveal a large soft tissue protruding from the abdomen, occasionally demonstrating the umbilicus at its apex associated with an abnormal gas pattern (Fig. 3-28). Surgery is mandatory and primarily consists of

returning the omphalocele's contents to the peritoneal cavity. A patch may be necessary to close the anterior abdominal wall.

Gastroschisis   The stomach, midgut, and occasionally portions of the urinary tract may protrude through a paraumbilical defect in the ventral abdominal wall (left) lateral to or right at the midline. This entity, gastroschisis, occurs twice as often as an omphalocele. The peritoneal covering of the protruding viscera is absent, and the umbilicus position is normal. Malpositioning and shortening of bowel may be present, but overall there is a low incidence of associated anomalies. Children with this condition often are born prematurely.

Imaging with US often reveals this condition in utero, but on *conventional abdominal* radiographs a soft tissue mass can be seen protruding paramedially that can be confused with an omphalocele (Fig. 3-29). Clinically the normally located umbilicus is the key. The differentiation from an omphalocele may be difficult radiographically. Contrast studies may demonstrate that because the peritoneum was in contact with amniotic fluid prenatally, the myenteric plexus may be damaged, possibly resulting in disordered motility of the bowel, especially as the child grows.

Atresia and stenosis   Duodenal atresia occurs in approximately one in 4000 live births. It is considered a failure of the recanalization that occurs at 10 weeks gestation. Duodenal atresia occurs in 50% of patients with duodenal obstruction; partial failure at recanalization of the gut may result in stenosis (40%) or a web (10%). Duodenal stenosis also may be caused by an

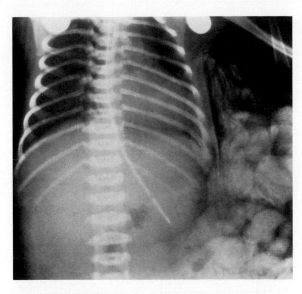

Fig. 3-29   Gastroschisis. Intestinal loops projecting outside the abdominal cavity.

Differential Diagnosis of "Double Bubble" Appearance (Few Dilated Loops)
Duodenal/jejunal atresia
Midgut volvulus
Malrotation (Ladd bands)
Annular pancreas
Duodenal web
Preduodenal portal vein

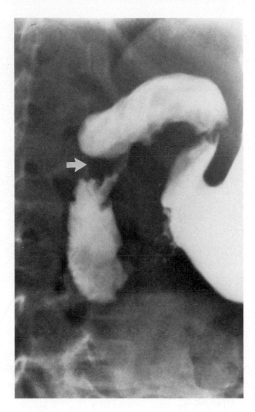

Fig. 3-30   Annular pancreas. Persistent circumferential narrowing (*arrow*) in the proximal descending duodenum.

annular pancreas when the two anlage of the pancreas fuse prematurely or by a preduodenal portal vein. A duodenal web (diaphragm) may be stretched by peristalsis, resulting in an intraluminal diverticulum. The nearly constant location of these anomalies in immediate proximity to the ampulla of Vater lends further strength to embryopathy as the cause. Furthermore, CHD, TEF, and imperforate anus are congenital anomalies associated in 20% to 30% of these patients. Down syndrome is found in up to 33% of patients, and approximately 50% of cases are associated with malpositioning of the bowel. The degree of bowel obstruction determines the presence and severity of symptoms. Clinically, bile-stained vomiting within the first 24 hours of life is the hallmark of atresia or severe stenosis. Prenatal US may show polyhydramnios proportional to the amount of obstruction to passage of bowel contents. *Conventional radiographs* may show the classic double-bubble appearance (see Fig. 3-1 and

the box). In theory this appearance occurs only if there is total atresia. If the duodenum is stenotic, a varying amount of distal bowel gas may be noted.

Upper GI evaluation may demonstrate varying degrees of obstruction. These may range from total obstruction (atresia), relative obstruction due to a (circumferential) mass (Fig. 3-30), or occasionally the classic windsock deformity is identified when an intraluminal diverticulum is present.

Atresia is much more common than stenosis. Atresia more distal in the small bowel is twice as common as in the duodenum. These distal atresias are equally distributed between the jejunum and the ileum.

Jejunal or ileal atresia is associated with other GI tract anomalies in up to 25% of cases and almost always present in the first 24 to 48 hours of life. Approximately 10% of cases are associated with cystic fibrosis. The probable cause is a fetal vascular accident precipitated by either embolus, volvulus, or intussusception, corroborated by the presence of mesenteric defects at the site of atresia in many of these cases.

Four types can be recognized. Type 1 (least common) consists of a web occluding the lumen. Type 2 consists of two blind-ending pouches connected by a fibrous cord (Fig. 3-31). There is no gender predilec-

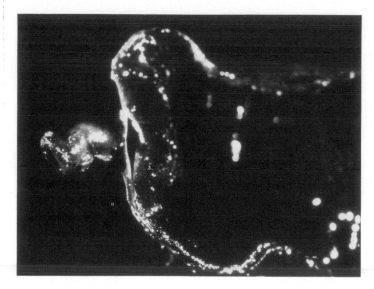

Fig. 3-31 Pathologic specimen of ileal atresia (type 2) illustrated in Fig. 3-1.

tion, and a quarter of these patients is premature. Clinically, these patients experience vomiting in the neonatal period.

There is a familial variant of jejunoileal atresia. In patients with the apple peel small bowel atresia (type 3), the atresia is located near the ligament of Treitz with absence of the mesentery and SMA. It is inherited as an autosomal recessive trait. Type 4 consists of multiple atresias.

Prenatal US imaging reveals polyhydramnios in 25% of affected infants, depending on how proximal the atresia is. Conventional abdominal radiographs classically show dilated loops of small bowel proximal to the atretic or stenotic segment (see Fig. 3-1).

If a contrast enema is performed, the colonic caliber depends on how proximal the stenosis is. With more proximal (jejunal) atresia, sufficient succus entericus is produced to stimulate development of a normal-caliber colon. Conversely, a more distal (ileal) atresia often results in a microcolon. The former occurs late in gestation, the latter early on. A hyperosmolar contrast agent is preferred as the contrast agent of choice. Because both meconium ileus and meconium plug are differential diagnostic possibilities, the hydrophilic properties of this contrast agent can be both curative and diagnostic (see box on p. 89).

Treatment consists of excision of the atretic (stenotic) segment and reanastamosis.

Colonic atresia is very rare (1:40,000 live births). Because the incidence of colonic atresia is uniform throughout the colon, an intrauterine vascular insult is the likely cause.

Duplication anomalies Frequently discovered during infancy, duplication anomalies (cystic lesions) are

lined with intestinal mucosa and are located on the mesenteric side of the GI tract. They rarely communicate with the true lumen. At least 15% contain gastric mucosa. They arise most commonly in the ileum (35%), esophagus (20%), stomach (5%), and duodenum, and often at multiple sites.

Clinically, an abdominal mass is palpable in one third of these patients, intussusception occurs in 15%. Vomiting caused by obstruction is common.

Conventional radiographs may show a mass, obstruction, or both but are usually normal. Calcification is rare, and associated bony vertebral anomalies seldom occur. US shows a cyst lined by interstitial mucosa and can be diagnostic (see Fig. 3-20). The differential diagnostic possibilities include an omental cyst, choledochal cyst, mesenteric cyst, giant Meckel diverticulum, and ovarian cyst.

Meckel diverticulum After the extraperitoneal counterclockwise rotation of the midgut (week 6), the omphalomesenteric (vitelline) duct usually regresses and becomes the umbilicus. Failure of this obliteration can result in a sinus, a fistula, an omphalomesenteric duct cyst, or most commonly a Meckel diverticulum (Fig. 3-32).

Meckel diverticula account for 90% of all omphalomesenteric duct abnormalities, are commonly found in 2% of autopsies and are situated approximately 2 feet from the ileocecal valve. Complications occur before age 2 years in 2% of all patients. Approximately 20% of Meckel diverticula contain ectopic gastric or pancreatic tissue.

The diverticulum is located on the antemesenteric border of the ileum, contains ileal mucosa, and may be large. Clinically, GI hemorrhage is the most common

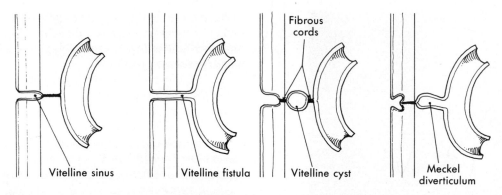

Fig. 3-32 Fate of the omphalomesenteric (vitelline) duct.

Differential Diagnosis of GI Bleeding

Anal fisssures—inspection will exclude
Meckel diverticulum—*only* if gastric mucosa present;
  ulcer
Juvenile polyp—one third of patients have more than
  one polyp
Inflammatory bowel disease—Crohn disease,
  ulcerated colitis
Peptic ulcer disease—medical diagnosis
Portal hypertension—cavernous transformation of
  portal vein, cirrhosis, ascites

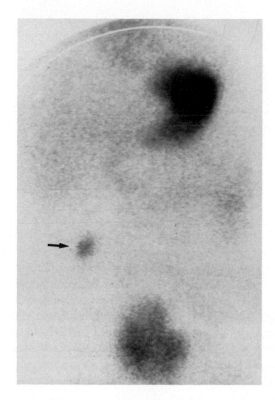

Fig. 3-33 Meckel scan shows uptake of radionuclide in the right lower quadrant (*arrow*) indicating hemorrhaging gastric mucosa within the diverticulum.

presentation when the patient is symptomatic, and the amount of bleeding can vary from hematochezic to hemocult levels. The cause for bleeding is ulcerating ectopic gastric mucosa, which is present in nearly 100% of cases that do bleed (see box). A Meckel diverticulum can be the lead point in intussusception and can be the focal point of a volvulus or obstruction.

Imaging with *conventional abdominal* radiographs may show obstruction, which, if it has lead to volvulus and infarction, may appear as air in the bowel wall or portal vein or even as intraperitoneal free air.

Contrast studies, including techniques such as enteroclysis, are of little use and are frequently only diagnostic in retrospect.

The most sensitive and specific evaluation is a Meckel scan using ^{99m}Tc pertechnetate. This study is positive only if gastric mucosa is present (20%), but in that instance it has a 95% sensitivity (Fig. 3-33). *Angiography* is rarely, if ever, indicated. In addition to requiring anesthesia, detection by angiography requires a blood loss of at least 0.5 ml per minute. If the diverticulum is diagnosed, surgery is curative.

Meconium Meconium consists of succus entericus that is composed of bile salts, bile acids, and debris from the intestinal mucosa collected in utero. It usually

is evacuated within 6 hours after birth or, because of perinatal stress, in utero as the result of a (probably) vagal response.

Radiographically meconium has a "mottled" appearance within the viscus during the first 2 days of life.

Four common problems are associated with meconium: meconium *peritonitis*, meconium *ileus*, meconium-*ileus equivalent*, and meconium *plug*.

Meconium peritonitis Meconium peritonitis occurs when there is antenatal bowel perforation, which can occur as early as the second trimester. It is often associated with obstructive lesions such as atresias and

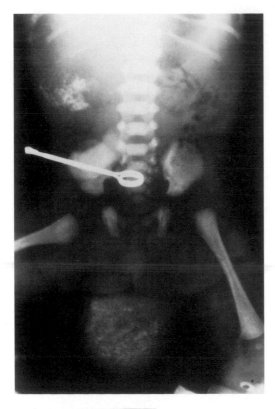

Fig. 3-34   Meconium peritonitis. Flocculent calcification location in the right hemiabdomen, as well as in the scrotum.

volvulus. The meconium spillage into the peritoneal cavity causes a sterile chemical peritonitis, resulting in dystrophic calcifications that may be radiographically evident in as few as 24 hours. Clinically, these patients come to attention because of bowel obstruction caused by fibroadhesive bands. The bowel itself most often is intact, with the perforation healed. If the processus vaginalis was patent at the time the perforation occurred, there may be involvement of the scrotum with calcification or hernias. Ascites also may be present.

Imaging is most often diagnostic on conventional radiographs. There may be evidence of obstruction or ascites. Calcification can be of various types and may be present anywhere in the peritoneal cavity, including the diaphragm (Fig 3-34).

Meconium ileus Meconium ileus occurs when meconium inspissates and obstructs the distal ileum, practically always (>99%) in patients with cystic fibrosis. Approximately 20% of patients with cystic fibrosis are initially seen with meconium ileus. Its symptoms frequently are vomiting and abdominal distention seen within hours in the newborn infant.

Conventional abdominal radiographs reveal a low obstruction with dilated loops (often of different caliber) of bowel, and air-fluid levels may occur.

A contrast enema with a hyperosmolar agent (Gastrografin or Cysto-Conray) is diagnostic. In 30% to 50% of cases of meconium ileus the water-soluble contrast medium is therapeutically useful. A true microcolon is always present.

US may demonstrate multiple characteristic echogenic foci separated by this bowel wall both prenatally and postnatally (Fig. 3-35).

Meconium-ileus equivalent Meconium-ileus equivalent, a misnomer, actually is a distal small bowel obstruction syndrome. In 15% of adolescents and adults with cystic fibrosis viscous bowel contents become impacted in the distal small bowel.

Recurrent bowel obstruction (often correlated with poor therapeutic compliance) evident as recurrent colicky abdominal (RUQ) pain is the clinical presentation. Radiographically mottled stool is seen in dilated loops of small bowel (Fig. 3-36).

Meconium plug This radiographic appearance may actually be seen in two different age groups. A long plug of thick meconium may lodge in the distal colon, probably as a result of neuronal underdevelopment (maturing cranial caudad progression of bowel innervation) and resultant suboptimal peristalsis. These children are usually *full term* and will have a distal obstruction with clinical signs, including abdominal distention, failure to pass meconium, and vomiting at 2 to 3 days of life.

Conventional radiographs of the abdomen may show distention of the bowel. Enemas using a contrast agent such as Gastrografin usually reveal a small to normal left colon with a proximally distended transverse and occasionally right colon and the meconium plug .

In *premature* infants there is often functional immaturity of the colon, especially in infants of diabetic mothers. In addition, there may be functional obstruction caused by inspissated feedings. This condition most often is seen in premature infants who are fed powdered milk formulas but can be the result of any feeding entering the hypoperistaltic bowel. A contrast enema usually reveals a small descending colon and normal-caliber transverse and right colon. This condition resolves spontaneously with the passage of several stools.

The *differential diagnosis* includes long-segment Hirschsprung disease, described below, and the megacystis–microcolon–intestinal hypoperistalsis syndrome, which include a dilated bladder, a microcolon, and hypoperistalsis of the colon. This latter entity is occasionally familial and occurs in girls but is very rare (30 described cases).

Hirschsprung disease Hirschsprung disease, or congenital megacolon, occurs in one in 4500 live (term) births. It is characterized by the absence of ganglion cells in the myenteric plexus, probably as a result of failure of craniocaudal migration of neuroblasts

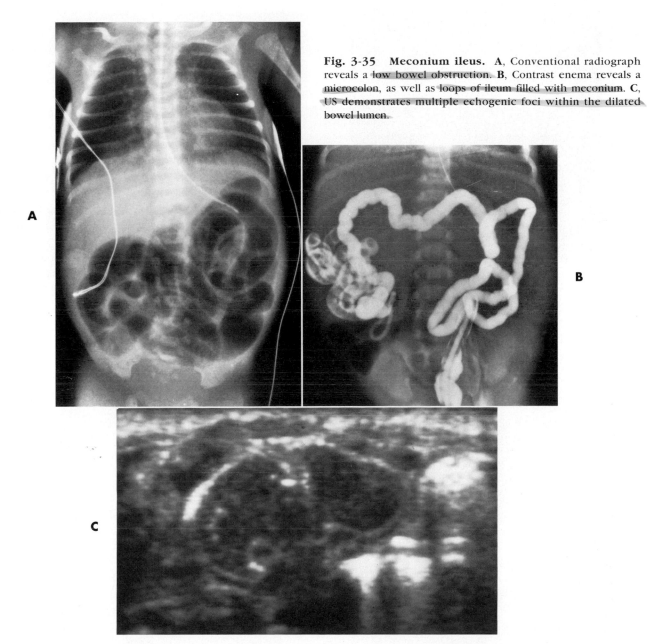

Fig. 3-35   Meconium ileus. **A**, Conventional radiograph reveals a low bowel obstruction. **B**, Contrast enema reveals a microcolon, as well as loops of ileum filled with meconium. **C**, US demonstrates multiple echogenic foci within the dilated bowel lumen.

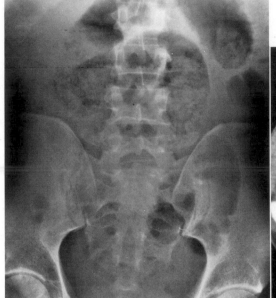

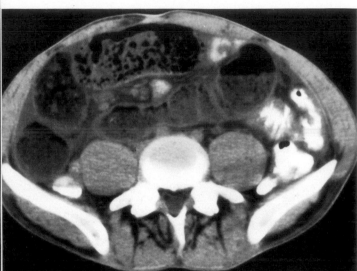

Fig. 3-36 Meconium ileus equivalent. **A**, Small bowel stool impaction in a 16-year-old patient with CF. **B**, CT confirms stool within dilated loops of small bowel with a normal caliber colon.

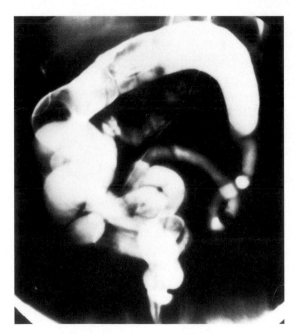

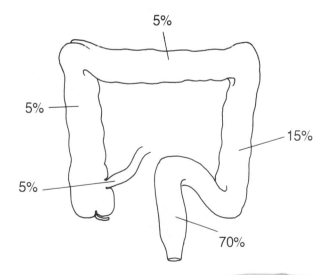

Fig. 3-37 "Meconium plug." Small caliber descending colon and a normal caliber transverse and ascending colon.

Fig. 3-38 Relative incidence of the transition zone in Hirschsprung disease.

between the seventh and twelfth week of gestation. Most commonly, the aganglionosis involves the distal sigmoid colon and rectum (80%), whereas in 15% the colon lacks ganglion cells distal to the hepatic flexure (Fig. 3-38). The disease occurs four times more often in boys, and there is an increased incidence of the disease in children with Down syndrome. When there is entire colonic and occasional terminal ileum involvement (total aganglionosis), there is an equal male and female prevalence and an occasional family history.

Clinically, the diagnosis often is made within the first month of life (80%). There is often (90%) failure to pass meconium within 24 hours, and abdominal distention is common. In 15% of patients these is development of enterocolitis (Clostridium difficile), which presents as explosive watery stools, fever, and sometimes shock. These patients have a mortality rate of 20% to 30% unless prompt treatment is instituted.

Imaging by conventional abdominal radiographs typically reveals low obstruction in the newborn, with multiple air-fluid levels and distention of the bowel. In older children there may be abundant stool in the distended colon.

The differential diagnosis in infants or young children with conventional radiographs showing low bowel obstruction includes meconium ileus, neonatal left colon syndrome, meconium plug, or atresia or stenosis of the small bowel (or colon).

Contrast examination of the colon using barium is used to evaluate for the presence of a transition zone.

Low Intestinal Obstruction With Many Dilated Loops
Imperforate anus
Colonic atresia (very rare)
Hirschsprung disease
Meconium plug syndrome
Ileal atresia
· Meconium ileus

Care is taken not to manipulate the rectum digitally, and a straight, small catheter is used. Delayed radiographs (24 hour) are necessary to confirm poor propulsion.

The transition zone is identified best on the initial lateral rectal view taken during early filling. It may be abrupt or gradual and often is not identified. If a transition zone is identified, there is no need to continue administering the contrast enema, for it may present a risk for retention (Fig. 3-39).

The rectosigmoid index can also be used. In the healthy patient the rectum is usually wider than the sigmoid colon (AP), whereas the opposite is true in patients with Hirschsprung disease. A ratio greater than 0.9 excludes the diagnosis of rectosigmoid Hirschsprung disease. However, this index may be useful when no transition zone is identified. Irregular, spiculated contractions may be noted in the aganglionic

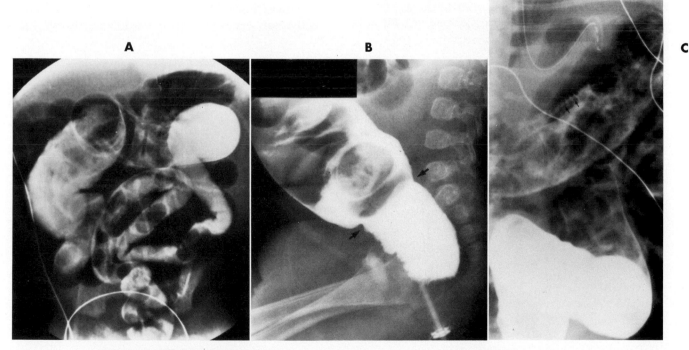

A   B   C

Fig. 3-39 Hirschsprung disease. **A**, Neonatal Hirschsprung with a transition zone in the proximal descending colon mimicking meconium plug. **B**, Lateral radiograph demonstating a rectosigmoid transition zone (*arrows*). **C**, Hirschsprung colitis as evidenced by spiculated edematous transverse colonic mucosa (*arrows*).

segment, a finding that must be differentiated from those of enterocolitis. The contrast enema may be normal in up to a third of patients.

The imaging evaluation, if inconclusive, is followed by rectal manometry and suction biopsy. If this does not establish the diagnosis, a full-thickness biopsy specimen is taken at least 2 to 3 cm above the dentate line.

Surgical management initially consists of constructing a defunctionalizing colostomy. Subsequently, there are three possible surgical interventions for the definitive treatment:

- The most common technique is that developed by *Duhamel* in which, after resection of the aganglionic segment, an end-to-side anastomosis is performed just above the rectum. It preserves innervation of the rectum, has few postoperative complications, and is easier to perform than the Swenson operation.
- The *Soavé* pull-through procedure consists of permanently intussuscepting the normal colon through the aganglionic segment. The radiographic appearance eventually returns to normal.
- The *Swenson* operation consists of forming an end-to-end anastomosis after removing the aganglionic segment. This is often accompanied by increased incidence of fecal and urinary incontinence.

Variants of Hirschsprung disease include total colonic aganglionosis and neuronal intestinal dysplasia. The former may be seen after 1 month of age (35%), with vomiting and abdominal distention, and imaging may reveal a normal colon (75%) or a microcolon (25%). In the latter condition hyperplasia of neuronal plexuses results in a megacolon, mimicking Hirschsprung disease (pseudoobstruction). It may be an isolated condition or exist in association with neu-

rofibromatosis, type 1, or multiple endocrine neoplasia (MEN) type 2 syndrome.

Anorectal malformations   Major anomalies of anorectal structures occur in one of 5000 live births, appearing slightly more commonly in boys. Most common are an imperforate anus and anal atresia, both presenting as low obstruction with marked dilation of the bowel in the neonate. The underlying cause most likely involves abnormal separation of the genitourinary (GU) and hindgut structures (urogenital septum or perineal body) during fetal development.

Classification of these malformations as high (supralevator), intermediate (partially translevator), and low (fully translevator) is based on the location of the *patent* portion of the rectum in relation to the puborectalis muscle. In most infants with a high or intermediate imperforate anus the rectum may rupture into the neighboring structures: the urethra and bladder in males (Fig. 3-40) and the vagina in females or the skin in both. All of these infants are treated with a colostomy at birth because their anorectal malformations will be repaired at a later date.

Low malformations may also develop fistulas to the skin but do so less often. This variant is primarily repaired through a perineal approach.

The role of imaging is to delineate the level of the pouch and evaluate the presence of fistulas and associated anomalies. Anomalies of the lower spinal cord are found in 30% to 40% of these patients (most commonly associated with tethering of the cord); thus US screening is necessary.

Urinary tract abnormalities occur in 25% of patients with a low malformation and in 40% of patients with a

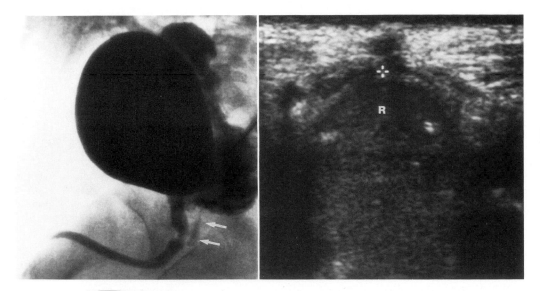

Fig. 3-40 Imperforate anus. **A**, Communication between the posterior urethra and the rectum (*arrows*). **B**, Transperineal US illustrating the distance from the pouch (*R*) to the anal dimple (*x*), as well as calcific densities within the meconium in the rectal pouch.

Differential Diagnosis of Thickened "Wet" Small Bowel Loops

Enteric infections: *Yersinia, Campylobacter, Salmonella* or *Shigella, Escherichia:* and parasites (*Ascaris lumbricoides*).

Protein-losing enteropathy (with peripheral eosinophilia).

Celiac disease (gluten enteropathy): most common chronic malabsorptive syndrome in children; onset at approximately 1 yr with diarrhea. Thickening of the valvulae conniventes is variable; lumen is always dilated.

Graft-versus-host disease (GVHD): almost 50% of bone marrow transplant recipients develop GVHD 2 wk to 2 mo after transplantation.

Henoch-Schönlein purpura: characterized by submucosal hematomas that occur in children with anaphylactoid purpura. It is caused by angiitis (capillaries or small arterioles). Similar findings occur in hemophilia.

Lymphangectasia either primary (congenital) or secondary, caused by obstruction of lymphatics (e.g. inflammatory lesion, malrotation). The protein loss causes diarrhea.

---

high malformation. Thus a voiding cystourethrogram is recommended as the initial imaging modality.

Calcification may be noted in the GI tract on the initial abdominal radiograph. It is the result of urine and meconium mixing because of a fistula between the colon and the urinary system. US also may demonstrate it and may delineate the distance from the anal dimple to the pouch through a transperineal approach (see Fig. 3-40). MRI is reserved for postoperative evaluation of the pull-through operation.

Acquired Anomalies

Gastroenteritis   Gastroenteritis is a very common condition affecting children and can be bacterial, viral, or parasitic in origin.

Viral causes include human rotavirus in almost half the cases of diarrhea occurring between ages 2 and 6 years. Adenovirus and other viruses also have been implicated.

Bacterial gastroenteritis (occurring in approximately 10% to 15% of patients with diarrhea) is most commonly caused by *Salmonella, Shigella, Escherichia coli, Yersinia*, and *Campylobacter*.

Parasitic gastroenteritis is most commonly caused by *Ascaris lumbricoides* (roundworm). *Strongyloides* is seen less frequently, as is *Trichuris trichiura* (whipworm).

Giardiasis, caused by the protozoa *Giardia lamblia*, is especially common in children with dysgammaglobulinemia, and frequently results in malabsorption.

In all of these instances, imaging by conventional supine and upright abdominal radiographs may be normal or reveal air-fluid levels in the small and large bowels that can mimic obstruction or ileus. These are all manifestations of the diarrhea with which these patients most often present.

Contrast (barium) studies may show increased transit time, nodular or thickened folds (Fig. 3-41), or dilution of the contrast ("wet") while the medium passes

---

Differential Diagnosis of Thick (Nodular) Folds of Small Bowel

Nodular lymphoid hyperplasia (see Fig. 3-3)

Lymphoma

Polyposes syndromes

Amyloidosis, chronic granulomatous disease, cystic fibrosis, Crohn disease

---

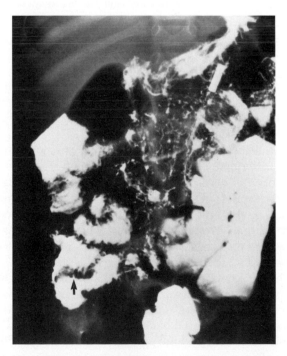

Fig. 3-41   Thickened (*arrow*) and "wet" small bowel loops in a contrast examination of a patient with protein-losing enteropathy.

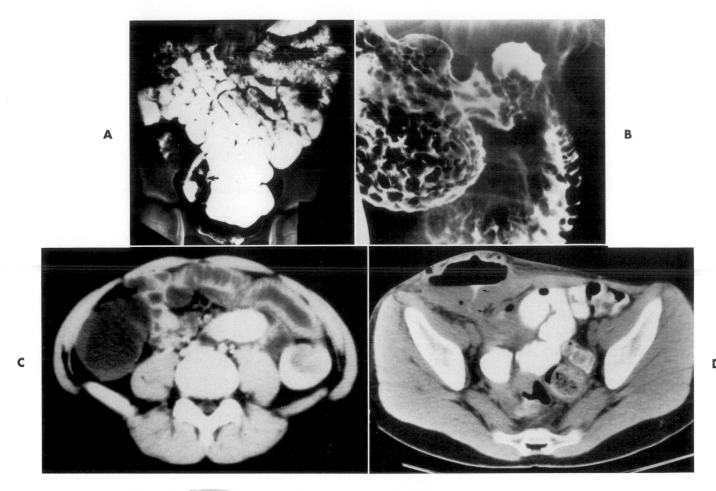

Fig. 3-42   Crohn disease. A, Thickened, fixed terminal ileum and cecum (*arrow*) on UGI. **B**, Edematous antral wall and duodenal folds with "cobble stoning." **C**, CT confirming the findings in **A**. **D**, CT demonstrating an abscess with a fistulous tract (*arrows*).

the small bowel. However, these are nonspecific findings, and their differential diagnosis is presented in the accompanying boxes.

Crohn disease

Crohn disease, or regional enteritis, has no known cause, although infection, altered immunity, and stress have been implicated. It is characterized by segmental full-thickness granulomatous involvement, with inflammation of the bowel wall. Imaging hallmarks include skip lesions, irregular stenosis with loss of normal mucosal landmarks, increased separation of bowel loops, and fistula formation.

The incidence is six per 100,000 children. In children less than 10 years of age the disease is rare (3.5%). Peak incidence is between 20 and 40 years of age, with 20% of cases diagnosed in childhood. The disease has a familial tendency, and the patient with this disease clinically often is seen initially with failure to thrive, symptoms similar to those of appendicitis, or recurrent vague abdominal pain. There is often diarrhea and bleeding per rectum, and perirectal fistulas may occur.

In 10% of children sacroiliitis or arthritis of large joints is present. The most common (although rare) skin manifestation is erythema nodosum.

Conventional radiographs suggest IBD in three quarters of patients. Obstruction, bowel wall thickening, or a mass and ascites may be present.

US may illustrate thickening of the terminal ileal wall but is more useful in excluding appendicitis, ovarian pathology, and ascites.

Contrast evaluation of the small bowel reveals the involvement of the terminal ileum (TI), fistulas, cobblestoning (transverse ulcerating fissures), or a mass. Unfortunately, in children 15% of patients with Crohn disease have a normal TI. The colon may be similarly involved: normal areas alternating with involved areas ("skip lesions").

CT is useful to evaluate recurrence of disease and to evaluate better the extraluminal involvement (phlegmon, fistula, abscess) (Fig. 3-42).

Surgery is avoided as long as possible because the procedure may exacerbate the disease. Recurrences

A   **B**   **C**

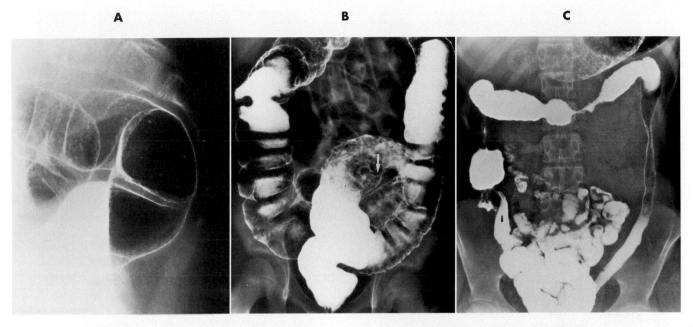

Fig. 3-43 UC. A, Double contrast view of the lateral rectum reveals fine granularity of the mucosa. **B,** Postinflammatory (filiform) polyps in the sigmoid (*arrow*). **C,** An ahaustral left colon, "back wash" ileitis (*i*), and generalized foreshortening in chronic UC.

have been related to stress, with flare-ups common, for instance, during examination periods, pregnancy, or onset of menses, or pregnancy.

Ulcerative colitis Ulcerative colitis (UC), an idiopathic, mucosal, disease occurs more commonly in adults 30 to 60 years of age. In 15% of cases UC is diagnosed in childhood, with diarrhea, abdominal pain, and rectal bleeding as symptoms. In less than 5% these symptoms develop before the age of 10 years. There is an increased incidence of UC in first-degree relatives of affected patients and in patients with human leukocyte antigen (HLA)-B27.

The most common clinical feature in children is diarrhea, often accompanied by rectal bleeding. The latter can be copious and acute in 30% of patients. Failure to thrive is present in 15% of patients. Common adult clinical presentations such as stomal aphtha, arthritis, uveitis, and toxic megacolon are rare in children. In one third of patients abnormal liver function test results and fatty liver infiltration are seen. Toxic dilation of the (transverse) colon (megacolon) occurs in 1% to 3% of children with UC.

Imaging by *conventional* abdominal *radiographs* may show bowel wall thickening or loss of the normal haustral pattern. A toxic megacolon may be evident. In this case contrast enema evaluation is contraindicated. In all other cases the next imaging method of choice uses a double-contrast barium enema technique. Diagnostic findings early in the disease include granularity of the mucosa, beginning at the rectum and extending proximally to a variable extent. More severe disease is heralded by punctuate ulceration progressing

to submucosal tracking ("collar button" ulcer). UC is confined to the rectosigmoid area in 25% of patients and to the transverse and left colon in 50%. The entire colon is involved in 25%. Backwash ileitis is seen in 10% of patients. As the disease progresses, ulceration becomes more obvious. Areas of regenerating colonic mucosa and focally spared mucosal islands result in the appearance of pseudopolyps. Postinflammatory (filiform) polyps are seen in the healing phase. Chronic disease results in fibrosis and foreshortening of the colon that appears ahaustral (Fig 3-43).

Because the overall death rate can be as high as 2% per year after the first 10 years (a factor 20 times the normal incidence) and because there is an increased incidence of adenocarcinoma of the colon as compared with the general population, total colectomy is often the treatment of end-stage disease.

The *differential diagnosis* includes other infectious causes as noted in "Other Colitides" below. A unique additional consideration in children is the hemolytic uremic syndrome that has been closely linked to *Shigella* and *E. coli* infections, with symptoms of hemolytic anemia, renal failure, and thrombocytopenia. Bowel involvement is not common, but a prodromal colitis occurs in 80% of patients up to weeks before the renal symptoms appear (Fig. 3-44).

Other colitides A variety of organisms (*E. coli, Salmonella and Shigella, Yersinia, Campylobacter,* and *Entamoeba histolytica*) and cytomegalovirus (CMV) in immunosuppressed patients can cause colitis with symptoms of diarrhea and abdominal pain, with or without bleeding. Conventional radiographs often

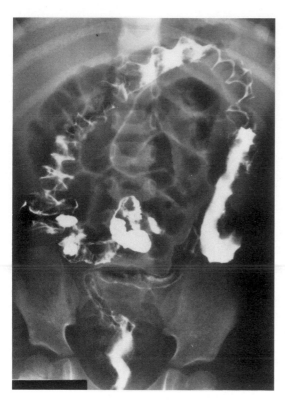

Fig. 3-44 Hemolytic uremic syndrome. Thickened colonic wall that is consistent with colitis 7 days before renal symptons appeared.

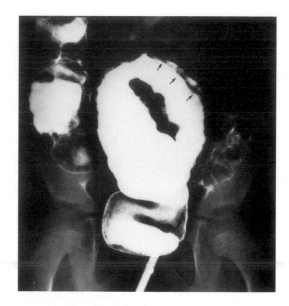

Fig. 3-45 Pseudomembranous colitis. A pseudomembrane is illustrated in the sigmoid colon (*arrows*).

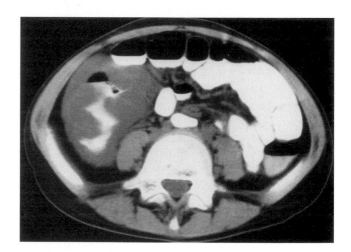

Fig. 3-46 Typhlitis. Cecal wall thickening in a patient treated for ALL.

reveal air-fluid levels and dilated bowel loops. Barium enema findings, mimic those of IBD in patients with colitis caused by *Campylobacter* and *Yersinia*, those of Crohn disease in amoebic or CMV colitis.

Pseudomembranous colitis occurs in patients who have received antibiotics. Alteration of normal flora by the antibiotic results in colonization by C. *difficile.* Symptoms typically begin 4 to 10 days after the start of antibiotic therapy with severe diarrhea. A similar infection can occur in infants without previous exposure to antibiotics.

Conventional radiographs of the abdomen reveal dilation and air-fluid levels in the colon. A contrast enema can demonstrate the pseudomembrane (Fig. 3-45), but is contraindicated in severe cases; endoscopy is diagnostic.

Typhlitis is a necrotizing colitis in young adults that may occur in children who are neutropenic, and usually is associated with lymphoma, aplastic anemia, or acute lymphoblastic leukemia. *Pseudomonas*, CMV, and *Candida* are the most common pathogens.

Conventional abdominal radiographs may show a thickened cecal wall, a mass, or occasionally pneumatosis. A contrast enema is contraindicated. CT/US may be diagnostic (Fig. 3-46).

Appendicitis This difficult-to-diagnose condition is the most frequent entity requiring abdominal surgery in the pediatric age group. Inflammation causes obstruction of the lumen, resulting in retention of secretions, bacterial invasion, and vascular compromise. It is unusual in children less than age 7 years, and the peak incidence occurs during the teenage years. Perforation at the tip occurs in one third to one half of infants and young children with appendiceal inflammation, often leading to abscess formation. In older children the omentum is thought to prevent abscess formation from occurring.

Clinically, there may be abdominal tenderness migrating around McBurney's point. "McBurney's sign"

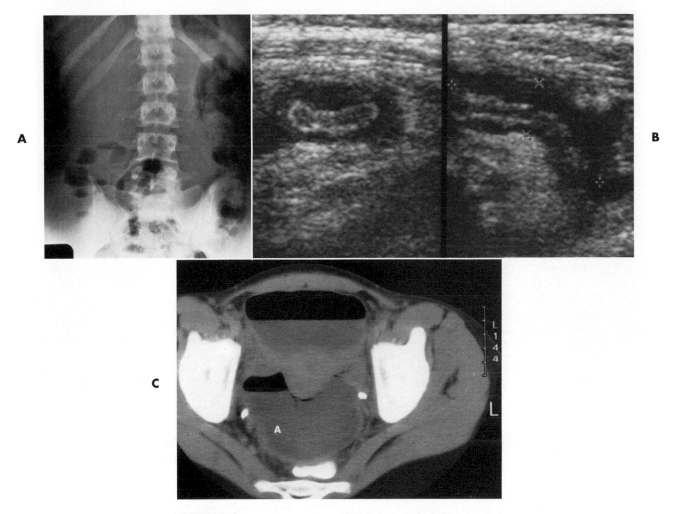

Fig. 3-47 **Appendicitis.** **A**, Conventional radiograph reveals splinting and a localized ileus in the lower right quadrant. **B**, US demonstrates a thickened (> 6mm), inflamed appendix. **C**, CT demonstrates a periappendical abscess (*A*).

consists of tenderness over the inflamed appendix, often elicited on US examination. Nausea, vomiting, fever, and diarrhea also occur frequently.

Conventional abdominal *radiographs* may show a localized ileus in the RLQ (70%), small bowel obstruction (43%), splinting of the lumbosacral spine, a mass (25%), obliteration of the psoas shadow (15%), or an appendicolith (10%) (Fig. 3-47, *A*). An appendicolith is presumably due to post-inflammatory precipitation of calcium salts in inspissated feces. If an appendicolith is noted, prophylactic laparotomy is advocated. Air in the appendix, especially in a retrocecal one, has been thought to indicate appendicitis but may be a normal finding.

US evaluation may demonstrate the inflamed appendix (>6-mm wall thickness and noncompressible). This technique is highly accurate (93%), with a specificity and sensitivity of 95%. US also rules out other causes of RLQ symptoms such as ovarian cyst, IBD, or endometriosis. CT is the modality of choice in complex cases to demonstrate the extent of the presence of an abscess (Fig. 3-47, *B* and *C*). Both CT and US are used in percutaneous drainage of an abscess.

A *contrast* (barium) *enema* is used seldom with the experience gained by US and CT and is often noncontributory. Nonfilling by barium of a normal appendix may be seen in up to 30% of healthy children.

Neoplasms

Except for the premalignant polyposis syndromes such as Gardner's syndrome and including Peutz-Jeghers syndrome, a *malignant* lesion of the small or large bowel in children is extremely rare. Lympho(sarco)ma, including Burkitt's lymphoma, is the most frequently seen primary malignancy of small bowel in the pediatric age group. Children with this entity frequently present with intussusception or hema-

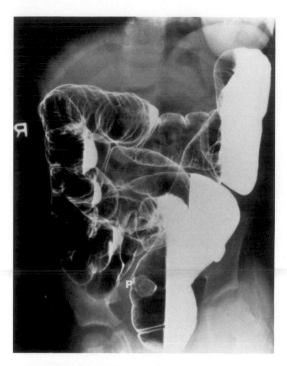

Fig 3-48 Juvenile polyp. Air contrast enema demonstrates a juvenile polyp in the rectosigmoid (*p*).

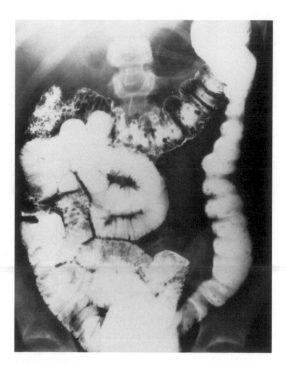

Fig. 3-49 Familial polyposis with polyps throughout the colon and distal small bowel.

Table 3-4 Polyposis syndromes

Syndrome	Type	Location	Inheritance*	Malignancy
Juvenile polyposis	Juvenile	Colon (100%)	AD	No
Familial polyposis	Adenoma	Colon (100%), small bowel (SB), stomach (70%)	AD	Yes
Gardner	Adenoma	Colon (100%), SB, stomach (70%)	AD	Yes
Turcot	Adenoma	Colon	AR	Yes
Peutz-Jeghers	Hamartoma	SB (95%), stomach (30%)	AD	Maybe

•AD, Autosomal dominant; AR, autosomal recessive.

tochezia. Adenocarcinoma is the next most common lesion; again it is extremely rare but occurs in teenagers.

The most common *benign* lesions are juvenile polyps. Occurring most commonly between 2 and 6 years of age, their probable origin is a primary hamartomatous process. Eighty percent are located in the rectosigmoid and are often solitary entities (25% multiple), and there is a slight male predominance. There is no inheritance or malignant potential (Fig. 3-48). Other benign colonic lesions include neurofibroma, hemangiomas (Osler-Weber-Rendu disease), lipomas, and leiomyomas.

The polyposis syndromes, all occurring more commonly in adults, are summarized in Table 3-4.

Familial polyposis occurs in one in 8000 live births and two thirds of patients have a family history; the condition usually is present by the teenage years. Commonly sheets of small polyps cover the entire colon, occur in the stomach in 70% of patients, and occur less commonly in the rest of the small bowel (Fig. 3-49).

Siblings of patients with familial polyposis coli should undergo yearly colonoscopic surveillance from 10 to 15 years of age.

Only 20% of patients with Gardner's syndrome have the triad of soft tissue hamartomas and osteomas of the mandible and facial bones. Mesenteric fibromatosis (desmoid tumor) occurs in 5%. It is avascular and may lead to adhesions.

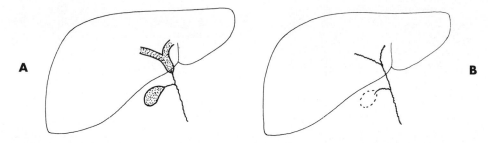

Fig. 3-50 Biliary atresia. The main right and left hepatic ducts down to their junction may be normal (**A**) or abnormal (**B**), with many variations possible. The former comprises 10% to 15% of all cases and is correctable; the latter is not.

Peutz-Jeghers syndrome is the most common small bowel polyposis syndrome, but only 15% of cases are seen before patients reach their twenties. There is accompanying pigmentation of all mucocutaneous surfaces, especially the lips and buccal mucosa. Approximately 50% of patients have a family history of the syndrome.

Liver and Biliary Tree

Anatomy and Developmental Anomalies
  Biliary atresia
  Choledochal cysts
  Congenital hepatic cysts
  Cystic disease of liver and kidneys
Acquired Lesions
  Inflammation
  Intrahepatic calcifications
  Fatty infiltration of liver
  Air over the liver
    Portal venous air
    Air in biliary tree
Neoplasms
  Malignant lesions
    Hepatoblastoma
    Hepatocellular carcinoma
    Rhabdomyosarcoma
    Metastatic lesions
  Benign lesions
    Hemangiomas
    Hemangioendotheliomas
    Focal nodular hyperplasia
Gallbladder
  Cholelithiasis
  Cholecystitis
    Calculous cholecystitis
    Acalculous cholecystitis
  Hydrops

Anatomy and Developmental Anomalies

The liver, gallbladder, and biliary tree develop from the hepatic diverticulum of the foregut. The larger cranial division (pars hepatica) gives rise to the liver, which initially comprises 10% of body weight. At birth it represents 5% (200 g) of body weight. The smaller caudal part (pars cystica), initially solid and connected to the foregut, develops into the gallbladder and cystic duct (see Fig. 3-4, *A*). Bile secretion starts at week 12. Congenital anomalies, infection, and acquired conditions can affect the liver's size, shape, and position.

Biliary artresia Biliary atresia enters the differential diagnosis spectrum when cholestatic jaundice persists in an infant beyond 4 weeks of age. Neonatal jaundice may be due to sepsis, hemolysis, infection (CMV, hepatitis A and B, rubella), and metabolic abnormalities (e.g. α-antitrypsin deficiency, cystic fibrosis). When such other causes have been excluded, neonatal hepatitis or biliary atresia accounts for more than two thirds of remaining cases of conjugated hyperbilirubinemia in the neonate. It is postulated that both biliary atresia and neonatal hepatitis are part of the same spectrum of cholestatic jaundice and hepatomegaly. This might explain the variations encountered in the types of biliary atresia (Fig. 3-50) and the fact that surgical results to repair biliary atresia are significantly better before 2 months of age, suggesting that early intervention may slow the progression of the disease.

The differentiation between biliary atresia and neonatal hepatitis depends on imaging to a large and significant degree. Differentiation is important because surgery is the treatment for the former but not the latter and because liver biopsy results are falsely negative in up to 40% for either condition—further proof these entities are part of the same cholangiopathy.

Imaging evaluation by *US* can reveal either a normal liver or an inhomogeneous parenchymal pattern in both entities and a visualized (1.5 to 2 cm) gallbladder in up to 25% of patients with biliary atresia. Nonvisualization of the gallbladder thus is not diagnos-

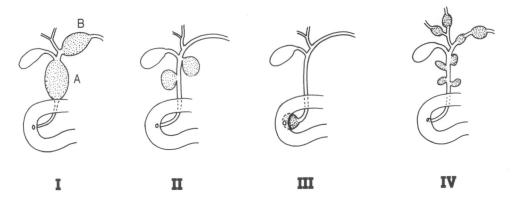

Fig. 3-51 Types of cystic malformations of the biliary tree.

tic. Biliary duct dilation, when seen, is characteristic of atresia. Periportal fibrosis may be seen early in infants with biliary atresia as increased periportal echogenicity. US primarily serves to *exclude* choledochal cysts, choledocholithiasis, or other destructive liver lesions.

Nuclear scintigraphy using ^{99m}Tc imino-diacetic acid derivatives (IDA) are more reliable in differentiating the two entities. Visualization of the radionuclide in the duodenum essentially excludes biliary atresia. If the radionuclide (1) does not appear in the gallbladder at 15 minutes or (2) does not appear in the proximal small bowel at 30 minutes and (3) disappears from the liver by 6 hours with a significant concomitant increase in renal excretion, the diagnosis of biliary atresia may be entertained, and delayed imaging is considered necessary. The sensitivity of radionuclide studies to detect biliary obstruction is 100% and the specificity approximately 80%. Administering phenobarbital before the procedure is essential. In contrast, the hallmark of neonatal hepatitis is normal or slow uptake but significantly *delayed* clearance from the liver and GI tract.

After radionuclide imaging confirms the diagnosis of biliary atresia, further imaging of the biliary tree is performed at laparotomy because a preoperative percutaneous cholangiogram is difficult to obtain in neonates and infants and requires the use of anesthesia. Therefore an intraoperative cholangiogram often is obtained to identify the anatomy to assess whether primary anastomosis, feasible in 10% to 15% of biliary atresia patients, should be attempted. The main right and left hepatic ducts down to at least their junction must be of normal caliber for a Roux-en-Y anastomosis to be successful (Fig. 3-50).

The Kasai hepatic portoenterostomy is used when this favorable anatomy is not present. The jejunum is anastomosed to the under surface of the liver, allowing bile to drain into it. Operative success depends on the presence of microscopic biliary structures at the hilus and is inversely proportional to the age of the patient. Liver transplantation is an option when the Kasai opera-

tion fails or if progressive neonatal hepatitis has resulted in cirrhosis.

Choledochal cysts   Choledochal cysts are rare, occur four times more frequently in girls than boys, and are more common in Orientals. Fifty percent of patients have symptoms before the age of 10, including abdominal pain (50%), fever, obstructive jaundice (80%), and a mass (50%). The classic triad of episodic abdominal pain, jaundice, and a right upper quadrant mass on the right side is present in 15% to 20%.

Choledochal cysts are considered cystic malformations of the biliary tree. Their cause has been ascribed to an obstruction at the sphincter of Oddi or to abnormal insertion of the common bile duct (CBD) into the pancreatic duct. Another theory is that biliary atresia, choledochal cysts, and neonatal hepatitis have a common viral cause. A weakness in the bile duct wall has also been suggested.

These are four types of choledochal cysts (Fig. 3-51):
- Type IA
    fusiform or concentric dilation of the CBD below the cyst duct
- Type IB
    fusiform dilation of the CBD above the cyst duct
- Type II
    eccentric diverticulum of the CBD
- Type III
    dilation of the CBD at the level of the sphincter of Oddi (choledochocele); rarest form
- Type IV
    multiple fusiform dilations of the intrahepatic bile duct (Caroli's disease) without evidence of obstruction; very rare. Type IV may be a distinct entity, an autosomal recessive inherited disorder. In fact there may be two forms, the pure form (type 1), consisting of intrahepatic biliary dilation, and type 2, associated with hepatic fibrosis. The former presents with stone formation, the latter with portal hypertension and varices.

The *differential diagnosis* includes hydrops of the gallbladder, pancreatic pseudocyst, renal cyst, enteric duplication cyst, ovarian cyst, or omental cyst.

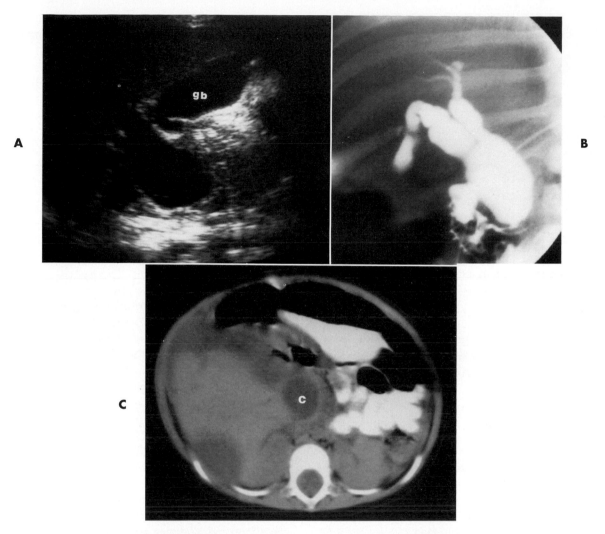

Fig. 3-52 Choledochal cyst. A, US evaluation demonstrates a cystic structure communicating with the gallbladder (*gb*). **B,** ERCP confirms the fusiform dilation of the distal common bile duct. **C,** CT confirms the choledochal cyst (*C*) and the biliary ascites with which the patient presented.

Conventional radiographs and contrast (barium) studies may show evidence of a mass but are usually normal.

US provides information about the size, contour, position, and character of the choledochal cysts. Calculi and wall calcification are rare. Hepatic fibrosis is uncommon, and associated renal cysts seldom occur.

Endoscopic retrograde studies can futher delineate the type of cystic dilation.

The CT appearance can be specific in cases of choledochocele and often clearly demonstrates the other types of choledochal cyst (Fig. 3-52).

Radionuclide studies using the ^{99m}Tc-IDA derivatives may also be useful when US or CT does not document communication between the cyst and the biliary tree. These studies may show accumulation, occasionally delayed, of the radiopharmaceutical in the cyst.

The treatment consists of total excision with direct enteric drainage of a biliary tree, for treatment delay may result in cirrhosis, portal hypertension, cholangitis, and pancreatitis. There is a twentyfold increase in the risk of biliary tract carcinoma in patients with choledochal cyst as compared to the normal population.

Cysts *Congenital hepatic cysts* Congenital hepatic cysts are extremely rare, are more common in the right lobe, probably arise from aberrant bile ducts, and may be multilocular in 20% of cases.

Cystic disease of liver and kidneys Hepatic involvement in autosomal recessive polycystic kidney disease (ARPKD) manifests as periportal fibrosis and hepatic cysts. The perinatal and neonatal forms of ARPKD usually result in death in infancy, and their hepatic involvement is minimal. Patients with the infantile and juvenile forms have nephromegaly and renal symptoms, but

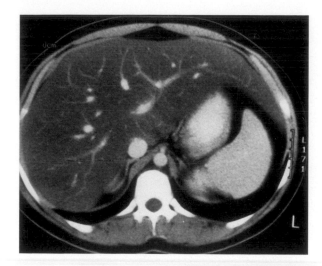

Fig. 3-53 Fatty infiltration of the liver in a patient on steroid therapy. Note the normal spleen.

the clinical picture is influenced by the degree of hepatic involvement with cysts, periportal fibrosis, and subsequent impairment of liver function, resulting in portal hypertension.

Acquired Conditions

Inflammation   Inflammation of the liver can be caused by viral (most common, CMV; hepatitis B), bacterial (*E. coli*), and fungal (*Candida*) organisms, the latter in immunocompromised patients. Parasitic abscess formation by *Echinococcus* results in the formation of cysts in the liver (80%), which may calcify in 30%, whereas amoebic abscesses (*E. histolytica*) are most prevalent in patients less than age 3 years. Chronic granulomatous disease of children (CGDC) is a congenital X-linked defect of leukocytes that also causes granuloma and abscess formation in the liver. Scintigraphy is very useful, although it is nonspecific in detecting inflammation. US is the screening modality of choice in detecting abscess cavities greater than 1 cm in diameter. CT also is useful, and either modality is useful for percutaneous drainage guidance, the therapy of choice.

Intrahepatic calcifications   The differential diagnosis for intrahepatic calcifications includes primary tuberculosis or histoplasmosis, hemangiomas, hamartomas, neoplasms, biliary calculi secondary to furosemide (Lasix) therapy, and CGDC.

Fatty infiltration of liver   The *differential diagnosis* for fatty infiltration of the liver includes cystic fibrosis, malnutrition or hyperalimentation, glycogen storage disease, and steroid therapy.

Although conventional radiographs may suggest fatty infiltration, CT and MRI are diagnostic (Fig. 3-53).

Air over the liver   *Portal venous air* (peripheral in location) Differential diagnosis of portal venous air includes NEC, bowel obstruction, sepsis, and iatrogenic (e.g., umbilical catherization) causes.

Air in biliary tree (central in location). Differential diagnosis of air in the biliary tree includes fistulas, trauma, and infection.

Conventional radiographs are often diagnostic (see Fig. 3-5, *B*). US with Doppler is sensitive for air bubbles in the portal vein but lacks specificity.

Neoplasms

Malignant lesions

Hepatoblastoma   Hepatoblastoma most commonly occurs in children less than age 3 years, with a 2:1 male predominance, and 50% to 60% of cases occur before the child is 1 year of age. The right lobe is more frequently involved, and approximately one third of lesions occurs in both lobes. Calcifications occur in approximately 40% of these lesions. Metastatic disease to the lungs occurs in 10% of affected children. Serum levels of α-fetoprotein are elevated in two thirds. There is an association of hepatoblastoma with biliary atresia, hemihypertrophy, polycystic kidneys, diaphragmatic hernia, and neonatal hepatitis.

Conventional radiographs of the abdomen may show a large hepatic contour. US may show an inhomogeneous hyperechogenic lobulated mass. Its highly vascular nature can be documented on color-flow Doppler studies. Coarse liver calcifications can be noted on abdominal radiographs, and US may reveal shadows.

CT with IV contrast delineates the extent of an inhomogenous, hypodense lesion preoperatively. Disease extending across the falciform ligament precludes operative resection. CT also evaluates the most common site of metastatic involvement, the chest.

MRI confirms CT findings as a hypointense area on T1 and a hyperintense and inhomogeneous lesion on T2.

Hepatocellular carcinoma   Hepatocellular carcinoma is rare in children less than age 5 years and can be divided into two subtypes: hepatocellular carcinoma and fibrolamellar hepatocarcinoma. The latter occurs in late teenage years, equally in both sexes, and has a better prognosis. In children with hepatocellular carcinoma there is a slight male predominance. The tumor is particularly likely to arise in children with underlying liver disease: α1-antitrypsin deficiency, biliary atresia, glycogen storage disease, and chronic hepatitis.

Clinically, children with hepatocellular carcinoma are seen with an abdominal mass, nausea, vomiting, and weight loss. Serum α-fetoprotein levels are elevated in almost all cases, although not as high as in hepatoblastoma.

Conventional abdominal radiographs show hepatic

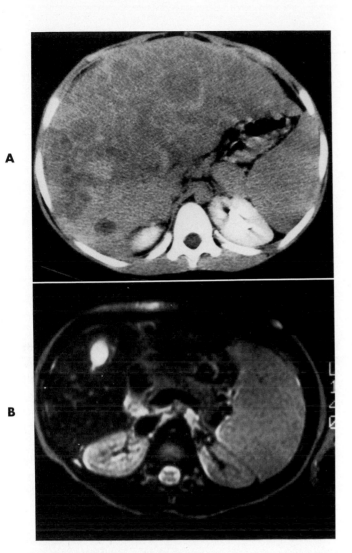

Fig. 3-54 Hepatocellular carcinoma in a 4-year-old patient with chronic hepatitis. **A**, Contrast enhanced CT; **B**, MR. Hepatoblastoma can look identical.

calcification and hepatomegaly in 15% to 25% of these children, and US is highly sensitive in detecting an often homogeneous, slightly hyperechogenic liver mass that can extend into the portal or hepatic vessels. Arteriovenous (AV) shunting can be documented on color-flow Doppler studies.

CT with IV contrast enhancement more accurately defines the extent of an often multicentric mass and evaluates the presence and extent of regional spread and chest metastases.

MRI has sensitivity and specificity similar to that of CT. The T1- and T2-weighted images can look exactly like those of hepatoblastoma. The "satellite" lesions, if present, are diagnostic (Fig. 3-54).

Rhabdomyosarcoma Rhabdomyosarcoma of the biliary tree is a rare lesion that presents with jaundice in children less than age 5 years. Most rhabdomyosarcomas occur in the urogenital or skeletal systems. Most

commonly in the liver this lesion is associated with bile duct dilation. It occurs equally in both genders with a uniformly poor prognosis.

US and *CT* reveal the dilation of the biliary tree and may define the mass. Differentiation from other hepatic tumors is almost impossible. The mass resembles "Swiss-cheese" on US. On cholangiography the botryoidal (grapelike) quality of this tumor is evident.

Metastatic lesions A variety of neoplasms can invade the liver parenchyma. The differential diagnosis includes infantile neuroblastoma (stage IV-S in children less than age 1 year), Wilms tumor, and lymphoma or leukemia. US is the screening modality of choice, although a 15% to 20% false negative rate occurs. CT is the better modality to delineate the preoperative or pretreatment extent of these lesions. The MRI appearance is nonspecific.

Benign lesions These predominately mesenchymal and vascular lesions often present with hepatomegaly in the first 2 years of life. Hemangiomas (cavernous) and hemangioendotheliomas can be difficult to distinguish on the basis of pathology (immature endothelioid cells) or on CT (peripheral enhancement), MRI, or US imaging. Classically, nuclear imaging shows a characteristic early appearance and inhomogeneity of the radiopharaceutical in children with hemangioendotheliomas. Hemangiomas are more definitively documented (high T2) on MRI. Color-flow Doppler may be helpful as well. Treatment often includes embolization.

Hemangiomas are more common in adults but also represent the most common benign hepatic neoplasm in children, are asymptomatic, and are often detected incidentally as a well defined echogenic mass on US (<2 cm).

Infantile *hemangioendotheliomas* may be the cause of congestive heart failure (CHF), as well as hepatomegaly or a bruit in neonates and infants. Levels of α-fetoprotein are often normal, and there are cutaneous hemangiomas in 50% of these patients.

Hemangioendothelioma is the most common symptomatic vascular liver tumor of infancy. Often multiple, 90% are seen before the infant is 6 months old and girls outnumber boys 2:1. The condition tends to regress spontaneously over the next several months of life. Fine nodular calcifications can be seen in 40% on CT (Fig. 3-55). US may show hypoechoic or hyperechoic lesions similar to those of cavernous hemangiomas. Enlarged celiac feeding vessels may be diagnostic.

Focal nodular hyperplasia Focal nodular hyperplasia is uncommon in the pediatric age group. It is a benign epithelial tumor located in the subcapsular region and occurs much more commonly in young women taking oral contraceptives. Uptake of radioisotope peripherally in Kupffer cells around a central scar

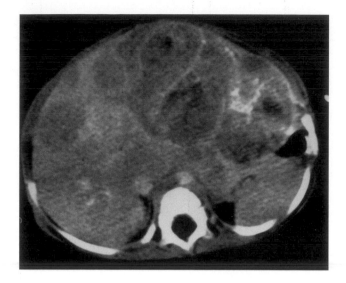

Fig. 3-55 Hemangioendothelioma. Contrast enhanced CT demonstrates an enlarged heterogeneous liver with area of enhancement as well as necrosis.

is diagnostic. Results from CT, US, or MRI often are difficult to interpret because the lesion blends into the normal liver tissue.

Gallbladder

Cholelithiasis Cholelithiasis is often idiopathic or may have nonhemolytic or hemolytic causes. Girls are more commonly affected than boys, whereas familial incidence, obesity, estrogen therapy, and diabetes may predispose the individual to their formation.

In *infants* immature physiologic mechanisms for gallstone or sludge formation include the lower secretory rate of bile acids as compared to that of adults (50%), the immature biliary conjugation pathways, lack of oral feeding, and the use of diuretic therapy (furosemide) in premature infants with HMD. Prenatal gallstones are extremely rare.

Hemolytic disease such as sickle cell disease, thalassemia, and hereditary spherocytosis or sepsis can lead to gallstone formation secondary to cholestasis.

Conventional abdominal *radiographs* reveal up to 50% of gallstones. US imaging, on the other hand, is almost always sufficient for diagnostic purposes (95% accuracy). In the spectrum of cholelithiasis, sludge, sludge balls, and echogenic densities that change position with gravity are all well identified on US. In patients receiving total parenteral nutrition, sludge develops within 10 to 14 days. Biliary duct dilation (cholestasis) also can be assessed reliably. The upper limit of the normal dimension of the CBD is 4 mm up to the teen years and is 7 mm thereafter.

In approximately 40% of older *children*, cholelithiasis is idiopathic. A hemolytic cause (e.g., sickle cell disease, thalassemia) or Wilson disease is responsible in approximately 30%. Abnormal enterohepatic circula-

tion is the proposed cause in children with IBD affecting the ileum; cystic fibrosis, obesity, and short-gut syndrome after surgery have also been associated with increased gallstone (cholesterol) formation.

In contradistinction to the infant, older children with cholelithiasis more often have symptoms: RUQ pain, nausea, and vomiting. The *differential diagnosis* should include renal, appendiceal, and ovarian considerations. Treatment is cholecystectomy. Extracorporeal shock-wave lithotripsy in children remains under study.

Cholecystitis

Calculous cholecystitis Acute *calculous* cholecystitis represents inflammation of the gallbladder, often with gallstones present that obstruct the cystic duct. An organism is seldom recovered, and the condition occurs more commonly in adolescent girls. Repeated self-limited episodes of calculous cholecystitis may lead to chronic cholecystitis.

Acalculous cholecystitis Acute acalculous cholecystitis occurs in the absence of gallstones, possibly secondary to increased bile viscosity as seen in children receiving total parenteral nutrition or who have experienced trauma. Viral and bacterial organisms rarely have been isolated. RUQ pain, jaundice (40% of patients), and nausea are the most common clinical symptoms.

US demonstration of an anechoic gallbladder with a thickened (>3 mm) often hyperreflective irregular gallbladder wall or occasionally sludge or gallstones, as in the adult, signifies true cholecystitis. A hypoechoic halo often is present. However, it also is seen in patients with ascites or hypoalbuminemia or who have eaten a recent meal, causing physiologic thickening of the gallbladder wall.

Hydrops Hydrops is an acute distention of the gallbladder and may be idiopathic (sepsis, burns) or occur

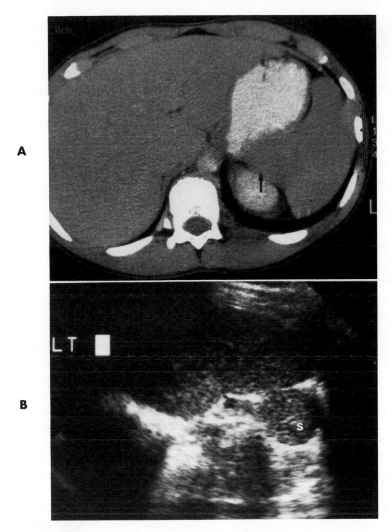

Fig. 3-56 The spleen. **A**, CT demonstrates the medial lobe of the spleen (*arrow*). **B**, US demonstration of a splenule (*s*).

as part of Kawasaki disease (mucocutaneous lymph node syndrome). Mesenteric adenopathy or a vasculitis in the absence of stones is the presumed cause. US demonstrates a gallbladder that is longer than the ipsilateral kidney.

Spleen

Anatomy and Developmental Anomalies
    Anatomic variations
        Asplenia
        Polysplenia
Infection or Abscess
Neoplasms
    Malignant lesions
    Benign cysts

Anatomy and Developmental Anomalies

Congenital variations of the spleen include accessory spleens (10% to 15%), ectopic spleen, variation in shapes, asplenia, and polysplenia (Fig. 3-56). The latter two are part of the heterotaxy syndrome. The spleen develops rapidly near the fifth week of gestation as a mesenchymal bulge. Erythropoiesis is maximal by 20 weeks gestation. Spleen ectopia is due to an absent lienorenal ligament. Accessory splenic tissue may result from abnormal budding of the mesenchymal bulge.

Radioisotope scanning using 99mTc-sulfur colloid is useful to assess splenic anatomy and function. US is the screening modality of choice, although it may be difficult to image the entire spleen on US, and splenic measurements are not very reliable. However, if the tip of the spleen reaches lower than the lower pole of the left

Differential Diagnosis of Splenomegaly

Infection (tuberculosis, bacteremia)
Hemolytic anemias (sickle cell, thalassemia)
Leukemia or lymphoma
Cysts, either of traumatic or congenital origin
Portal hypertension (US: omental thickness > 1.7
  times the size of the aorta and splenomegaly)

kidney on US, splenomegaly is strongly suggested (see box).

Asplenia Asplenia is associated with bilateral trilobed ("right") lungs and eparterial bronchi. In addition, GI anomalies such as situs inversus and a centrally located symmetric liver occur (3% to 5%). Severe congenital cardiac abnormalities (e.g., atrial septal defects, atrioventricular canal, transposition) are associated as well. Most patients are boys. There is increased susceptibility to infection and most of these children die before 1 year of age.

Polysplenia Polysplenia is associated with bilateral bilobed ("left") lungs and hyparterial bronchi. The GI anomalies are similar in incidence as in patients with asplenia, but the cardiac anomalies are less severe (ASD, VSD). Interruption of the hepatic portion of the inferior vena cava with azygous continuation occurs in 60% to 70%. Most patients are girls, and CHF is the most common clinical finding.

Infection or Abscess

An abscess may form because of a variety of causes, including as a complication of systemic sepsis, and is most commonly noted in immunocompromised hosts (leukemia). Fungal infections are most common in these cases. Often microscopic in size, these cystic lesions must be larger than 1 cm to be identified on US or CT. Most splenic abscesses, however, are multiple and small and may be difficult to image. *Candida* infection occasionally presents a specific "Swiss-cheese" appearance.

Neoplasms

Malignant lesions Lymphoma and leukemia most frequently affect the spleen primarily; metastatic disease from many primary causes can involve the spleen, but the causes are usually diagnosed at autopsy.

Benign cysts
Aside from a splenic cyst (epidermoid), benign cysts are rare. Splenic cysts can be divided into true epidermoid cysts (lined by epithelium) or secondary cysts,

resulting from hemmorhage, infection (hydatid disease), or infarction.

The most common cause for a splenic cyst is trauma, followed by hydatid disease (Fig. 3-57). Other lesions (lymphangioma, hamartoma) are rare.

Percutaneous drainage usually is not successful, for there is a high rate of recurrence. Injection (slerosis) of the cyst may be curative.

Pancreas

Anatomy and Developmental Anomalies
  Cystic fibrosis
  Pancreatitis
  Neoplasms

Anatomy and Developmental Anomalies

In two thirds of patients the main pancreatic duct (Wirsung) and the accessory duct (Santorini) fuse in direct apposition or in the wall of the duodenum (week 10). In approximately one fifth of cases the accessory duct does not reach the lumen, and in 10% the two ductal systems do not connect, resulting in pancreas *divisum*, associated with an increased incidence of pancreatitis. When the two anlagen of the dorsal and ventral pancreas fuse too early (week 6), an *annular* pancreas may result, encircling and thus possibly obstructing the second portion of the duodenum. This variant is associated with esophageal atresia, tracheoesophageal fistula, Down syndrome, and malrotation or duodenal atresia stenosis in 75% of cases. Uncommonly, a preduodenal portal vein, situs inversus, and Hirschsprung disease also have been associated. Annular pancreas is slightly less common than a pancreas divisum (see Figs. 3-4 and 3-30).

Ectopic pancreatic tissue can be seen along the entire GI tract. It most commonly is seen in the stomach (70%), duodenum, and in a Meckel diverticulum. The greater antral curve is the most common location.

Cystic fibrosis In all patients with cystic fibrosis pancreatic insufficiency of some degree is present. The severity varies widely. Eighty-five percent have steatorrhea, whereas the remaining 15% will have normal fat absorption but still have deficient pancreatic enzyme secretion. A mixture of inflammatory changes, obstructive secretions, and/or debris leads to progressive fibrosis and atrophy of the pancreas; calcification may occur, but cysts are rare.

Pancreatitis There are severe distinct causes for acute pancreatitis in childhood. (Occult) trauma is the most common cause. Other causes include generalized conditions such as sepsis or hemolytic uremic syndrome, biliary tree obstruction, or inflammation and

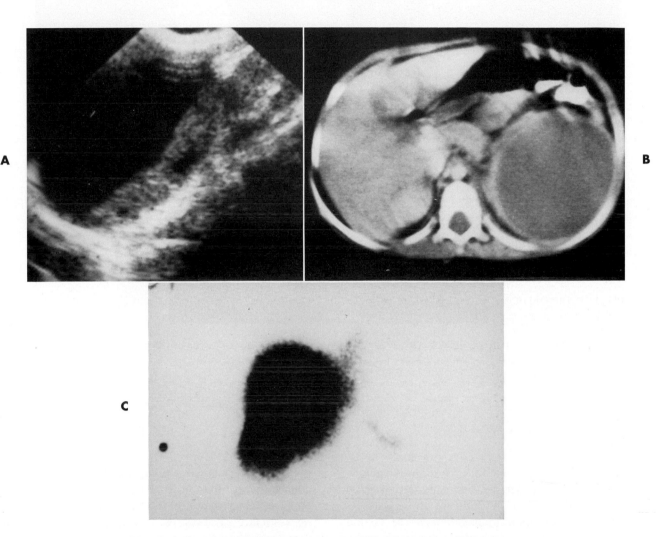

Fig. 3-57   Posttraumatic splenic cyst. A, US demonstration of a cystic structure in the upper left quadrant with internal echoes. **B,** CT confirmation of same. **C,** Radionuclide study confirming the internal echoes on **A** to be residual functional splenic tissue compressed by the cyst.

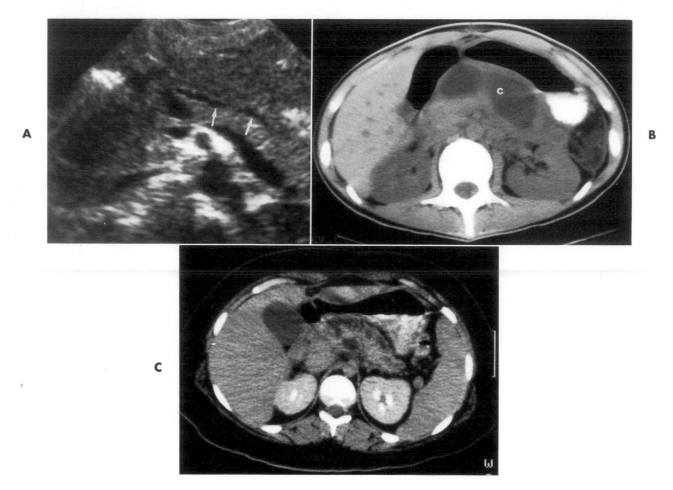

Fig. 3-58   Pancreatitis. A, Transverse abdominal US reveals diffuse enlargement of the pancreas with a dilated pancreatic duct (*arrows*). **B,** CT demonstrates a multiloculated pseudocyst (*c*). **C,** Contrast enhanced CT of chronic pancreatitis with areas of necrosis.

hereditary pancreatitis. Metabolic conditions such as cystic fibrosis, hyperlipidemia, and long-term steroid use are also known causes. Clinically, these patients most often have abdominal pain after eating, lasting several days and associated with nausea and vomiting.

Imaging of the pancreas has improved enormously since the advent of cross-sectional imaging.

Conventional radiographs of the abdomen occasionally show calcification (10% to 15%), usually occurring in the teenage years of patients with cystic fibrosis or chronic pancreatitis. A pseudocyst (occurring in 5% of all cases) is suspected if a mass is identified. Effective imaging centers around US, which is 95% accurate in detecting pancreatic abnormalities, as the initial diagnostic procedure. In patients with pancreatitis there may be focal or diffuse enlargement of the entire gland accompanied by decreased echogenicity. If the pancreatic duct is visualized, it should be less than 2 mm in diameter when normal. US findings in children with cystic fibrosis include an echogenic pancreas with occasional cysts detected. There may also be associated gallstones. CT is more useful in the demonstration of pancreatic pseudocysts, particularly in assessing the wall thickness, which is an important factor in deciding whether surgical or percutaneous drainage should be attempted. CT, like US, assists in guiding the therapeutic approach (Fig. 3-58).

Endoscopic retrograde cholangiopancreatography (ERCP) can delineate the pancreatic duct structure and can be useful in determining the need for pancreatectomy in cases of pancreatic trauma.

Neoplasms   Neoplasms are exceeding rare but may consist of islet cell (functional) tumors (insulinoma) and nonfunctional exocrine derivatives (adenocarcinoma).

Trauma

General Considerations
Liver
Spleen
Pancreas
Bowel and Mesentery

General Considerations

Traditionally, peritoneal lavage was the method that, in addition to physical examination, was used to assess whether intraperitoneal bleeding has occurred after trauma. False negative results were few and were probably the result of retroperitoneal injuries. False positive studies probably resulted from traumatic insertion of the trocar. Peritoneal lavage seldom is used in children today.

The availability of CT has had a considerable impact on the choice of imaging techniques commonly used in determining extent of intrabdominal trauma in pediatric patients. It is the single best imaging method currently available and is at least as accurate as scintigraphy and US and, in certain instances, more accurate. It can be performed safely and accurately in the severely injured child and therefore does *not* delay the diagnostic process but speeds it along if done properly. Anatomic detail is superior to that provided by scintigraphy and US; the extent of injury is imaged more completely; and it illustrates associated injuries 17% or 18% better than US or EU. However, a negative result from an abdominal CT scan does not mean absence of injury, and it also should not preclude additional tests when deemed clinically necessary.

Prompt evaluation with CT will determine the presence or absence of intraperitoneal or retroperitoneal hemorrhage and the integrity of the major solid organs. Furthermore, CT may detect a bleeding source, and contusions or superficial lacerations of the solid organs and the bowel may be demonstrated. Enhancement of the bowel wall and a small IVC compared to the aorta may suggest shock.

Peritoneal lavage should not be performed before the CT scan because retained lavage fluid can simulate intraperitoneal fluid and the presence of air can suggest visceral perforation.

Scintigraphy does have an advantage over CT in that it is affected less by patient motion, does not necessitate the use of sedation, and does not require contrast media. Conversely, scintigraphy takes as long or longer than CT to perform, and its radiation dose to the patient is higher. However, it is quite organ-specific to the liver and spleen.

Imaging should be postponed or tailored if significant hypoxemia or clinical instability necessitates immediate laparotomy.

Liver

The appearance of the typical hepatic laceration is that of a low attenuating lesion that is focal, peripheral, and most commonly located in the right lobe. It often is associated with a right pleural effusion and possibly contusion in the right lung, with or without rib fractures (Fig. 3-59, A). Acute hepatic hemorrhage usually is hyperdense because of the high protein content of the retracted clot or sedimented blood, whereas bile collections have lower attenuation. The evolution of findings in hepatic trauma can be exquisitely demonstrated on CT, obviating other studies. CT therefore is the imaging modality of choice, and its use contributes to the trend to more nonoperative management of this injury in the child.

When deep trauma has occurred, the injury often is associated with a biloma, hematobilia, and, over time, pseudoaneurysms of the hepatic artery and bile duct disruption.

Left-lobe lesions are more severe and harder to detect and often are associated with trauma to the pancreas and duodenum (Fig. 3-59, B). The caudate lobe, as a result of its posterior location, is only rarely involved in trauma.

Gallbladder injuries from blunt abdominal trauma are extremely rare.

When the clinical course is stable, a follow-up scan in 7 to 10 days with either CT or US is most useful to assess for resolution regardless of the initial imaging modality used (Fig. 3-59, C).

Spleen

In approximately 10% to 20% of patients the diagnosis of splenic injury is not obvious. Other injuries may overshadow its symptoms, and rupture can be delayed (48 to 72 hours after trauma). In addition, US and radionuclide evaluation both have a false positive rate of approximately 7% and a false negative rate of approximately 2%. Because there has been a tendency over the last 20 years to treat splenic trauma conservatively, it is important that the modality used to diagnose it has a high sensitivity. CT's sensitivity in splenic abnormalities is assessed as near 100%. The ability to image the rest of the intraabdominal structures concurrently provides a distinct advantage over organ-specific radionuclide imaging. The detection of subcapsular hematomas and lacerations make IV contrast administration essential (Fig. 3-60). Anatomic variants of splenic anatomy may contribute to false positive inter-

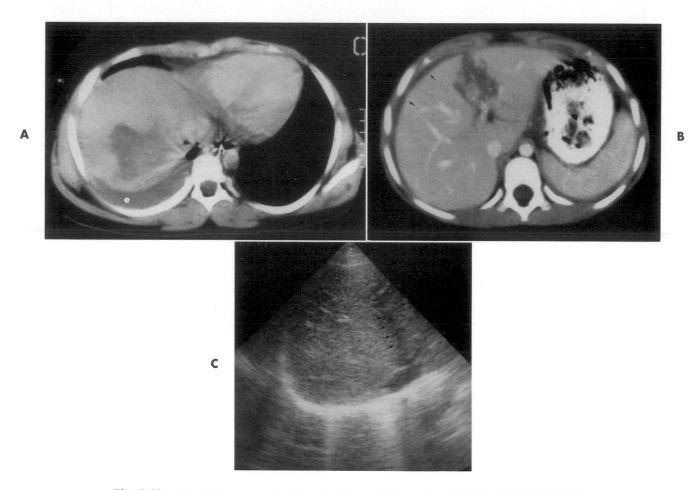

Fig. 3-59   Hepatic trauma.   A, Contrast enhanced CT reveals a right lobe hepatic laceration with an associated pleural effusion   (*e*). **B,** Enhanced CT demonstrates a left lobe hepatic laceration with subcapsular fluid (*arrows*). **C,** Follow-up US demonstrates a healing laceration (*arrows*).

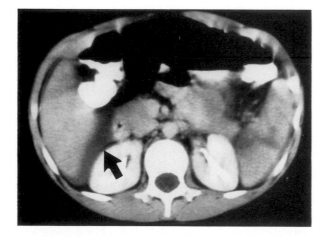

Fig. 3-60   Splenic trauma. Enhanced CT demonstrates splenic laceration with fluid in Morison's pouch (*arrow*).

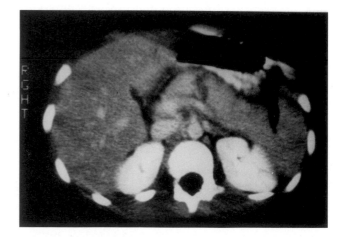

Fig. 3-61   Pancreatic trauma. Enhanced CT demonstrates a transverse fracture of the body of the pancreas.

Indications for Emergency Abdominal CT
Severly injured but stable patients suspected of having injuries to multiple intraabdominal organ systems
Patients whose abdomens cannot be examined with US (e.g., ones with open wounds or extreme abdominal tenderness)
Unstable patients or those with severe head trauma who need an evaluation of the abdomen (physical examination unsatisfactory)
Patients with abdominal trauma in whom the results of other modalities are either equivocal or do not fit the clinical impression

pretation. Long-term sequelae include splenic abnormalities and pseudocyst formation. US is the modality of choice for follow-up imaging.

Pancreas

Pancreatic injuries often escape early detection in children. However in early childhood trauma is the most common cause of pancreatitis, which may be complicated by sepsis, shock, and the later development of pseudocysts.

In children the CT delineation of the pancreatic outline may be difficult to determine without meticulous oral and IV contrast enhancement because of the lack of retroperitoneal fat. It is unusual to see the slightly obliquely situated gland in the upper abdomen on one CT slice. The dimensions of the pancreas depend on the age of the patient, and their use is not very practical.

CT can demonstrate transection of the pancreas and pancreatitis (Fig. 3-61). Posttraumatic pancreatic pseudocysts can be detected within 72 hours. CT is the recommended initial study in complex cases.

US is the screening modality of choice for the pancreas. It can demonstrate peripancreatic fluid, assess the other solid organs, and identify pseudocysts more reliably than CT. Overlying dressings and/or air may be a limiting factor. ERCP may be needed to confirm the integrity of the pancreatic duct.

Bowel and Mesentery

Trauma to the mesentery can involve any part of the colon or small bowel. It can be detected on CT but usually only retrospectively, and the lacerated viscus is only rarely identified. Intraperitoneal blood or gas also can be detected, but an intramural hematoma is identified in only approximately 50% of patients.

The primary indications for performing emergency abdominal CT in the pediatric age group are summarized in the box.

Suggested Readings

Texts

Daneman A: *Pediatric body CT*, London, Springer-Verlag, 1987.

Kirks DR, editor: *Practical Pediatric Imaging*, Little, Brown, and Co, 1992, pp 724-895.

Siegel MJ, editor: *Pediatric Sonography*, 1991, Raven Press, pp 115-256.

Silverman FM, Kuhn JP, editors: *Caffey's Pediatric X-Ray Diagnosis*, ed 9, vol 1, St Louis, Mosby, 1992, pp 893-1144.

Silverman FM, Kuhn JP, editors: *Caffey's Pediatric X-Ray Diagnosis*, ed 9, vol 2, St Louis, Mosby, 1992, pp 2029-2100.

Stringer DA: *Pediatic Gastrointestinal Imaging*, 1991, Decker.

Sty JR, Wells RG, Starshak RJ et al: *Diagnostic Imaging of Infants and Children*, vol 1, Aspen Publishers, 1992, pp 139-326.

Swischuk LE: *Imaging of the Newborn, Infant and Young Child*, ed 3, 1989, Williams & Wilkins, pp 355-588.

Teele RL, Share JC: *Ultrasonography of Infants and Children*, Philadelphia, 1991, WB Saunders, pp 214-461.

Welch KJ, Randolph JG, Ravitch MM et al, editors: *Pediatric Surgery*, ed 4, vol 2, St Louis, 1986, Mosby, pp 731-1126

Articles

Abramson SJ, Berdon WE, Baker DH: Childhood typhlitis: its increasing association with acute myelogenous leukemia, *Radiology* 146:61, 1983

Amodio J, Berdon WE, Abramson J et al: Microcolon in prematurity: a form of functional obstruction, *AJR* 146:239, 1986.

Amodio JD, Abramson J, Berdon WE et al: Pediatric AIDS, *Semin Roentgenol* 22:66, 1987.

Berdon WE, Slovis TK, Campbell RB et al: Neonatal small left colon syndrome: its relationship to aganglionosis and meconium plug syndrome, *Radiology* 125:457, 1977.

Bisset GS III, Kirks DR: Intussusception in infants and children: diagnosis and therapy, *Radiology* 168:141, 1988.

Blumhagen JD, Maclin L, Krauter D et al: Sonographic diagnosis of hypertrophic pyloric stenosis, *AJR* 150:1367, 1988.

Bowen A: The vomiting infant: recent advances and unsettled issues in imaging, *Radiol Clin North Am* 26:377, 1988.

Eklöf O, Hugooson C: Post evacuation findings in barium enema treated intussusceptions, *Ann Radiol (Paris)* 19:133, 1976.

Franken EA Kao SCS, Smith WL et al: Imaging of the acute abdomen in infants and children, AJR 153:921, 1989.

Haller JO, Cohen HL: Hypertrophic pyloric stenosis: diagnosis using US, *Radiology* 161:335, 1988.

Haller JO: Sonography of the biliary tract in infants and children, *AJR* 157:1051, 1991.

Kirks DR, Caron KH, Bissett III GS: CT of blunt abdominal trauma in children: an anatomic "snapshot in time," *Radiology* 182:631, 1992.

Markowitz RI, Meyer JS: Pneumatic versus hydrostatic reduction of intussusception, *Radiology* 183:623, 1992.

Nowicki P: Intestinal ischemia and necrotizing enterocolitis, *J Pediatr* 117:S14-S19, 1990.

Sivit CJ, Newman KD, Boenning DA et al: Appendicitis: usefulness of US in diagnosis in a pediatric population, *Radiology* 185:549, 1992.

Taylor GA, Eichelberger MR, O'Donnell R et al: Indications for CT in children with blunt abdominal trauma, *Ann Surgery* 213:212, 1991.

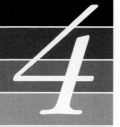

CHAPTER 4

Genitourinary Tract

Imaging Techniques

Voiding Cystourethrography
Excretory Urography
Ultrasonography
Nuclear Medicine
Computed Tomography
Magnetic Resonance

Voiding Cystourethrography

A voiding cystourethrogram (VCUG) is the most frequently used and optimal method to demonstrate vesicoureteral reflux (VUR) and to evaluate bladder anatomy and function.

Urinary tract infection (UTI) is the most common indication for VCUG, followed by dilation of the renal collecting system (hydronephrosis), detected either prenatally or postnatally by ultrasound (US) screening. Because genitourinary (GU) tract anomalies can be associated with anorectal malformations, myelodysplasia, and prune-belly (Eagle-Barrett) syndrome, a VCUG is needed in these instances to delineate anatomic and functional relationships. Voiding dysfunction and enuresis in boys are also common indications for a VCUG.

Labial adhesions are considered a relative contraindication—relative because after medical or surgical release of these adhesions, a VCUG is still performed. The usual contrast medium, chosen because it is least irritating to the bladder wall, is an 18% to 25% ionic contrast agent (e.g., Cysto-Conray). Sterile catheterization of the bladder (no. 8 Fr pediatric feeding tube) is a benign procedure, for complications such as reinfection or false passage are extremely rare.

After catheterization of the bladder, the contrast is dripped in by gravity, with the reservoir suspended

Tailored Imaging Sequence (see Fig. 4-1)

Early filling film: confirms catheter position; may show noncompressed ureterocele (one exposure)
Filled Bladder: both oblique views to visualize ureterovesical juntion (two exposures)
Both renal beds: exposed at this time only if vesicoureteral reflux (VUR) is present
Urethra while voiding: two oblique views in a boy; one anteroposterior view in a girl
Postvoid bladder: to estimate residual urinary volume (one exposure)
Renal beds: to stage "high pressure" VUR or to confirm that VUR did not occur (two exposures)
"Cyclical voiding" views: may be useful in child with suspected ectoptic insertion of the ureters; allows contrast to enter (reflux) into ectopic ureter *during* voiding

approximately 3 feet above the table top. Cessation of flow heralds a full bladder and the beginning of the imaging sequence. The rule of thumb for estimated bladder volume (in milliliters) for children less than age 6 years follows: age (in years) plus 2 times 30 (see box; Fig. 4-1). A basic, *normal* VCUG entails seven (eight in boys) exposures, resulting in approximately 25 mrad of gonadal radiation exposure (50% less if digital fluoroscopy is used).

Excretory Urograph

Urography visualizes the entire urinary tract by means of an excreted, intravenously administered contrast agent. It demonstrates anatomic detail and is a semiquantitative estimate of renal function.

Indications include abnormal US examination of the upper tracts, suspicion of urinary tract calculus, incontinence (in girls), and suspected neurogenic dysfunc-

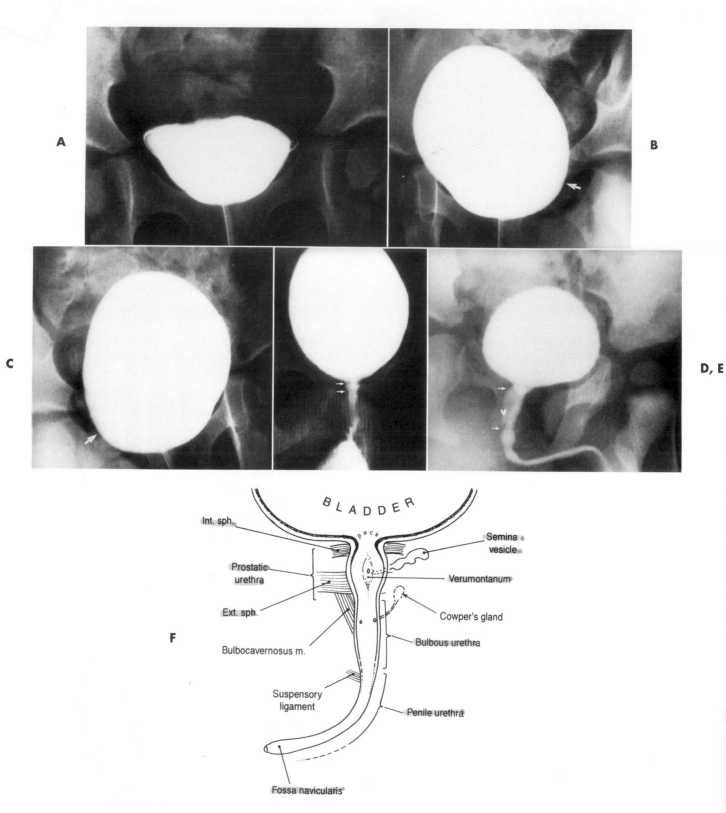

Fig. 4-1 A, Early filling film verifies catheter position and excludes a ureterocele. **B, C,** Oblique view to evaluate ureterovesical junction (*arrows*). **D,** Normal female urethra: internal and external sphincters (*arrows*). **E,** Normal male urethra (*V,* verumontanum); internal and external sphincters (*arrows*). **F,** Schematic representation of the male urethra.

Directed Excretory Urography Imaging Sequence

Preliminary abdominal radiograph: to evaluate proper technique, identify urinary tract calculi, and evaluate bony structures (dysraphism) (one exposure)

One-minute and 5-minute exposure of the upper abdomen: to evaluate symmetry of excretion (nephrographic phase), renal contours, and the calyces (pyelogram) (two exposures)

Twenty-minute radiograph of the abdomen: evaluates collecting systems and the course of the ureters. Prone positioning is useful to take advantage of the contrast's being heavier than urine and to delineate the extent of a dilated collecting system and/or ureter (one exposure)

Other views: obtained at the discretion of the managing radiologist; tomography seldom necessary to settle diagnostic dilemmas

tion of the bladder. Use of the "one-shot" excretory urogram in trauma settings is discouraged in favor of CT evaluation.

Dehydration and shock are absolute contraindications to performing excretory urography. Knowledge of previous allergic reactions to contrast agents or shellfish constitutes a relative contraindication.

In the neonatal age group the glomerular filtration rate (GFR) increases from 20% of the adult value at birth to 50% of the adult GFR value at 10 days of age; therefore an excretory urogram is less useful than nuclear renography in the first month of life. The GFR is at adult levels by 18 months of age.

The contrast media that are used include ionic (1300 to 1400 mOsm/L) and nonionic or low-osmolar (600 to 700 mOsm/L) compounds. The latter's advantages include less irritation to the extravascular soft tissues and a major adverse reaction rate that is less than one tenth that for ionic contrast agents. In children less than 10 years of age, approximately 1 cc/lb is a reliable contrast dose for intravenous (IV) enhancement, up to 50 cc maximally (see box).

Four exposures often suffice, thus exposing the child to an average 7 to 8 mrad (boys; slightly higher in girls) of gonadal radiation.

Ultrasonography

US does not use ionizing radiation and provides exquisite delineation of renal and (retro) vesical anatomy but is fairly operator dependent. Duplex Doppler and color-flow Doppler imaging allow the evaluation of vascular structures, particularly those of renal transplant patients. Determination of resistive indices has not yet proved clinically reliable in evaluating obstruction or rejection in patients with transplants.

The use of prenatal US has significantly influenced the indications for postnatal screening because hydronephrosis, infravesical obstruction, and the anatomy of the kidneys can be exquisitely imaged in the fetus from 18 weeks gestation onward. Prenatal hydronephrosis of a mild degree will have resolved in 97% of neonates at birth. Moderate-to-severe hydronephrosis must be reevaluated postnatally. VUR, a multicystic dysplastic kidney, and ureteropelvic junction (UPJ) obstruction are the most common underlying conditions of neonates with severe hydronephrosis. Furthermore, the postnatal real-time US is the screening method of choice in infants and neonates with urosepsis or an abdominal mass and in children at high risk for renal anomalies and tumors, ambiguous genitalia, and genital tract anomalies. Mechanical sector and phased-array real-time US is performed with either 3.5- or 5-MHz medium-focused linear or sector transducers. Occasionally, in the very premature a 7.5-MHz transducer also is used.

The normal US appearance of the kidney changes with increasing age (Fig. 4-2). In neonates the kidney and liver are of equal echogenicity in the vast majority of infants. It is thought that more glomeruli occupy the

Fig. 4-2 Neonatal kidney reveals lobulations and the relatively echofree renal pyramids (*p*).

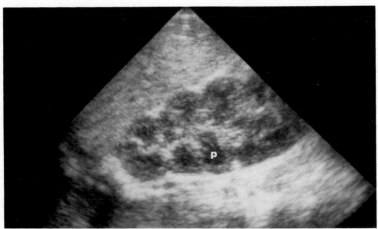

renal cortical volume in infants up to 6 months of life. In addition, the renal pyramids are as prominent as they are hypoechoic, a condition attributed to a relatively larger medullary fluid volume (more loops of Henle) with little supporting stroma. This feature may persist for up to 18 months. Fetal lobulation may also remain apparent up to 1 year of age. The interrenicular septum (junctional defect) is seen posterosuperiorly and more often on the right side; it can be confused with renal scars. This septum is believed to represent the site of fusion of metanephric reniculi.

There are no contraindications to US evaluation of the kidneys, and sedation seldom is used.

Nuclear Medicine

In radionuclide (RN) examinations technetium ^{99m}-diethylenetriaminepentaacidic acid (DTPA), the most commonly used isotope used as a renal medium, is neither absorbed or excreted by the collecting tubules in the kidney. It is used to evaluate differential renal function, GFR, renal plasma flow, and renal clearance. After an initial flow phase (perfusion), the second functional phase, with time activity curves, identifies and quantifies lesions such as UPJ or ureterovesical junction (UVJ) obstruction. A rough estimate of renal size and shape may also be obtained. Depending on the clinical circumstance, a diuretic may help elucidate certain aspects of a RM renogram.

Technetium ^{99m}-dimercaptosuccinic acid (DMSA) and ^{99m}Tc-glucoheptonate are concentrated by the tubular cells; therefore their use results in a better assessment of renal morphology such as in assessment of scars, malposition of kidneys, a column of Bertin, or a local inflammatory process.

To evaluate for VUR, ^{99m}Tc-pertechnetate is used as a contrast agent in a fashion similar to that for the VCUG and is instilled into the bladder by catheter before imaging commences. Although the radiation dose to the gonads and bone marrow is much less with scintigraphy (5% of a conventional VCUG) and the sensitivity for VUR is higher, the specificity for lower urinary tract anatomic abnormalities is significantly lower than on a conventional VCUG.

There are no contraindications to these studies. Sedation occasionally is needed. The time needed to perform renal RM studies limits their usefulness in trauma settings.

Computed Tomography

The strength of computed tomography (CT) lies in cross-sectional depiction of anatomy without an adverse effect on the image by gastrointestinal (GI) gas, bone, or extracorporeal bandages or casts. CT ampli-

fies information gathered by US or excretory urography, especially after the administration of an IV contrast agent; thus it is used in special circumstances such as trauma or tumor staging. It is particularly useful in assessing renal injury and the extent of trauma to the other intra-abdominal structures.

The dosage of IV contrast is the same as in excretory urography (1 cc/lb up to 50 cc at age 10 years), and the *contraindications* are identical. If there is intracranial hemorrhage noted on the cranial CT, it is suggested IV contrast agent not be administered to avoid the reported increased incidence of seizure activity caused by the disruption of the blood-brain barrier.

Magnetic Resonance Imaging

In the GU tract the main advantage of magnetic resonance imaging (MRI) over CT lies in better resolution of anatomic information and its multiplanar capabilities. Some disadvantages of using MRI in children include the occasional need for sedation because of the long data acquisition times and occasional anxiety from claustrophobia.

Normal Anatomy

Upper Urinary Tract
Lower Urinary Tract

Upper Urinary Tract

The development of the kidneys differs from that of the viscera. Organs such as the liver or pancreas evolve by a direct, continuous process beginning with and incorporating the primordium. In the case of the kidneys, three sets of structures appear successively, and only the last one differentiates into the full-grown organ.

The set of structures that appears in the first two embryonic weeks is called the *pronephros*. In humans it is only rudimentary and disappears by the fifth embryonic week. It consists of several tubules formed from mesodermal cells of the intermediate cell mass in the cervical region. It is nonfunctional, and glomeruli do not develop; tubules do not open into excretory ducts. The first formed tubules regress before the more caudally placed last ones are formed, leaving the pronephric duct as their only remnant.

The *mesonephros* then is formed, overlapping the caudal part of the pronephros. It originates from the mesodermal cells of the intermediate cell mass in the thoracic and lumbar regions, and it consists of 30 to 40 nephrons that have primitive glomeruli and no loop of Henle and drain into the mesonephric (or wolffian)

Table 4-1 Fate of mesonephric structures

	Male structures	Female structures
TUBULES	Epididymis Efferent ductules of testes	Mesosalpinx
DUCTS	Vas deferens Seminal vesicles Ejaculatory ducts	Complete involution

duct, which in turn opens into the cloaca. The mesonephric blood supply comes through small arteries from the ventrolateral aorta. The mesonephros disappears completely during the third month except for a few caudal mesonephric tubles that become associated with the genital system in the male (Table 4-1).

The *metanephros* develops (around the fifth embryonic week) from two sources: the ureteric bud from the mesonephric duct and the metanephrogenic cap from the intermediate cell mass of the lower lumbar and sacral regions (the nephrogenic blastema). The ureteric bud elongates and penetrates the metanephric blastema at the end of the nephrogenic ridge. The ureteric bud forms the primitive ureter of the metanephric kidney and dilates at its upper end to become the renal pelvis, which is enveloped by the metanephrogenic cap. Once this occurs, caliceal branches subdivide and form minor calyces and collecting tubules. This process is completed toward the end of the fifth month of gestation. The metanephrogenic cap forms Bowman's capsule, the proximal and distal convoluted tubules, and the loop of Henle. This development is intimately associated with the development of the ureteric bud so that each new tubule has its own cap of mesoderm. This explains why the fetal kidney is at first lobulated with the developing units visible until these lobulations disappear after birth (see Fig. 4-2).

There are usually seven anterior and seven posterior lobes, which are separated by a fibrous longitudinal band that may be visible as the interrenicular septum or, if it is incomplete, the junctional parenchymal defect. This "band" is identified for most of the first year of life (on the right side 3:1).

As this "renal ascent" progresses, the nephrogenic mass starts its 90-degree medial rotation into the renal fossa. This ascent up the posterior abdominal wall is not really due to the renal ascent but is the result of the growth of the lumbar and sacral regions of the body and straightening of its curvature. Concomitantly, the ureter elongates until the kidneys eventually reach their normal position in the renal fossae.

Renal blood supply is furnished by successively higher levels of splanchnic arteries off the aorta. The venous drainage is for a large part derived from the supracardinal anastomoses.

Thus there are three critical events in the development of the normal kidney: (1) the appearance of the ureteric bud at the end of the fifth week; (2) the ureteric bud's invagination of the nephrogenic blastema during the sixth week; and (3) the ascent of the kidney during the sixth and seventh weeks. Failure to develop properly at either of the first two stages results in absence, aplasia, or hypoplasia of the kidney. Splitting of the ureteric bud results in various duplications of kidney and ureter. Failure or arrest of ascent results in ectopia of the kidney.

Lower Urinary Tract

In contradistinction to upper tract structures, which are formed from mesoderm, the structures of the lower urinary tract are formed from endoderm. The development of these structures is intimately tied to that of the anus, rectum, and lower reproductive tract.

At approximately the thirteenth day of development, the future bladder can first be identified as the allantois, a ventral outgrowth of the hindgut. This structure reaches the chorion through the extraembryonic mesoderm of the body stalk. At the end of the fourth week, the cloacal membrane forms the medioventral wall of the cloaca. The mesonephric (wolffian) ducts enter the bladder laterally, just caudal to the allantoic stalk. The urorectal septum then starts to divide the cloaca in a transverse coronal direction. The cloacal membrane ruptures, and the anal and urogenital orifices are formed. The ventral aspect of the cloaca then elongates and forms the following structures in the male: (1) the prostatic and membranous part of the urethra (formed from the pelvic portion of the urogenital sinus); (2) the distal or phallic part of the urethra; and (3) the urachus.

In the female the pelvic portion of the urogenital sinus develops into the urethra.

The urachus descends into the pelvis, leaving a fibrous remnant at term, which may be identifiable in the adult as the medial umbilical ligament, the former connection of the allantoic stalk to the cloaca. Failure of this descent can lead to a patent urachus. Obliteration of the stalk at the ventral and dorsal ends only results in a urachal cyst, and incomplete fusion can leave a urachal remnant at the dome of the bladder.

If the cloacal membrane does not form correctly, the spectrum of abnormality ranges from classic bladder extrophy to epispadias.

Pseudodiverticula of the bladder, "bladder ears," may occur where the bladder protudes into the internal os of the inguinal canal, a more common occurrence in infancy. They disappear with full distention of the bladder (Fig. 4-3). Ninety-five percent of true bladder diverticula are congenital (Hutch) diverticula, which arise at the UVJ with herniation of the bladder mucosa through a bladder wall muscular defect. They may cause secondary VUR because they distort the UVJ and also may predispose the child to infection and stone formation. Some diverticula are seen only after voiding, and they may be associated with Menke's (kinky-hair) syndrome, Ehlers-Danlos syndrome, cutis laxa, and prune-belly syndrome (Fig. 4-4).

The ureteric bud of each side arises near the termination of the corresponding mesonephric duct. With

the development and growth of the bladder, the ureters migrate laterally and cranially to open at the lateral angles of the trigone, and the mesonephric (wolffian) ducts remain midline and migrate distally.

In the male the remaining mesonephric duct forms the epididymis, vas deferens, and the common ejaculatory duct. In the female the duct totally regresses (see Table 4-1).

The gonads initially appear as a genital tubercle, a slight midline protuberance just cephalad to the distal end of the cloaca. Cloacal folds are located on both sides; they evolve into a labioscrotal swelling with a central phallus. In the *absence* of stimulation by androgens this complex forms the female external genitalia. However, under the influence of androgens, the labioscrotal folds swell and fuse to form the scrotum. The ridges of urethral folds fuse to form the cavernous urethra by 12 to 14 weeks.

CONGENITAL ANOMALIES

Renal Agenesis
Renal Hypoplasia
Renal Ectopia
Renal Dysplasia
    Duplex systems
    Multicystic dysplastic kidney
Hydronephrosis
    Ureteropelvic junction obstruction
    Posterior urethral valve
    Anterior urethral valve
    Ureterocele
      Simple ureteroceles
      Ectopic ureteroceles
    Prune-belly syndrome
    Primary megaureter
    Epispadias and cloacal exstrophy
Hypospadias

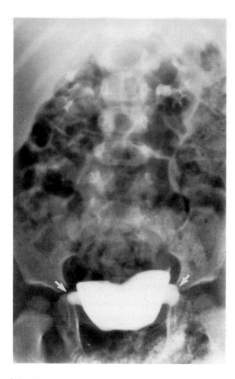

Fig. 4-3 Excretory urogram. Bladder ears *(arrows).*

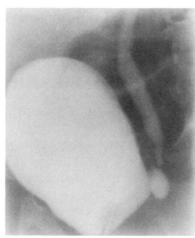
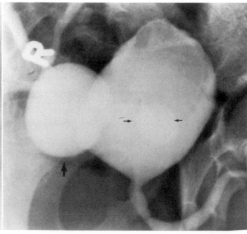

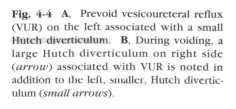

Fig. 4-4 A, Prevoid vesicoureteral reflux (VUR) on the left associated with a small Hutch diverticulum. **B,** During voiding, a large Hutch diverticulum on right side *(arrow)* associated with VUR is noted in addition to the left, smaller, Hutch diverticulum *(small arrows).*

Renal Agenesis

Bilateral renal agenesis is incompatible with life. It occurs in one of 8000 births, with a male-to-female ratio of 3:1. The characteristic clinical presentation consists of oligohydramnios, prematurity, and a characteristic Potter facies, with low set, floppy ears, prominent epicanthal folds, and micrognathia. Concomitant pulmonary hypoplasia occasionally is associated with a pneumothorax. No functioning renal tissue is demonstrable on isotope or contrast imaging.

Unilateral renal agenesis is a fairly common congenital anomaly, occurring in approximately one in 500 births. It may be due to lack of development or disappearance of the ureteric bud or the nephrogenic blastema. The ipsilateral adrenal gland is present in 85% of these patients and is discoid in shape. There is ipsilateral absence of the hemitrigone and ureter. The solitary (contralateral) kidney usually undergoes compensatory hypertrophy. The anatomic splenic flexure of the colon may occupy the renal fossa in patients with left renal agenesis (or ectopia), or the duodenum may relocate into the empty right renal fossa (Fig. 4-5). Renal agenesis is associated with genital malformations; in girls these malformations include hydrometrocolpos, vaginal atresia, or a septum. The association of unilateral agenesis and müllerian abnormalities (absent uterus) is known as Mayer-Rokitansky-Küster-Hauser syndrome. In boys, genital abnormalities associated with unilateral renal agenesis include cryptorchidism, hypospadias, and absent testes.

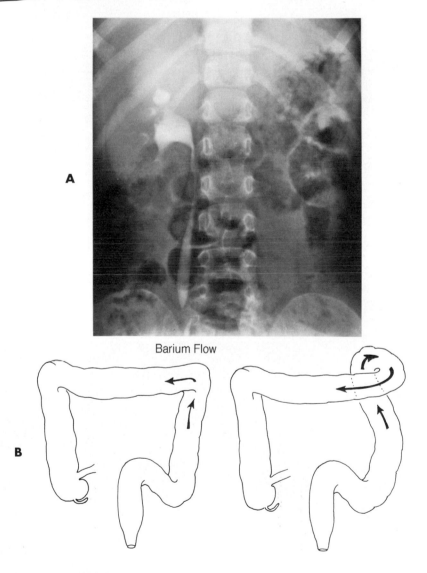

Barium Flow

Fig. 4-5 A, Left renal agenesis with the splenic flexure relocated into the empty left renal fossa. Note the compensatory enlargement of the solitary right kidney. **B,** Schematic diagram of the colonic anatomy in left renal agenesis (ectopia).

Hypoplasia

Hypoplasia may occur as a focal, global, unilateral, or bilateral condition. All renal structures (reduced number of calyces, pyramids, and lobes) are smaller than normal (miniature kidney). If the hypoplasia is segmental, the reduced number of calyces may result in cortical loss. An Ask-Upmark kidney contains a unilateral or bilateral characteristic area of parenchymal thinning at the poles, with such thinning occasionally occuring in the midportion. This thinning is pathologically seen as a groove in the capsule. A similar finding of parenchymal thinning is seen associated with VUR: focal reflux nephropathy (Fig. 4-6).

Renal Ectopia

Renal ectopia denotes an abnormal position of the kidney. It occurs more often in boys than girls. The kidney migrates too far cranially (a thoracic kidney) or, more commonly, does not ascend completely, coming to rest anywhere from the pelvis to the renal fossa. One kidney (or both) may cross the midline to locate on the opposite side of the abdomen, almost always fusing to the orthotopic kidney (crossed-fused ectopia). More commonly (one in 500 newborns), if midline renal fusion occurs, a "horseshoe" kidney results. In more than 90% of these fused kidneys, the lower poles are fused across the midline, creating an isthmus com-

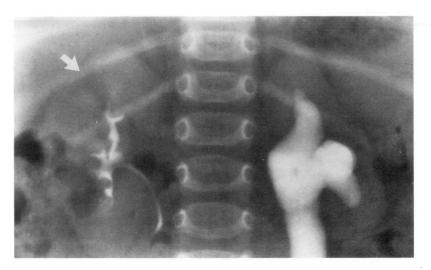

Fig. 4-6   Reflux nephropathy. Excretory urogram demonstrates focal scarring due to VUR on the right (*arrow*), renal hypoplasia on the left.

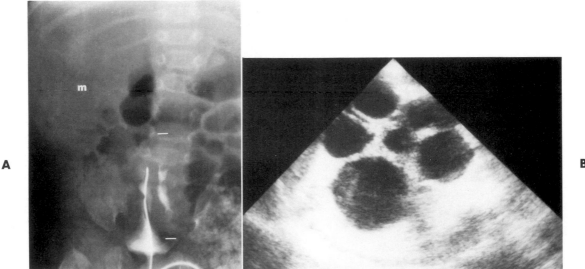

Fig. 4-7 A, Excretory urography with a catheter in the bladder reveals an ectopic pelvic left kidney. Mass (*m*) occupying the right renal fossa shows no function. **B,** US of right renal fossa reveals a multicystic dysplastic kidney with multiple noncommunicating renal cysts and virtually no parenchyma.

posed of either renal tissue or fibrous tissue or a mixture of both. Any kidney that is ectopic in location will fail to undergo the 90-degree rotation along its longitudinal axis that is necessary for the renal pelvis to have its normal anteromedial orientation. This anteriorly oriented pelvicaliceal system can cause relative obstruction to efflux of urine, leading to a hydronephrotic appearance of this malrotated pelvis, which may predispose to stone formation and infection. In addition, there often is an anomalous arterial supply in addition to an anomalous venous drainage pattern. In a patient with a horseshoe kidney, Wilms and transitional cell tumors have an increased frequency. Hypertension develops more often in patients with anomalously positioned kidneys.

US may suggest ectopia, but excretory urography and occasionally CT are necessary to confirm the location, structure, and function of renal ectopia (Fig. 4-7).

Renal Dysplasia

Dyplex systems   Duplication occurs in approximately one in five patients, and its spectrum ranges from a bifid renal pelvis to complete duplication to the level of the bladder, with the ureters entering through separate orifices. It is the sequella of premature branching of the metanephric duct. Duplication is the most common abnormality of the upper tracts, occurs more often unilaterally (five times as common), and is more often incomplete than complete. It occurs four times as frequently in girls than boys. When duplication is complete, the Weigert-Meyer rule applies: the lower pole moiety, usually larger in size, inserts in its

normal trigonal position (orthotopically) (Fig. 4-8, the ureteral orifice of the upper pole moiety ins medially and caudal to this location (ectopically) it bladder or, less often, into the uterus, vagina, epididymis, or urethra. The incidence of VUR in the normally located ureter is the same as in the general population or may be higher if there is distortion of this ureteric orifice by the ectopic ureter's inserting nearby. The upper pole associated with the ectopically inserting moiety often is obstructed and almost always is associated with a ureterocele.

US will demonstrate a dilated (obstructed) upper pole and may suggest an unobstructed duplex system. It and excretory urographic findings are described under "Ectopic Ureteroceles" later in this chapter.

Multicystic dysplastic kidney   Next to hydronephrosis, a multicystic dysplastic kidney is the second most frequently occurring cystic abdominal mass in the neonate. It usually is discovered on the first day of life or by prenatal US. It is not heritable. The incidence is approximately 0.03% at autopsy, and the probable cause is atresia of the UPJ. There is an equal gender incidence. Two forms are recognized:

- Pelvoinfundibular: most common; involves atresia of ureter and pelvis, resulting in multiple cysts
- Hydronephrotic: may occur less frequently with a dominant cyst in the region of the renal pelvis; if the infant survives, the condition must be unilateral

A small, hypoplastic renal artery will be present in both types, along with the total absence of functioning renal tissue. In approximately 20% of patients with unilateral multicystic dysplastic kidney, there is a contralateral abnormality, most commonly a UPJ obstruction (see Fig. 4-7). Approximately 50% of these patients have congenital heart disease and facial anomalies.

A multicystic dysplastic kidney previously was believed premalignant and thus was removed surgically. Current practice suggests that there is little need to

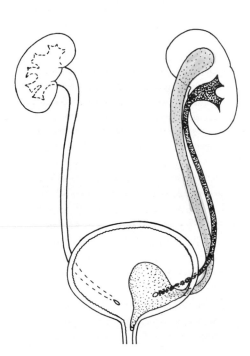

Fig. 4-8   Weigert-Meyer rule. The upper pole ureter inserts medially and caudal to the ipsilateral normal ureteric orifice and is often associated with a ureterocele.

remove an asymptomatic one. US criteria supporting this clinical decision include no enlargement of the lesion during the 3 years of follow-up (at 6-month intervals) after diagnosis, disappearance of all recognizable renal (cystic) tissue, and absence of clinical hypertension or sepsis.

Excretory urography (see Fig. 4-7, *A*) and radionuclide scanning should show no function at all on the affected side. CT can exclude a cystic Wilms tumor. Antegrade pyelography is useful in that a patent connection between calyces and the renal pelvis is present with UPJ obstruction but is absent in children with multicystic dysplastic kidney.

Hydronephrosis

The most common cause for a neonatal abdominal mass is hydronephrosis. Overall, UPJ obstruction, posterior urethral valves, and ectopic ureterocele occur respectively approximately 20% of the time, whereas prune-belly syndrome and obstruction together account for 20%. Urinary tract dilation is not caused only by obstruction, however. VUR comprises the other 20%, and polyuria and infection may also cause dilation of the urinary tract.

In the neonatal age group hydronephrosis often is diagnosed prenatally. If the condition is moderate to severe, it may persist after birth. If it persists more than 3 months as shown by US, it needs further evaluation (by VCUG) to plan definitive therapy. This occurs in approximately 50% of neonates with significant hydronephrosis persisting after birth. In mild cases the prenatal hydronephrosis disappears, probably as a result of the neonate's emergence from the special environment of the uterus (gravity, improved GFR).

Ureteropelvic junction obstruction   The cause of this most common site of obstruction (UPJ) of the urinary tract ranges from intrinsic abnormalities such as abnormal musculature or increased fibrosis thought caused by extrinsic mechanical compression by either an aberrant vessel, a fibrous band, or inflammatory kinks. The majority of UPJ obstructions are on the left side, with an incidence of contralateral UPJ obstructions of approximately 20%. The severity of UPJ obstruction ranges from a mild hold-up of urine flow to a complete obstruction (Fig. 4-9).

Most often neonates present with a mass, and US may delineate a hydronephrotic renal pelvis, with or without associated dilation of the calyces that is often less severe than the pelvic dilation. Excretory urography or renal scintigraphy can confirm the diagnosis, with renal scintigraphy more diagnostic in the first 2 weeks after birth. Obtaining a VCUG is also necessary to exclude VUR as the cause for hydronephrosis. Grade 4 or 5 VUR can simulate, even exacerbate, an existing UPJ obstruction. This coexistence of VUR and a UPJ obstruction, although rare, must be excluded because therapy can be severely affected. The VUR must be repaired first. Mild obstruction at the UPJ often is treated by follow-up US (expectantly) in the first 6 months of life. Significant UPJ is treated by surgical excision of the narrowing and reanastomosis of the renal pelvis and ureter (dismembered pyeloplasty).

Young children with UPJ obstruction often have gross hematuria because the dilated renal pelvis is more prone to trauma. US evaluation of the retrovesical region is mandatory to exclude a primary megaureter or an ectopic ureterocele.

Variants of caliceal dilation can take several forms.
- Caliceal diverticula or pyelogenic cysts can be 1 cm or more in diameter and are incidental findings. They can become infected and are congenital outpouchings of the collecting system that rarely require surgical intervention.
- Fraley syndrome is a rare condition characterized by upper-pole caliceal dilation caused by compression by vascular structures of the infundibulum.
- Congenital megacalyces, very uncommon, are characterized by caliectasis caused by underdevelopment of medullary pyramids. They are often 20 to 25 in number, occur in boys more often than girls, and do not affect renal function. Their appearance can be confused with severe hydronephrosis with dilated, flat calyces, but their normal function is preserved, and they occur unilaterally.

Posterior urethral valve   Immediately distal to the verumontanum is the inferior urethral crest, which terminates in several plicae (folds) that are oriented caudally and encircle the urethra. When these folds are too prominent, they "become" membranous and resemble a valve. This posterior urethral "valve" occurs in approximately one in 5000 to 8000 boys. There are three types:
- *Type I* (most common): the anterior margins of the normal plicae colicularis fuse. The resulting membrane circumferentially obstructs the antegrade flow of urine.
- *Type II* (rarest): mucosal folds extend cranially from the verumontanum to the bladder neck.
- *Type III* (rare): a disk-like membrane just distal to the verumontanum.

Clinically, these patients may present with difficulty voiding, an abdominal mass (distended bladder), and UTI or hydronephrosis on prenatal US. A VCUG is the modality of choice to diagnose a posterior urethral valve because these valves are invisible to retrograde examination by imaging or endoscopically. Imaging findings are characterized by dilation and elongation of the posterior urethra. There is a distinct caliber change between the normal anterior and abnormal posterior urethra and visualization of the obstructing valve. VUR (30%), trabeculation, and/or enlargement of the bladder or urinary ascites may be associated with this condition

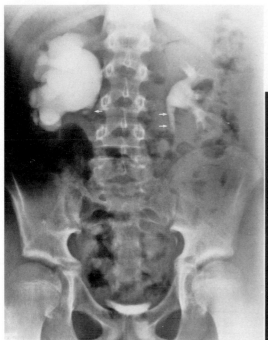

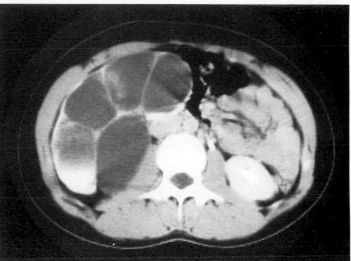

Fig. 4-9 UPJ obstruction. A, Excretory urogram demonstrates marked obstruction at the UPJ, with the suggestion of a crossing (fibrous) band (*arrow*). Normal ureteric striations are seen in the left proximal ureter (*arrows*). **B,** CT demonstrates the dilated right pelvicaliceal system with dependent layering of the contrast.

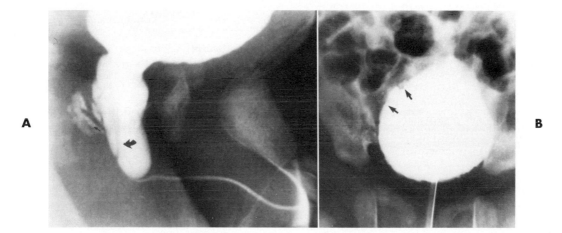

Fig. 4-10 Posterior urethral valve. A, VCUG illustrates dilation of the posterior urethra caused by the obstructing valve (*arrow*). There is reflux into the utricle (*small arrow*). **B,** Marked trabeculation of the bladder (*arrows*).

(Fig. 4-10). If the obstruction is severe, the neonate may have pulmonary hypoplasia (and a pneumothorax) as a consequence of oligohydramnios. Prenatal US may reveal the oligohydramnios. Approximately half the patients have a posterior urethral valve present in the first 3 months of life. Treatment consists of fulguration of the valve, and the prognosis depends on the degree of existing renal impairment secondary to the hydronephrosis.

Anterior urethral valve An anterior urethral valve is a semilunar fold, often the anterior lip of a urethral diverticulum, that occurs in the floor of the urethra near the penoscrotal junction. It is rare but constitutes the second most common obstructive urethral lesion in boys after strictures. This diverticulum may balloon with urine to such an extent that it obstructs the antegrade flow of urine or becomes infected. A VCUG delineates this lesion best.

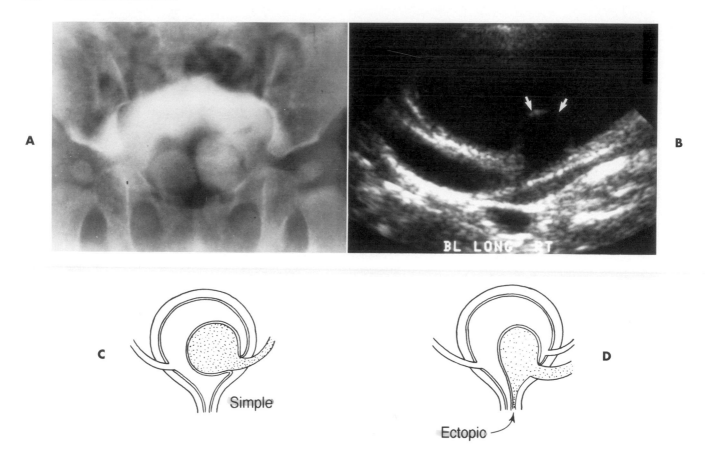

Fig. 4-11 **A,** Excretory urography of bilateral simple ureteroceles. Contrast-laden urine within the ureteroceles is separated from the contrast-laden urine in the bladder by the wall of the ureteroceles. **B,** US representation of an ectopic ureterocele (*arrows*). **C, D,** Schematic diagrams.

Ureterocele A ureterocele is a congenital dilation of the intramucosal portion of the ureter believed caused by delayed rupture of Chwalle's membrane during embryogenesis.

Simple ureteroceles Simple ureteroceles are located entirely within the bladder and are primarily an adult lesion. They are much less common than ectopic ureteroceles and occur equally in boys and girls. The ureteral orifice usually is normal in location and is stenotic. The lesion may be either unilateral or bilateral. Its characteristic appearance is a radiolucent filling defect in the bladder seen on either a VCUG or an excretory urogram. More commonly during excretory urography, contrast material within the ureterocele is surrounded by a radiolucent halo and, if bilateral, resembles the "cobra head" appearance. On US, the ureterocele often is clearly delineated in the urine-containing bladder (Fig. 4-11).

Ectopic ureteroceles Ectopic ureteroceles invariably are associated with the upper moiety of a duplex system and are usually unilateral, appear far more commonly in girls (5:1), and usually cause obstruction of the upper pole's collecting system and ureter. They may cause VUR into the lower pole's ureter by distort-ing the normally located ureteric orifice, and they are associated with a contralateral ureterocele in almost half of the patients. They often manifest in an infant before age 2 years as a UTI or hematuria or present prenatally as hydronephrosis. Ectopic ureters without a ureterocele can occur and become apparent as epididymitis or hydronephrosis in boys, with constant wetting or UTI in girls. As mentioned previously, these different presentations reflect the different embryology of the ectopic orifice in girls in whom the ectopic ureter may empty distal to the external bladder sphincter and anywhere along the uterus, vagina, and broad ligaments. In boys the ectopic ureter always drains proximal to the distal bladder sphincter but may termi-nate in the eipdidymis, vas, or spermatic cord (Fig. 4-12).

Imaging by VCUG may not demonstrate the ectopic ureterocele because it may be flattened and even evert-ed by the intravesical pressure of the instilled contrast medium. This can be avoided by obtaining the early filling film on a VCUG. An excretory urogram of the nonfunctioning, nonvisualized dilated upper moiety may reveal up to seven characteristic findings: (1) increased distance between the top of the nephrogram

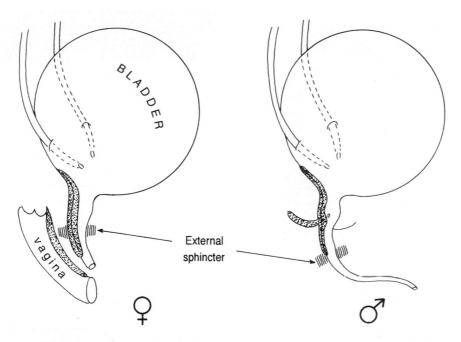

Fig. 4-12 Diagram of possible ectopic ureterocele orifice locations (*shaded area*).

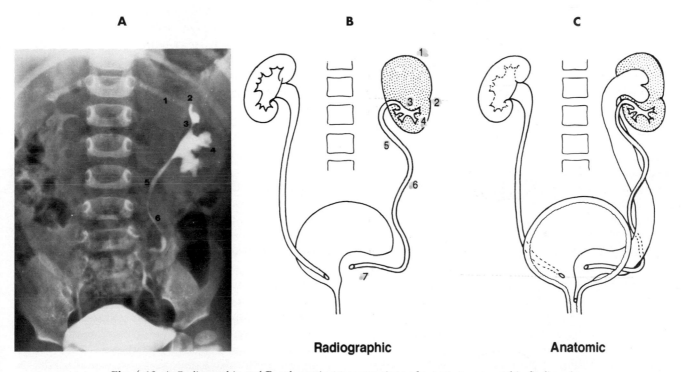

A   **B**   **C**

Radiographic   **Anatomic**

Fig. 4-13 A, Radiographic and **B,** schematic representations of excretory urographic findings in a nonfunctioning, nonvisualized dilated upper pole moiety associated with an ectopic ureterocele. For listed findings, see text.

and the top of the collecting system; (2) an abnormal caliceal axis, and (3) a concave upper border of the renal pelvis (all contributing to the "drooping lily" appearance); (4) fewer calyces than expected; (5) lateral displacement of kidney and ureter as a result of the obstructed, dilated, ectopic, upper-pole ureter; (6) a tortuous course of the ureter; or (7) a filling defect in the bladder (Fig. 4-13). US may show a characteristic dilated upper pole connecting with a dilated tortuous ureter and may demonstrate the ectopic ureterocele within the bladder or urethra (see Fig. 4-11, *B*).

Treatment in both instances ranges from transurethral unroofing of the ureterocele in emergent cases of sepsis to heminephroureterectomy.

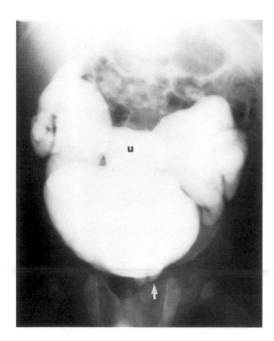

Fig. 4-14 Prune-belly syndrome. VCUG demonstrates an enlarged bladder with a urachus (*u*) and massive bilateral vesicoureteral reflux. Reflux into the utricle (*arrow*) also is noted.

Males >> females

Prune-belly syndrome Eagle-Barrett syndrome's classic triad consists of hypoplasia or absence of the abdominal musculature, cryptorchidism, and marked dilation of the urinary tract. The cause is either primary nondevelopment of the anterior abdominal musculature or hypoplasia of the muscles secondary to the marked dilation of the urinary tract. The syndrome occurs almost exclusively in males, has a frequency of one in 40,000 live births, and may have several associated clinical abnormalites (see box). Approximately 20% of patients die in infancy.

A VCUG may reveal a hypertrophied bladder, often with a urachal remnant (diverticulum). VUR, which can impede diaphragmatic motion and thus lead to pulmonary hypoplasia, is present in three quarters of patients. *Urachus* It occurs in tortuous, dilated, and poorly peristaltic ureters, and may lead to cystic dysplasia of the kidneys. There is marked dilation of the posterior urethra and often filling of a utricle (vagina masculina) (Fig. 4-14). Excretory urography documents the renal size, shape, and position and the residual renal function. Scintigraphy helps decide whether a surgical drainage procedure is useful.

L@sided most common

Primary megaureter A primary megaureter is dilated because it has a short juxtavesical segment that is normal in caliber but is aperistaltic and thus functionally obstructed. It is one of the major causes of obstructive hydronephrosis in children, is less common than UPJ obstruction, and is probably caused by fibrosis of

Associated Abnormalities With Eagle-Barrett Syndrome

Prune-Belly

Hypoplasia of the lungs
Polydactyly (syndactyly)
Malrotation
Scoliosis
Congenital heart disease
Pneumothorax
Microcephaly
Imperforate anus

the distal ureteral segment. That the aperistaltic segment does contain ganglion cells refutes the notion that this lesion is analogous to Hirschsprung disease. It is more common in boys than girls (2.4:1), varies in severity, is found at all ages, and usually is stable when uncomplicated. It is more common on the left side and is bilateral in 20% of patients. Imaging by excretory urography demonstrates columnization and dilation but no tortuosity of the ureter proximal to a normal distal juxtavesical segment (Fig. 4-15). Oblique views are useful to display the aperistaltic segment optimally. The aperistaltic segment can also be demonstrated on US, which may also illustrate ureteric peristaltic waves. Because the UVJ itself is normal, VUR may coexist and is demonstrable on VCUG (in approximately 10%). Treatment is either expectant or surgical. The latter consists of excision of the distal aperistaltic segment and reimplantation of the ureter. The dilated ureter and pelvicaliceal system often return to normal caliber after successful surgery.

Epispadias and cloacal exstrophy This rare spectrum of conditions, epispadias and exstrophy of the cloaca, is due to failure of the urogenital septum to induce fusion of the anterior abdominal wall. Normally the urorectal septum divides the GU and GI tracts. The cloacal membrane ruptures when it joins this urorectal septum, forming the normal GU and rectal openings. Failure of the septum to touch the cloacal membrane results in cloacal malformation. Failure of the cloacal membrane to regress interferes with normal closure of the anterior abdominal and pelvic walls and produces cloacal exstrophy.

Epispadias is the mildest form of this spectrum, and cloacal exstrophy is the most severe.

In children with epispadias/exstrophy radiographically there is separation of the pubic symphysis (>1 cm), and there may be an association with spinal dysraphism or intestinal malrotation (omphalocele) (Fig. 4-16). The upper urinary tracts are usually normal. Clinically, a low position of the umbilicus is noted. In male epispadias, the urethral meatus is located any-

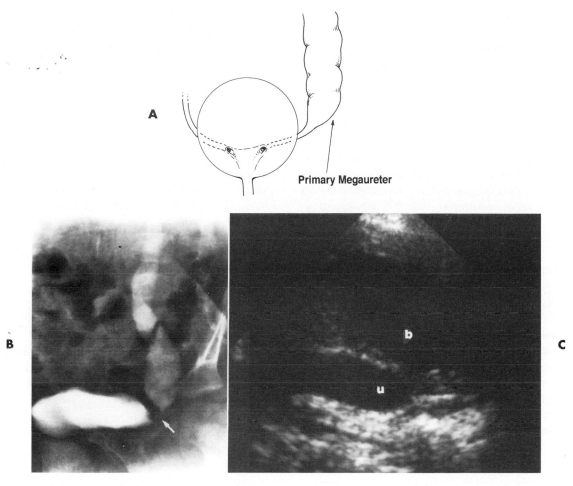

Fig. 4-15 **Primary megaureter.** A, Schematic diagram. B, Excretory urography illustrates the nonperistaltic juxtavesical segment (*arrow*). C, US demonstrates the dilated ureter (*u*) adjacent to the bladder (*b*).

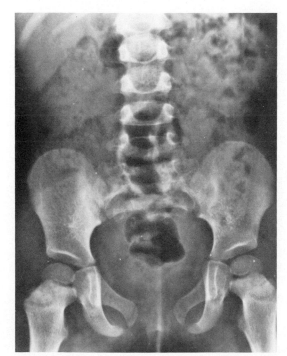

Fig. 4-16 **Exstrophy.** Conventional radiograph demonstrates separation of the pubic symphysis.

where along the dorsum of the penis. Urinary continence frequently is preserved. Female epispadias is very rare and is characterized by a divided clitoris and a short urethra with an absent bladder neck.

Bladder exstrophy, although rare in itself (1:30,000), is the most common anomaly of this spectrum and affects boys 2 1/2 times as often as girls. Because the bladder is not fused anteriorly, the trigonal and urethral openings are exposed. The margins of the everted bladder are continuous with the anterior abdominal wall. A septate vagina or short upward curving pelvis (dorsal chordee) may be evident. Unilateral or bilateral crypt-orchidism may be present. Upper tract abnormalities are rare.

On the other hand, *cloacal exstrophy* is very rare (1:200,000), with a slight male predominance. It is believed caused by a primary defect of mesodermal migration in the anterior abdominal wall. The cloaca becomes exstrophied, and the infant often is premature. In boys there is a hypoplastic, paired penis. In girls the vagina may be septate. Approximately 50% of these children have a myelomeningocele or an omphalocele. Renal dysgenesis frequently is present.

Cloacal malformation occurs in girls only and is characterized by the rectum and GU tract converging at different levels in the perineum and subsequently emptying through a small cloacal opening.

A VCUG, excretory urography, and occasionally MRI may all be used to elucidate the anatomy before surgical reconstruction.

Imaging by VCUG and catheterization of the skin's orifices will confirm physical findings and may be necessary to plan surgical reconstruction of the bladder and (temporary) ureteric diversion.

Hypospadias

Hypospadias in males is characterized by abnormal termination of the urethra on the ventral aspect of the penis. The glandular and coronal types account for 85%, and a horseshoe kidney may be associated. Female hypospadias often is seen in girls up to age 4 years on VCUG. Its hallmark, vaginal reflux, occurs because of (1) failure of complete descent of the urogenital septum; (2) plump labia; or (3) negative intrapelvic pressure during the voiding process. No matter what the cause, it resolves spontaneously in time (Fig. 4-17).

CYSTS AND CALCIFICATIONS

Autosomal Recessive Polycystic Kidney Disease
Autosomal Dominant Polycystic Kidney Disease
Simple Cysts
Medullary Cystic Disease
    Medullary sponge kidney
    Juvenile nephronophthisis
Calcifications
    Nephrocalcinosis
    Urolithiasis

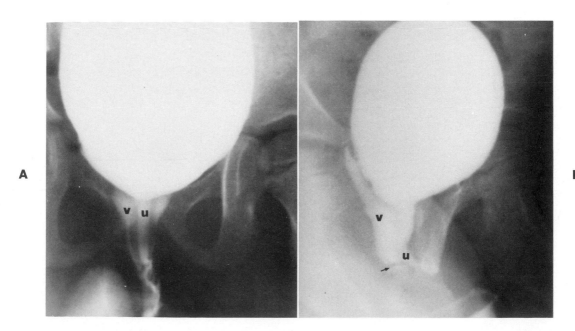

Fig. 4-17 Vaginal reflux seen on VCUG. A, Urethra (*u*) outlined against contrast-laden urine in the vaginal vault (*v*). **B,** Oblique view illustrating the hymen (*arrow*).

Autosomal Recessive Polycystic Kidney Disease

Infantile polycystic disease and *adult polycystic disease* are no longer considered useful terms because there is no clear-cut separation between the two entities. The relative severity of renal and hepatic involvement in infants with autosomal recessive polycystic kidney disease (ARPKD) results in a spectrum of clinical presentations. The majority of infants with ARPKD die shortly after birth, but some children survive for several years, even into adolescence, with slowly progressing renal insufficiency. The underlying defect consists of medullary ductal ectasia and has associated cellular hypoplasia. This condition leads to loss of concentrating ability, tubular atrophy, and systemic hypertension. There may be concomitant biliary duct hyperplasia and portal fibrosis, leading eventually to portal hypertension. The various forms of ARPKD are listed in the box.

Renal changes thus may be thought of as inversely proportional to periportal fibrosis and biliary ductal hyperplasia.

US is the imaging modality of choice and will demonstrate nephromegaly with increased occasionally inhomogenous echo texture and with obliteration of the central echo complex. An excretory urogram will be characterized by a prolonged pyelogram and may show brushlike tubules and linear contrast streaks radiating from the papillae into the cortex. Overall function depends on the degree of tubular involvement (Fig. 4-18). Stone formation, demonstrable on US or CT, may occur.

Classification of ARPKD

PERINATAL FORM

Most infants die within the first month of life and have large kidneys with 90% of renal tubules involved, along with *some* hyperplasia of the biliary ducts.

NEONATAL FORM

Most neonates die at 2 to 8 months of life, with approximately one half of renal tubules involved and with *mild* periportal fibrosis in addition to biliary ductal hyperplasia. They also have nephromegaly at birth.

INFANTILE FORM

Renal and hepatic failure is not evident until 5 to 10 years of age, although the nephromegaly is diagnosed before 1 year of age. Only approximately one fourth of the renal tubules are involved, but *moderate* periportal fibrosis and biliary ductal hyperplasia are present. Portal hypertension often develops.

JUVENILE FORM

Hepatomegaly and portal hypertension are diagnosed in the first year of life, but nephromegaly is seldom present because less than 10% of renal tubules is involved.

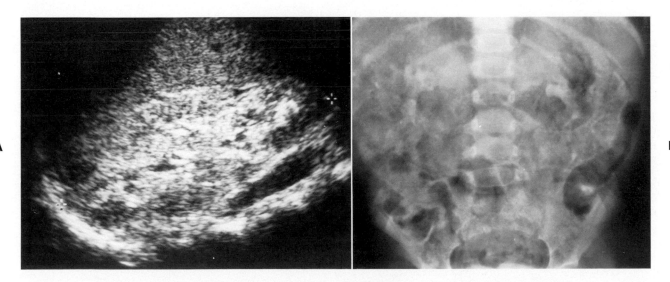

Fig. 4-18   Autosomal recessive polycystic kidney disease. A, US demonstrates increased echogenicity and loss of corticomedullary differentiation. **B**, Excretory urography demonstrates nephromegaly with poor excretory function.

Autosomal Dominant Polycystic Kidney Disease

Autosomal dominant polycystic kidney disease (ADPKD; adult polycystic kidney disease) is inherited as an autosomal dominant trait with variable penetrance. It usually manifests in late childhood or in adulthood and is constant among one family. The cysts are located anywhere along the nephron (glomerular, ductal, tubular) and when they enlarge will compress and destroy normal renal tissue with concomitant obstruction of the collecting system. Hepatic cysts occur in approximately one third of patients, but fibrosis is notably absent. Cysts also are noted in the spleen, ovaries, testes, pancreas, and lungs. Intracranial berry aneurysms are present in approximately 20% of patients.

The US appearance of ADPKD may be identical to that of ARPDK—nephromegaly with increased echo texture—whereas excretory urography shows normal function but the pelvicaliceal system is distorted as opposed to the delayed, prolonged nephrogram with the brushlike appearance and enlarged kidneys of ARPKD (Fig. 4-19). In neonates and young children the imaging findings often are initially normal.

Simple Cysts

Simple cysts in children are seen with increasing frequency (2% to 4%) and must be differentiated from renal cystic disease (see box). They must meet the US criteria for simple cysts; otherwise further workup to exclude pathology is mandatory (Fig. 4-20). They are not familial and seldom are associated with other urinary tract anomalies.

Medullary Cystic Disease

Medullary sponge kidney Medullary sponge kidney (precalyceal canalicular ectasia) is unusual in the pediatric age group. Microscopically, the anomaly consists of dilated (ectatic) collecting tubules. On US, echo texture is often normal, with occasional increased echogenicity in renal pyramids, the result of renal stone formation. An excretory urogram usually appears normal in children. With age, small, rounded contrast collections are seen radiating from the papillae.

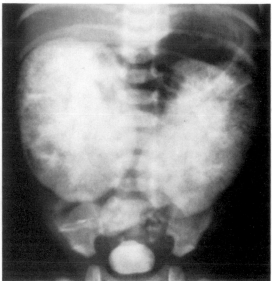

Fig. 4-19 Autosomal dominant polycystic kidney disease. Excretory urography demonstrates brushlike appearance of the collecting systems and bilaterally enlarged kidneys with good function.

Syndromes With Renal Cysts
SYNDROMES THAT MAY HAVE RENAL CYSTS
Tuberous sclerosis
von Hippel-Lindau disease
Ehlers-Danlos syndrome
Jeune syndrome
Zellweger (cerebrohepatorenal) syndrome
SYNDROMES CONTAINING MICROCYSTS OF THE KIDNEYS
Congenital cutis laxa syndrome
DiGeorge syndrome
Noonan syndrome
Turner syndromes
Ivemark syndrome
Goldenhar syndrome

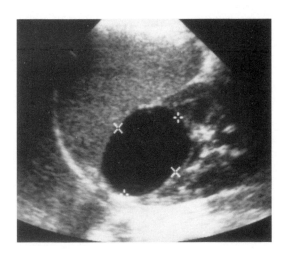

Fig. 4-20 Simple cyst. US demonstrates upper pole cyst with no internal echoes, posterior wall enhancement, and "beaking" of the renal cortex.

Juvenile nephronophthisis Juvenile nephronophthisis (autosomal recessive) is the juvenile-onset form of medullary cystic disease. These cysts are detected microscopically, and the child presents with polyuria or polydipsia and decreased concentrating ability. In adult-onset renal medullary cystic disease (autosomal dominant) these cysts can be seen macroscopically. The former is the most common cause for idiopathic renal failure in adolescents. Boys and girls are affected equally. Pathologically, the condition is characterized by medullary cysts associated with interstitial nephritis in overall small, scarred kidneys. It is characterized best on US that may reveal, in addition, a mildly echogenic cortex. Excretory urography may reveal small kidneys with poor function. The latter entity appears in adults and is associated with renal and retinal dysplasia and cone-shaped epiphyses (retinitis pigmentosa and Mindsner-Saldino syndrome).

Calcifications

The two main categories of calcification in the urinary tract are nephrocalcinosis and urolithiasis.

Nephrocalcinosis In general, deposition of calcium within the pyramids or parenchyma is uncommon in children. Nephrocalcinosis is the medullary deposition of fine (occasionally coarse) calcifications in the wall and lumen of the distal collecting tubles. The calcifications seldom cast a shadow on US. Their deposition has been described as the Anderson-Carr progression. The most common causes include renal tubular acidosis (RTA), hypercalciuria or hypercalemia of a chronic nature, or renal tissue damage and hyperoxaluria (see box). Opaque calcium stones account for 70% of all stones; Mg phosphate (struvite) stones account for 20% and are moderately opaque.

Imaging traditionally consists of conventional radiographs of the abdomen. Early detection of calcium, however, depends on density of the calcification. Early treatment may arrest the pathologic process and prevent renal damage. US exquisitely demonstrates this Anderson-Carr progression of calcium deposition in the renal pyramids (Fig. 4-21).

Urolithiasis In children calcific foci within the urinary tract are usually idiopathic (30%). Other causes may include chronic UTI, urinary stasis, proximal renal tubular acidosis, and enteric causes such as interruption of the enteropathic circulation (oxalate stones) and excessive enteric loss of fluid such as diarrhea (uric acid stones). In premature neonates prolonged furosemide therapy is a well-recognized predisposing condition.

Nephrocalcinosis

HYPERCALCIURIA OR HYPERCALCEMIA

Renal tubular acidosis (distal)
Drug induced (diuretics)
Immobilization, primary hyperparathyroidism
Milk-alkali syndrome
Hereditary hyperoxaluria
Cushing syndrome

TISSUE DAMAGE

Renal cortical necrosis
Renal papillary necrosis
Medullary sponge kidney
Chronic pyelo(glomerulo)nephritis

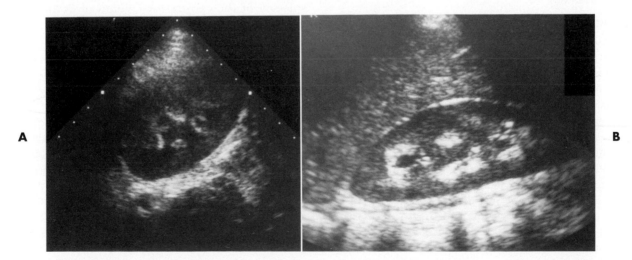

Fig. 4-21 Nephrocalcinosis. A, US illustrates rimlike deposition of calcium in the renal pyramids (*arrows*). **B,** Extensive pyramidal calcium deposition (Anderson-Carr progression).

US may demonstrate renal calculi, especially if they cast an acoustic shadow. Conventional radiographs often are sufficient (Fig. 4-22).

When imaging the sequellae of urolithiasis, excretory urography is the preferred modality in acute situations because it shows early obstruction of the renal pelvis and ureters (columnization) more reliably and earlier than US. US is useful for the follow-up of hydronephrosis but is limited in visualizing the entire urinary tract. Bladder stones are rare but are seen in patients with a neurogenic or hypotonic bladder or secondary to an intravesical foreign body. These stones are usually laminated.

Neoplasms

Renal Masses
 Benign mesoblastic nephroma
 Column of Bertin
 Multilocular cystic nephroma
 Angiomyolipoma
 Nephroblastomatosis/Wilms tumor
 Renal cell carcinoma
 Metastatic disease to the kidney
Adrenal Masses
 Benign: neonatal adrenal hemorrhage
 Malignant: neuroblastoma
 Opsoclonus/myoclonus syndrome
 Watery diarrhea with hypokalemia syndrome
 Pheochromocytoma
 Wolman disease
Bladder Masses (Rare)
 Benign lesions
 Malignant lesions

Renal Masses

Mesoblastic nephroma Mesoblastic nephroma (fetal renal hemartoma) is the most common neonatal mesenchymal neoplasm. It arises from the metanephric blastema like nephroblastomatosis and Wilms tumor. It is a solid renal lesion, occasionally diagnosed by prenatal US and presents in the neonate less than 3 months old with a large nontender abdominal mass. In the past it was considered an early form of Wilms tumor. Currently it is considered benign. There is no gender predilection. The lesion is characterized by a benign course without appearance of metastatic lesions.

On imaging, conventional radiographs of the abdomen are often normal but may show a mass, whereas on US there is evidence of a large solid hypoechoic slightly heterogeneous mass replacing most if not all of the renal parenchyma (Fig. 4-23). Cystic change

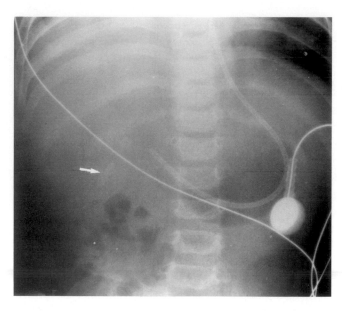

Fig. 4-22 Renal stones noted on an abdominal radiograph in a premature neonate receiving furosemide therapy (*arrow*).

may occur but is rare. Further imaging (i.e., MRI, CT) cannot differentiate this lesion from the (rare) neonatal Wilms tumor. Treatment is by surgical excision, which is curative.

Column of Bertin A column of Bertin consists of normal renal cortical parenchyma extending into the renal medulla, embryologically considered an infolding of the cortical renal tissue between adjacent renal pyramids. US may demonstrate an echogenic mass most commonly located between the upper and middle pole. Renal scintigraphy (DMSA) shows normal uptake in that area whereas on an excretory urogram slightly greater contrast density may appear in the portion of cortex invaginating the renal medulla. It may cause splaying of the calyces. A column of Bertin is of no clinical significance once differentiated from a neoplastic lesion or cyst.

Multilocular cystic nephroma Multilocular cystic nephroma (cystadenoma) is a benign unilateral, often solitary lesion that occurs in young (2 to 5 years of age) children and young (18 and over) adults. Boys predominate in childhood, women in adulthood. It represents 2% or 3% of all primary renal lesions and is initially seen as an abdominal mass. On imaging, this lesion resembles a cystic Wilms tumor, and the diagnosis of a benign lesion is made when there is no pathologic evidence for nephroblastomatosis. CT and US show multiple noncommunicating cysts of variable size. Nephrectomy provides the definitive diagnosis.

Angiomyolipoma Angiomyolipoma is a solitary yet rare tumor, but it can be seen in up to 50% of patients with tuberous sclerosis. In these patients the tumors

Fig. 4-23 Mesoblastic nephroma. A, US demonstration of a right upper quadrant, inhomogeneous renal mass in a 2-month-old infant. **B**, MRI confirms extent and character of the lesion.

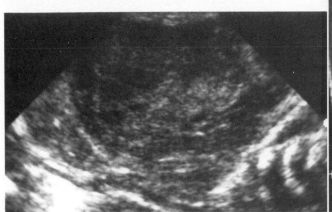

A

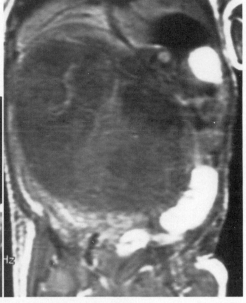

B

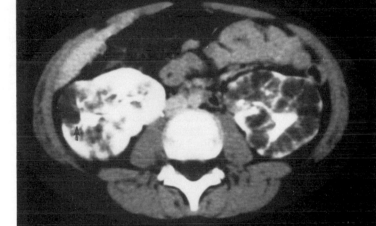

Fig. 4-24 Angiomyolipoma. Contrast-enhanced CT demonstrates multiple lesions containing fat (*arrow*) in a patient with tuberous sclerosis.

are multiple and often asymptomatic and occur bilaterally. There is an equal gender incidence. Renal angiomyolipomas not associated with tuberous sclerosis occur most commonly in middle age, with a 4:1 female predominance. These lesions are large, single, and often symptomatic because of hemorrhage within the tumor. Angiomyolipomas are extremely vascular and contain muscle and fat, the latter making imaging by CT with IV contrast characteristic. Approximately 20% are locally invasive (Fig. 4-24).

Nephroblastomatosis Nephroblastomatosis is considered a <u>precursor to Wilms tumor</u>, consisting of immature metanephric tissue (nephrogenic cysts) identified as <u>subcapsular nodules</u> in the renal cortex.

Microscopic cysts are seen in 1% of autopsies in neonates, whereas massive involvement is seen in the first 2 years of life. The risk for development of Wilms tumor varies. If nephroblastomatosis is present in a kidney removed for Wilms tumor, there is a 20% risk for developing Wilms tumor in the contralateral kidney. Nephroblastomatosis commonly is associated with trisomies 13 and 18 with Beckwith-Wiedemann and Drash syndromes. Imaging reveals enlarged kidneys with multifocal parenchymal masses of abnormal echogenicity on US. CT and excretory urography may confirm an irregular outline and the masses (Fig. 4-25, *A*). It may be difficult to differentiate this entity from ARPKD. The use of chemotherapy is controversial.

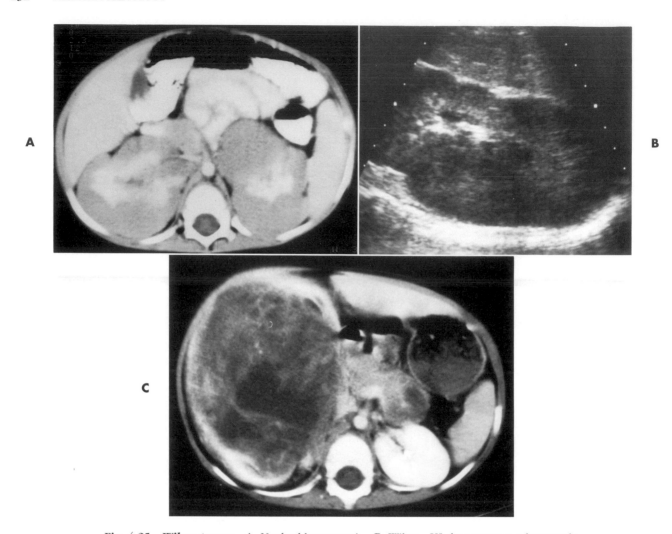

Fig. 4-25   Wilms tumor. A, Nephroblastomatosis. **B**, Wilms. US demonstrates a lower-pole, semisolid renal mass distorting the renal architecture. **C**, Contrast-enhanced CT illustrates a complex mass extending across the midline.

Wilms tumor   Wilms tumor accounts for approximately 10% of all childhood malignancies. It is the most common renal malignancy, with a peak incidence between 4 months and 4 years of age; 80% of cases occur in children 1 to 5 years of age. Males outnumber females by 1.2:1, and approximately 500 new cases occur each year in the United States. There is a 1% familial incidence, whereas associated congenital abnormalities occur in 15% of all children with Wilms tumor (see box).

Approximately 1% of all Wilms tumor patients have sporadic aniridia, and there may be a chromosomal basis, with deletion of the short arm of chromosome 11. Other associated chromosomal abnormalities have included various trisomies, translocations, and chromosome 45X.

Differential Diagnosis of Bilaterally Enlarged Kidneys (US)

Nephroblastomatosis
Nephrotic syndrome, glomerulonephritis, pyelonephritis
Polycystic kidney disease, angiomyolipoma
Glycogen storage disease
Lymphoma and leukemia

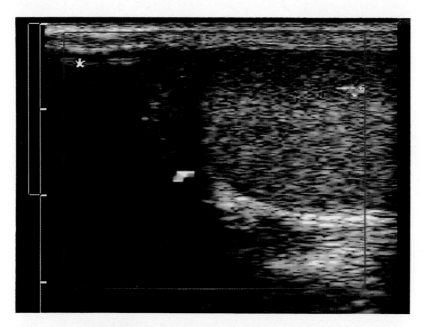

PLATE 1 Normal testicular echogenicity and flow.

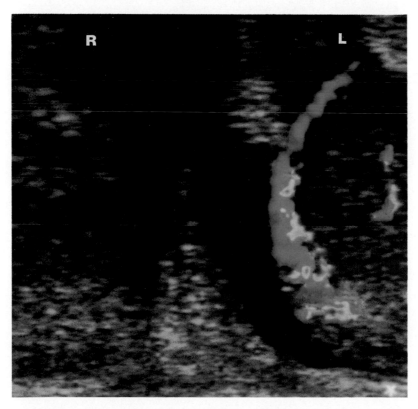

PLATE 2 Color-flow Doppler US demonstrating increased flow in the epididymis consistent with epididymitis.

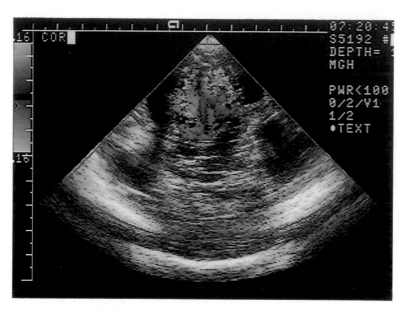

PLATE 3 Color-flow Doppler image.

Table 4-2 Anatomic staging of Wilms tumor

Stage	Description	2-Year survival rate (%)*
I	Confined to the kidney and totally resectable	95
II	Tumor extending beyond the kidney but totally resectable	90
III	Residual tumor but no hematogenous spread	85
IV	Hematogenous metastases to lung, liver, bone, or brain	55
V	Bilateral synchronous renal involvement	Individual stage dependent

When two lesions appear at different times, there is a 40% survival rate.

Most children are well at the time the abdominal mass is noted. The tumor often acutely enlarges dramatically as a result of hemorrhage. Hematuria and hypertension are common, and bilateral tumor lesions occur in approximately 5% of cases. Metastatic disease occurs preferentially locally, then spreads to the lungs and liver.

Imaging initially is accomplished by US, which reveals an often-large echogenic intrarenal lesion. It usually is sharply marginated and can be separated from the liver by its equal or slightly higher echogenicity. Necrosis and hemorrhage can result in mixed hypoechoic and hyperechoic areas within the tumor. The major advantage of US lies in Doppler evaluation of the vena cava. The tumor or clot extends into the renal vein and inferior vena cava in 15% of patients but may be difficult to assess if the tumor is large and bulky and compresses the vena cava. CT defines the location and extent of both the intrarenal and extrarenal components of the tumor better than US. Calcifications are noted in approximately 15% of patients; and necrosis or hemorrhage may be present. CT is also the optimal modality to evaluate the contralateral kidney, demonstrating metachronous tumors in up to 5% of patients. CT of the chest demonstrates pulmonary metastases in approximately 10% of patients at the time of initial diagnosis. On MRI, Wilms tumor has prolonged T1 and T2 relaxation times. The appearance is highly variable because of necrosis or hemorrhage, and the main advantage of MRI lies in the excellent tissue resolution that allows multiplanar staging and the exquisite visualization of the major abdominal vessels (Fig. 4-25, *B* and *C*). Staging is summarized in Table 4-2.

There are two major tumor types: favorable histology (90% survival rate) and unfavorable histology (54% survival rate) with anaplastic cells. The latter sarcomatous (clear cell) histology occurs in approximately 10% of patients. Liver metastases are present in 10% of

Malformations in Which Wilms Tumor Has a Tendency to Occur More Frequently

Beckwith-Wiedemann syndrome (5%)
Hemihypertrophy
Male pseudohermaphroditism and nephritis (Drash syndrome)
Sporadic nonfamilial aniridia
Neurofibromatosis-1
Cerebral gigantism (Sotos syndrome)

Abdominal Masses

NEONATES

Hydronephrosis
Cystic disease (multicystic dysplastic kidney)
Mesoblastic nephroma
Neuroblastoma
Adrenal hemorrhage
Ovarian cyst or torsion
Hydro(metro)colpos

OLDER CHILD

Hydronephrosis
Cystic disease (multicystic dyplastic kidney)
Wilms tumor
Neuroblastoma
Rhabdomyosarcoma of bladder or prostate
Ovarian cyst, torsion, or mass
Hematocolpos

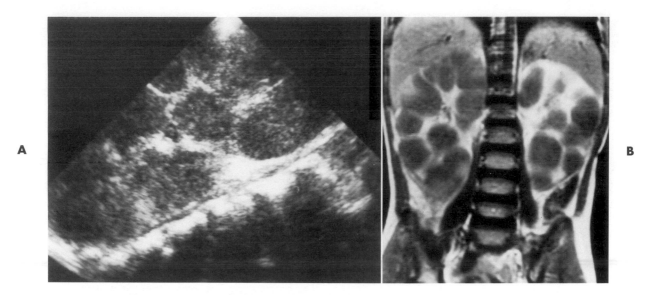

Fig. 4-26 Leukemia/lymphoma. A, Renal US demonstrates multiple solid nodules. **B,** MRI illustration of same.

patients, and bone metastases occur in another 5% and are osteolytic.

Surgical excision is by flank incision if no inferior vena caval (IVC) involvement is documented and by transabdominal incision if there is need for IVC resection.

Renal cell carcinoma Less than 1% of renal cell carcinomas occurs in the pediatric population, and occurrence is extremely rare before age 5 years. This lesion is most often a part of von Hippel-Lindau disease in which the renal cell carcinoma develops in the (bilateral) cysts.

Metastatic disease to the kidney The most common lesions metastasizing to the kidneys are neuroblastoma and leukemia and lymphoma. In 75% of patients with lymphoma, renal involvement is noted that is either nodular (masses) or, more often, diffuse in character (Fig. 4-26). In 50% of patients with leukemia, the infiltrative process is bilateral and diffuse. US, excretory urography, and CT imaging illustrate nephromegaly, increased echogenicity of the cortex, and occasional nodules. There may be some advantage to using IV contrast enhancement. Lymphadenopathy (spread) is seen better with CT.

Adrenal Masses (see box on p. 133)

Neonatal adrenal hemorrhage Neonatal adrenal hemorrhage is a relatively common abnormality that initially presents with anemia or jaundice, occurs on the right side 70% of the time, and is bilateral in 10% of neonates. Birth trauma, stress, anoxia, and/or dehydration has been implicated as a cause. US is the modality of choice for demonstrating the adrenal glands and

hemorrhage (Fig. 4-27). Hemorrhage is noted as an echogenic suprarenal mass, and US will document the shrinkage over time well. Clot extent, lysis, and calcification and the change from a solid to a cystic mass can be assessed reliably to differentiate hemorrhage from an adrenal neoplasm. Doppler evaluation may be useful in demonstrating the avascularity of a neonatal adrenal hemorrhage because a neuroblastoma usually is more vascular.

Neuroblastoma Neuroblastoma is, like Wilms tumor, the third most common malignancy of childhood after leukemia and primary brain neoplasms, accounting for 8% to 10% of all pediatric neoplasms. Approximately 500 new cases occur each year in the United States, an incidence of one in 10,000 children. The tumor arises from primitive neuroblasts in the neural crest of sympathetic ganglia and can originate anywhere from the cervical region to the pelvis. Approximately two thirds of the tumors are located in the abdomen, with two thirds of them in the adrenal gland. Of the remainder, 20% are in the chest, and the rest are in the head and neck region. Two thirds of patients are initially seen with an incidental abdominal mass, and two thirds of them are less than 4 years of age, with the majority between 2 months and 2 years of age. The tumor is slightly more common in boys than girls, with a familial incidence reported. At least two thirds of these children have disseminated disease at the time of presentation, with metastatic involvement of the skeleton, bone marrow, liver, lymph nodes, and skin reported. Dumbbell, extradural extension is common in the chest but is unusual in the abdomen. Neuroblastoma is unique because it can spontaneously transform into the more benign ganglioneuro(blast)-

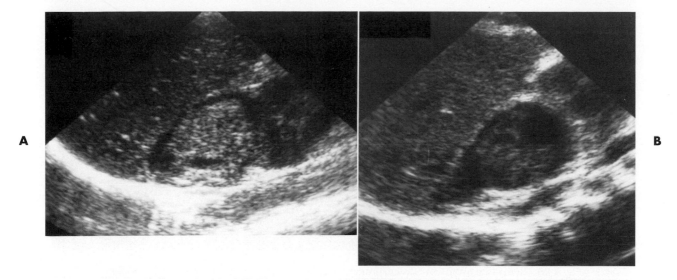

Fig. 4-27 Adrenal hemorrhage. A, US at day 1 of life reveals an echogenic suprarenal mass. **B**, After 5 days there are liquefaction and fragmentation of the clot.

oma.) Syndromes associated with neuroblastoma include Beckwith-Wiedemann, Klippel-Feil, and fetal alcohol. Hirschsprung disease also may be associated with it. Neuroblastoma is clinically silent until it invades adjacent structures. Symptoms then may include (bone) pain, fever, weight loss, and anemia, and approximately 10% of patients have hypertension. Two thirds demonstrate excess urinary catecholamine excretion and thus may initially present with flushing, sweating, and irritability.

Two paraneoplastic syndromes may occur in children with neuroblastoma.

Opsoclonus/myoclonus syndrome Opsoclonus/myoclonus syndrome, or "dancing eyes and dancing feet" and cerebellar ataxia, occurs in approximately 2% of patients with neuroblastoma. Up to one half of patients with myoclonic encephalopathy of children are thought to have associated neuroblastoma.

Watery diarrhea with hypokalemia syndrome Watery diarrhea with hypokalemia syndrome is caused by excessive secretion of vasoactive intestinal peptides (VIP) and catecholamines and occurs in 7% of patients with neuroblastoma. Occasionally there is periorbital tumor deposition resembling what has clinically been called *raccoon eyes.*

In children with myoclonic encephalopathy and neuroblastoma, there is equal gender incidence, higher frequency of thoracic lesions, and a better prognosis (90% survival). Staging of neuroblastoma and survival rates are summarized in Table 4-3.

The overall survival rate of children with neuroblastoma is 72% if the patient is less than 1 year of age, 28% for those 1 to 2 years of age, and 12% for patients more than 2 years of age.

Table 4-3 Staging of neuroblastoma and survival rates

Stage	Description	2-year survival rate (%)
I	Tumor confined to organ with complete surgical removal	75
II	Tumor extension beyond organ of origin; nodes may be positive; no crossing of the midline	75
III	Tumor crosses the midline	<25
IV	Distant metastases	<25
V (or 4S)	Metastatic disease confined to liver, skin, and bone marrow, with the primary tumor stage I or II	75

Imaging by conventional radiographs may reveal a mass that in two thirds of patients contains calcification; it may be stippled, diffuse, or amorphous. Metastatic lesions are often lytic and permeative and located in the metaphysis. An excretory urogram classically reveals displacement but not distortion of the pelvicaliceal system by the tumor. This modality has been replaced by US, CT, and MRI. US, particularly when used as the screening modality for suspected abdominal pathology, shows that the organ of origin is suprarenal, may reveal the inhomogeneous echo texture, may reveal the hypoechoic liver metastatic disease, and may identify tumor encasement of vessels. CT is superior to US in defining extent and retroperi-

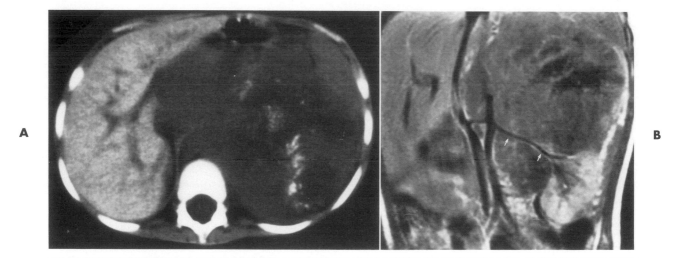

Fig. 4-28 Neuroblastoma. A, CT demonstrates a large left retroperitoneal mass containing multiple calcifications. **B,** MRI illustrates the extent of the mass, renal displacement, and vessel encasement (*arrows*).

toneal spread of the primary tumor. It is almost 100% sensitive and reveals calcifications in 85% of patients. MRI has an advantage over CT in that vertebral canal extension and vessel encasement can be demonstrated better without the need for intrathecal contrast administration (Fig. 4-28). MRI also demonstrates bone marrow involvement by metastatic lesions and encasement of the superior mesenteric artery (SMA) and other vessels to a greater extent because of its superior resolution and capability for multiplanar imaging. The tumor usually has prolonged T1 and T2 relaxation times and may be quite inhomogeneous as a result of necrosis.

Pheochromocytoma A pheochromocytoma arises from catechol-secreting (chromaffin) neural crest cells and usually is a benign lesion. Approximately 5% of these masses occur in childhood, 5% are malignant, and 5% are bilateral. Two thirds arise in the adrenal medulla. There may be a familial incidence, especially with an associated syndrome.

Associated syndromes occur in approximately 10% of patients with pheochromocytoma and include the multiple endocrine neoplasia (MEN) syndrome (higher likelihood of malignant lesions) and the phakomatoses (von Hippel-Lindau disease, Sturge-Weber syndrome, and neurofibromatosis). Clinically, these patients come to attention with signs of sympathetic overstimulation (flushing, tachycardia) and during evaluation for hypertension. Eighty percent of patients with a pheochromocytoma have hypertension, although this tumor accounts for only 10% of pediatric patients with hypertension.

Imaging (CT) with IV contrast should be used only with premedication with a blocking agent to avoid a hypertensive crisis. Currently under investigation are

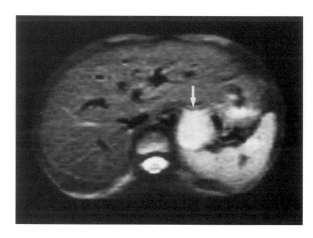

Fig. 4-29 Fast (hyperscan) MRI demonstrates a pheochromocytoma (*arrow*).

scintigraphy as a screening examination and fast (hyperscan) MRI (Fig. 4-29).

Wolman disease Wolman disease is a rapidly fatal inherited disorder of lipid metabolism. The classic imaging finding consists of calcification of both adrenal glands at birth.

Bladder Masses (Rare)

Benign lesions Benign entities include hemangiomas and neurofibromas in patients with neurofibromatosis. In half of these patients the mass is palpable. Bladder involvement with neurofibromas constitutes a pathognomonic finding for neurofibromatosis. Patients with hemangiomas of the bladder have other hemangiomas in the body in approximately 40% of cases.

Malignant lesions The most common malignant lesion is rhabdomyosarcoma. Of all rhabdomyosarcomas 20% occur in the lower urinary tract, especially the bladder (trigone) and prostate (40% in the head and neck, 20% in the extremities). Age at presentation usually less than 5 years, with boys more commonly affected than girls and African-Americans affected four times as often as Caucasians. Overall survival rate is near 75%, with metastatic disease occurring to lungs and liver.

VCUG may reveal a classic sarcoma botryoid (grapelike) pattern or a mass projecting from the dome in 25% of cases. US reveals nodularity and bladder wall thickening, whereas both CT and MRI are useful for staging the pelvic extent of this lesion (Fig. 4-30).

Metastatic disease to the bladder is uncommon but is seen in patients with leukemia or lymphoma as global masslike wall thickening.

URINARY TRACT INFECTION

Urinary Tract Infection and Vesicoureteral Reflux
Pyelonephritis
  Acute pyelonephritis
  Xanthogranulomatous pyelonephritis
Glomerulonephritis
  Nephritic syndrome
  Nephrotic syndrome
Hemolytic Uremic Syndrome

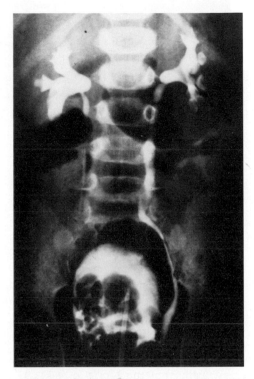

Fig. 4-30 Sarcoma botryoides as demonstrated on VCUG by grapelike filling defects in the bladder.

Urinary Tract Infection and Vesicoureteral Reflux

UTI is the second most common infection in childhood after upper respiratory tract infection. There is an incidence of 3% to 5%, which translates to 1.7:1000 boys and 3.1:1000 girls annually presenting with UTI. In children less than age 6 years UTI is an indicator of an anatomic and/or functional urinary tract disorder in 35% to 50% of these patients. VUR is present in 30% to 35% of them but is present in 85% of children with evidence of renal scarring. This scarring, in turn, is responsible for 20% to 40% of end-stage renal failure in patients less than 40 years of age.

There are many misconceptions about VUR and UTIs: a UTI causes reflux, or VUR causes a UTI; VUR is secondary to distal obstruction; cystoscopy is necessary in patients with UTI; and an excretory urogram or US is sufficient to rule out VUR. They are all false: VUR is a primary abnormality of the ureteric mucosal tunnel, and it most often presents with a UTI. Performing upper tract imaging only is insufficient; cystoscopy is outdated.

The objective of early diagnosis and treatment of VUR is prevention of damage and subsequent scarring of renal parenchyma. The younger the child, the greater is the risk for hypertension (20%) or renal failure (12% of adults less than age 50 years); the resultant incidence of scarring is estimated at 1% for boys and 0.5% for girls.

The key imaging questions are (1) after a documented UTI, is there an underlying anatomic abnormality (e.g., VUR, UPJ or UVJ obstruction, ureteroceles, posterior urethral valve); and (2) how should the imaging evaluation be structured most effectively.

Each child less than age 5 who has a well-documented UTI should be evaluated with a VCUG, followed by an US if the VCUG is normal and by excretory urogram if it is abnormal. A DMSA scan, particularly in patients less than 2 years of age, can be substituted for an excretory urogram because it is more sensitive to detect scarring.

"Abnormal" imaging in the presence of UTI most often occurs because of VUR, next most commonly because of UPJ or UVJ obstruction, and then, because of ureteroceles or a posterior urethral valve (PUV). VUR is *primary* and caused by a congenitally ineffec-

→ *Reflux is now thought to be a 1° abnormality of the UVJ (i.e., immaturity or maldevelopment*

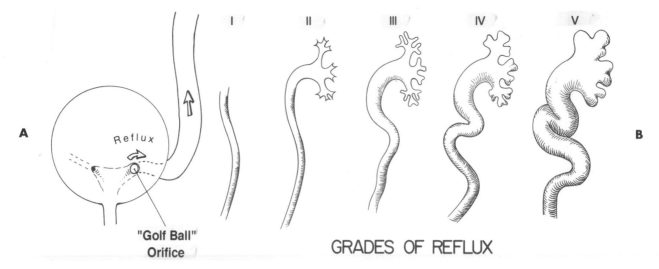

Fig. 4-31 VUR. A, Schematic representation of primary VUR. **B,** Grading of VUR according to the International Reflux Study Committee.

tive valve mechanism at the UVJ (Fig. 4-31, *A*); when the valve mechanism is distorted by anatomic abnormalities such as a Hutch diverticulum, a ureterocele, or cystitis it is considered *secondary* VUR. Primary VUR spontaneously disappears by age 6 years in 95% (25% per 2-year period) of these children and does so in lower grades more spontaneously than higher grades.

Grading of VUR is illustrated in Fig. 4-3, *B*. VUR occurring during bladder filling is called *low-pressure VUR*. VUR that occurs only during voiding is called *high-pressure VUR.* There is a well-established association between VUR and renal scarring. This scarring can be caused by sterile VUR alone but may be potentiated by a UTI. It has been established that intrarenal reflux (IRR) is necessary to cause scarring. IRR most often occurs in compound calyces that are found in the renal poles (Fig. 4-32).

For older children or adolescents who have UTI, US is the screening modality of choice. Any abnormality that is discovered is evaluated further with the appropriate modality. After treatment for VUR, DMSA (DTPA) and US are the preferred modalities to assure that scarring is monitored or arrested.

Medical management usually consists of low-dose chemoprophylaxis, which aims to maintain sterile urine while the VUR disappears with age. Follow-up (radionuclide) VCUGs and US (or excretory urogram or renal scan) are usually scheduled at 9- to 12-month intervals to monitor this. Surgical management of VUR currently is reserved for some of those patients with severe VUR (grades 4 and 5) in the presence of scarring or those resistant to medical therapy. Urodynamic evaluation may also be necessary in those

patients to rule out bladder-sphincter dyssynergia. If present, these patients can benefit from anticholinergic therapy.

Pyelonephritis

Acute pyelonephritis is an ascending infection that may occur in both the presence *and* absence of VUR. The former condition is more severe. The acute infection is caused most often by *Escherichia coli, Proteus,* and *Staphylococcus aureus* and becomes apparent as flank pain in 80% of cases. The infection is blood borne in neonates and in those with endocarditis. The kidney may be edematous and/or contain an inflammatory cellular infiltrate.

There is a paucity of imaging findings. US clues to acute pyelonephritis are as follows: (1) an indistinct corticomedullary junction of an enlarged kidney that shows either increased or decreased echogenicity; (2) impaired renal movement with respiration; or (3) a size discrepancy of more than 1 cm as compared to the contralateral kidney (Fig. 4-33). In the past excretory urograms were even less specific, most commonly showing decreased intensity of the nephrographic phase. Striations of the ureter may be evident. Scintigraphic evaluation with glucoheptonate (DMSA has a higher radiation dose to the kidneys) is the most reliable modality to demonstrate acute bacterial infection of the kidneys. It is more accurate than an excretory urogram or US and less accurate than CT if perirenal infection is suspected. A child with pyelonephritis may have complications such as perinephric abscess, pyonephrosis, or a renal carbuncle (most commonly

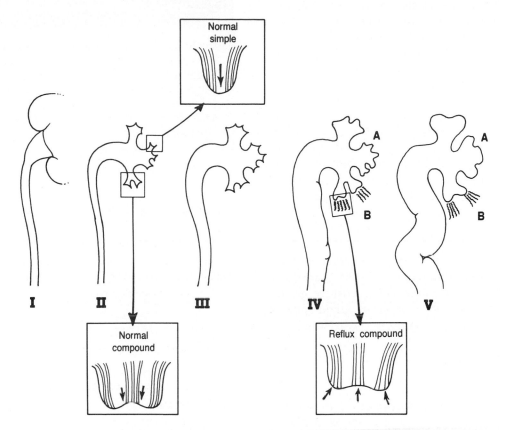

Fig. 4-32 Grading of reflux and illustration of its effect on simple and compound calyces. The orientation of the collecting tubules is oblique, preventing reflux in simple calyces.

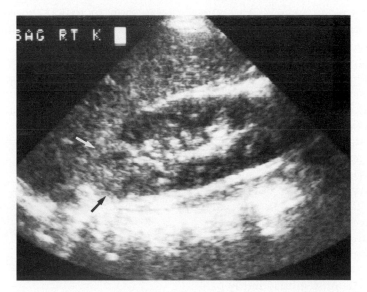

Fig. 4-33 US representation of acute pyelonephritis of the right upper pole with loss of corticomedullary differentiation and increased echogenicity (*arrows*).

caused by *S. aureus*). A focal area of pyelonephritis, also called lobar nephronia, may progress to a carbuncle (a spherical mass of increased echo texture) and then rarely to an abscess with central necrosis.

Pyonephrosis Pyonephrosis refers to an infected obstructed urinary tract. Both entities are imaged best by US but may need further delineation by CT. Both are initially treated best by percutaneous drainage.

Xanthogranulomatous pyelonephritis Xanthogranulomatous pyelonephritis is extremely rare in children and is associated with obstructing renal stones and resultant UTI. It is almost always unilateral and occurs more frequently in girls, with potential extension into the perirenal space. In children the localized form is more common than the generalized form. It is detectable on US, but CT is better suited to evaluate the perirenal structures.

Both modalities show a mass as a result of the destruction of normal architecture. No renal function is evident, which, in association with a positive gallium scan, confirms the diagnosis of xanthogranulomatous pyelonephritis. Nephrectomy is the treatment of choice.

Glomerulonephritis

The majority of patients that present with glomerular disease have either nephritic syndrome or nephrotic syndrome.

Acute nephritic syndrome Acute nephritic syndrome is defined as an abrupt onset of hypertension, oliguria, azotemia, hematuria, and proteinuria usually caused by poststreptococcal glomerulonephritis. The pathophysiology is immune complex related and occurs more commonly in boys than girls; it occurs most often in children 3 to 7 years of age. In 95% of patients total recovery is the rule. Three percent will develop chronic glomerulonephritis, and 2% will have a second episode. This syndrome can be associated with Henoch-Schönlein purpura (with rash, arthritis of knees and ankles, melena), Goodpasture's syndrome (with pulmonary hemorrhage), and hemolytic uremic syndrome (HUS; see below). For imaging, US is sufficient and, in the proper clinical setting, diagnostic. Increased echogenicity of the renal cortex associated with mild renal enlargement is common. The echogenicity is similar to that of the liver and spleen. Excretory urographic results are often normal.

Nephrotic syndrome Nephrotic syndrome is defined as hyperproteinemia, proteinuria, and hypercholesteremia and is predominantly a disease of young children (2 to 6 years of age). Most commonly, microscopic evaluation reveals that the underlying pathophysiology is the result of minimal change disease,

---

"Medical Renal Disease": Increased Renal Parenchymal Echogenicity on US
Nephrotic syndrome (minimal change disease, 85%)   Glycogen storage disease (type I; Gierke disease)   Hemolytic uremic syndrome (HUS)   Polycystic disease (autosomal recessive, autosomal dominant)   Glomerulonephritis, pyelonephritis   Lymphoma

which is treated with steroids. Associated entities are numerous.

Imaging by US usually is useful to rule out anatomic anomalies and may show increased echogenicity of the renal cortex (see box). Pleural effusions on chest radiographs are also seen frequently.

Hemolytic Uremic Syndrome

HUS is the most common cause of acute renal failure in infants. It occasionally occurs in older children and adults. Microangiopathy is the proposed mechanism. Clinically, diarrhea, vomiting, or respiratory distress is followed by acute renal failure, hemolytic anemia, hypertension, and GI hemorrhage. The kidneys are affected in most (90%) instances. Renal failure lasts up to 4 weeks, then gradually improves. Imaging by US may show increased echogenicity of the renal cortex and/or bowel wall thickening. This latter finding can be confirmed on barium contrast studies of the GI tract. On Doppler US imaging, the vasculitis cause is reflected in an increased resistive index. The majority of patients recover completely, with Doppler signal patterns returning to normal.

Trauma

Kidneys
Ureter
Bladder
Urethra

Kidneys

Blunt abdominal trauma, frequent in the pediatric age group, often involves the kidneys. Approximately 0.1% of pediatric hospital admissions are the result of renal injury.

The kidneys are more prone to trauma in children than adults because of their proportionally large size, reduced perirenal fat, and less-developed surrounding (protective) musculature, and they may be more delicate because of the presence of fetal lobulation.

Most injuries to the kidneys result in hematuria or flank pain. Twenty percent of all patients with renal injury also will have associated organ trauma.

Excretory urography (EU), the gold standard in evaluating the GU tract in previous decades, underestimates the extent of injury affecting the kidneys in 15% to 30% of cases. The "one shot EU" may be useful in assessing the pedicle integrity of the severely traumatized patient when there is no time for more extensive (CT) imaging evaluation. A kidney of uniform density that shows no distortion of the collecting system probably is free from significant injury. However, in the pediatric age group there should almost always be enough time to do a CT evaluation; therefore this modified excretory urogram is seldom used.

US is not very specific or sensitive to renal trauma because it does not give functional information.

Radionuclide evaluation is very organ specific but extremely time consuming, although it can be sensitive in the setting of renal trauma. Angiography has been largely abandoned. Therefore CT is the imaging modality of choice in patients with renal trauma. Peritoneal lavage is not generally performed on patients less than age 16 years except in rare cases in which CT is difficult to perform.

The classification of renal injury on CT (Fig. 4-34) is as follows:

- Group 1: minor (50%)—contusions; contained lacerations
- Group 2: major (25%)—extension of injury into the pelvicaliceal system
- Group 3: critical (25%)—fragmentation of the kidney, with or without vascular pedicle injury

Groups 1 and 2 are treated conservatively, and CT reliably identifies these groups of patients. In 15% of patients with traumatized kidneys and underlying abnormalities such as Wilms tumor, a UPJ obstruction or a horseshoe kidney is present.

Ureter

Injury to the pediatric ureter is uncommon. UPJ avulsion or a tear associated with renal trauma is the most frequent occurrence.

Bladder

Rupture of the bladder often is associated with blunt pelvic fractures and may be intraperitoneal (20%) or extraperitoneal (80%) (rarely both). Cystography is the

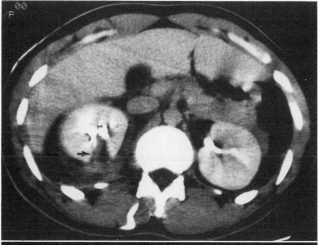

A

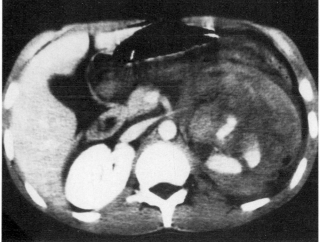

B

Fig. 4-34 Renal trauma. A, Major trauma: renal laceration extending into the collecting system with perirenal extravasation (*arrow*). **B,** Critical trauma: fragmented left kidney with few remaining areas of function.

modality of choice; extraperitoneal rupture at the bladder neck often results in elevation of the bladder floor. CT more accurately defines soft tissue and osseous injury.

Urethra

Uretheral injuries occur almost always in boys. They consist of tears, most commonly of the pendulous and posterior urethra, and are usually identifiable on retrograde contrast study. If a complete tear has occurred at the level of the pelvic floor, CT can be diagnostic because it shows elevation of the bladder floor within the pelvis.

Table 4-4 Common "female" pediatric abdominal and pelvic masses by age

	Neonate <1 mo	<2 yr	>2 yr
GENITOURINARY (50%)	Hydronephrosis Ovarian cysts Hydro(metro)colpos	Hydronephrosis Wilm tumor	
GASTROINTESTINAL (20%)	Duplications	Intussusception Appendix	Visceromegaly Leukemia or lymphoma
RETROPERITONEAL (20%)	Neuroblastoma Adrenal hemorrhage	Neuroblastoma Teratoma	

GENITALIA

Female Genitalia
- Uterus
    - Hydro(metro)colpos
- Ovaries
    - Cysts
    - Torsion
    - Ectopic pregnancy
    - Tuboovarian abscess
    - Cloacal malformation
    - Ovarian tumors

Male Genitalia
- Penile urethra
- Scrotum
    - Masses
        - Painless
        - Painful
    - Neoplasms

Female Genitalia (Table 4-4)

Uterus The neonatal uterus is quite large in relation to the bladder because of the presence of maternal estrogens. In the first month of life its measurements range from 2.3 to 4.6 cm in length, and in the subsequent months regression totaling approximately 1 cm in length occurs (prepubertal uterine length, ±3 cm). There is a very limited range of abnormalities of the uterus in infants and young children, and they usually do not present until menarche. The infantile cervix (triangular in shape on sagittal images) is larger than the uterus. After about 5 years of age, the uterus becomes bigger than the cervix and remains so until puberty when hormonal secretory changes result in the normal adult imaging relationship. A hypoplastic uterus occasionally is identified. Anatomic variants (i.e., duplex uterus, cloacal exstrophy, or retroverted uterus) may be identified by US (Fig. 4-35). Congenital absence of the uterus and upper two thirds of the vagina is diagnostic of the Mayer-Rokitanski-Küster-Hauser syndrome.

Hydro(metro)colpos Hydro(metro)colpos is defined as a dilated uterus and vagina. The causes of the obstruction range from (segmental) vaginal atresia (1:4000 live births) to imperforate hymen to a vaginal diaphragm. Infantile hydrometrocolpos often presents as an abdominal mass

Hydro(metro)colpos often is accompanied by imperforate anus, urinary tract abnormalities such as solitary kidney, and renal ectopia and by other congenital abnormalities of the vertebrae (12%) and various cardiac malformations.

Most cases of hydrometrocolpos caused by imperforate hymen are not discovered until menarche and then present as an abdominal or pelvic mass.

US again is the screening modality of choice (Fig. 4-36).

Ovaries The adnexa consists of the ovaries, fallopian tubes, and supporting ligaments. In infants less than the age of 2 years ovaries are not seen well by US. In this age group ovarian volume (0.5 x width x thickness x length) is less than 0.7 cm^3, but the volume increases to 1 to 3.5 cm^3 in girls 2 to 12 years of age. Normal volume of postmenarchal girls ranges from 4 to 6 cm.

US is the diagnostic modality of choice. The girl must have a full bladder for US to evaluate fully the retrovesical structures. The normal ovarian appearance is a solid, ovoid structure with a mildly heterogeneous texture in girls less than age 2 years (Fig. 4-37, *A, B*). Between ages 2 to 12 years, microcysts become apparent. With puberty, the number and size of physiologic (<0.9 cm) cysts increase. A corpus luteum cyst should be less than 3 cm in diameter.

Neonatal ovarian *cysts* are fairly common and are probably caused by maternal hormonal overstimulation. These ovarian cysts can be quite mobile in the peritoneal cavity (Fig. 4-37, *C*).

When a normal mature follicle fails to involute and

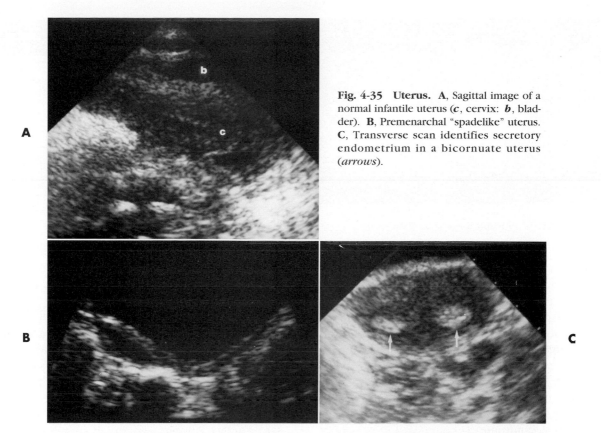

Fig. 4-35   Uterus. A, Sagittal image of a normal infantile uterus (*c*, cervix: *b*, bladder). **B**, Premenarchal "spadelike" uterus. **C**, Transverse scan identifies secretory endometrium in a bicornuate uterus (*arrows*).

Fig. 4-36   Hydrocolpos. Sagittal US demonstrates a fluid-fluid level in a markedly dilated vaginal vault and a normal uterus (*markers*).

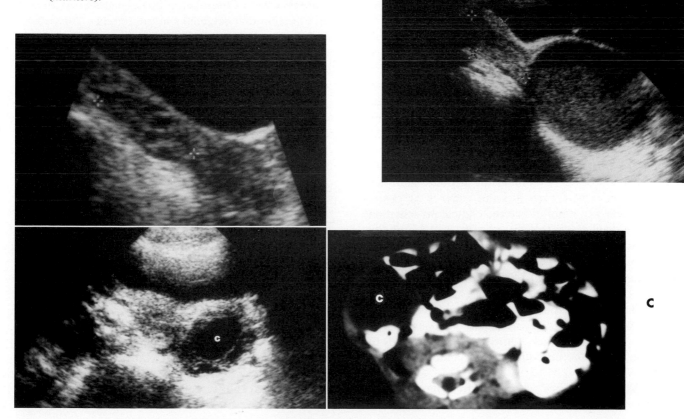

Fig. 4-37   A, Normal ovoid ovary with functional cysts. **B**, Corpus luteum cyst (*C*). **C**, CT demonstrates ovarian cyst in the right flank of a neonate.

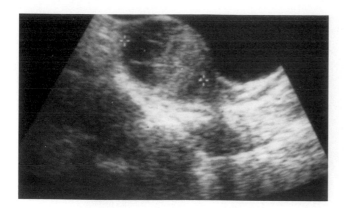

Fig. 4-38 US of hemorrhagic cyst of the ovary.

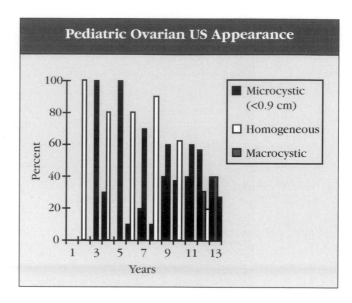

continues to enlarge, a functional ovarian cyst results. Since normal physiologic cysts are less than 3 cm, any 4- to 10-cm follicular or corpus luteum cyst deserves serial imaging over two to three menstrual cycles. Failure of the cysts to involute may necessitate aspiration to relieve symptomatology, exclude malignancy, or prevent torsion.

Polycystic ovary disease   Polycystic ovary disease (Stein-Leventhal syndrome) is common and is associated with amenorrhea, infertility, and hirsutism. Decreased levels of follicle stimulating hormone and luteinizing hormone are diagnostic. On US, there is bilateral ovarian enlargement (>14 cm³) with multiple small cysts.

Hemorrhagic *cysts*   Hemorrhagic cysts can present difficult differential diagnostic problems in the teenage patient. They can be confused with endometriosis, ectopic pregnancy, or a tuboovarian abscess (TOA). Internal debris in an ovarian cyst suggests minimal hemorrhage; an echogenic cyst results from extensive hemorrhage (Fig. 4-38). Fluid often is present in the cul-de-sac.

Ovarian torsion   Ovarian torsion is uncommon before 2 years of age except in the neonate and may then be associated with ovarian tumors or cysts. Imaging findings are not unlike the clinical presentation and are nonspecific. Arterial, venous, and lymphatic stasis results in congestion and/or necrosis. Duplex Doppler and color-flow Doppler imaging have had mixed success in distinguishing between torsion hemorrhagic cysts and TOA. The most reliable set of findings is a larger-than-expected size of the ovary, associated with fluid in the cul-de-sac, and small cysts around the periphery of the ovary. Untreated, torsion leads to infarction, shrinkage, and occasional calcification of the affected ovary.

Ectopic pregnancy   Ectopic pregnancy, like intrauterine pregnancy, is not an unusual ocurrence in teenage girls. Almost all ectopic pregnancies are located in the fallopian tubes and present by the seventh postmenstrual week by transabdominal US on transvaginal US. An extrauterine fetal pole is seen 10% to 15% of the time. More often, it is a nonspecific echogenic, complex, adnexal mass, often with fluid in the cul-de-sac. Duplex Doppler imaging, if showing ectopic fetal cardiac activity, is quite specific.

Tuboovarian abscess   TOA is a sequella of pelvic inflammatory disease (PID) often caused by *Neisseria gonorrhoeae* or *Chlamydia*. PID consists of an ascending infection that originates in the cervix. The diagnosis is made clinically, with symptoms of pain, vaginal discharge, and fever. US may detect a pyosalpinx, a TOA, or cul-de-sac fluid or abscess. CT may be required in complicated cases.

Cloacal malformation   Uncommonly (1:40,000 females), the rectum, vagina, and ureters converge in the pelvis into a common outflow channel, the cloaca (Latin for sewer). This occurs if there is persistence of the cloacal membrane, which interferes with normal closure of the anterior abdominal wall. Normal external genitalia are the rule. There is absence of the anus because the rectum communicates with the often-septated vagina (cloaca). The single perineal opening that is present is catheterized, and the anatomy is elucidated by injecting contrast into the cloaca in a lateral projection. Cross-sectional imaging usually is not helpful preoperatively. Associated renal and spinal anomalies are common, and US can screen for them.

Ovarian tumors   Benign ovarian teratomas (*dermoid cysts*) account for two thirds of pediatric ovarian tumors. The ovarian teratoma is the second most common teratoma after sacral teratoma. These tumors derive from totipotential cells that differentiate into ectodermal, mesodermal, and endodermal elements.

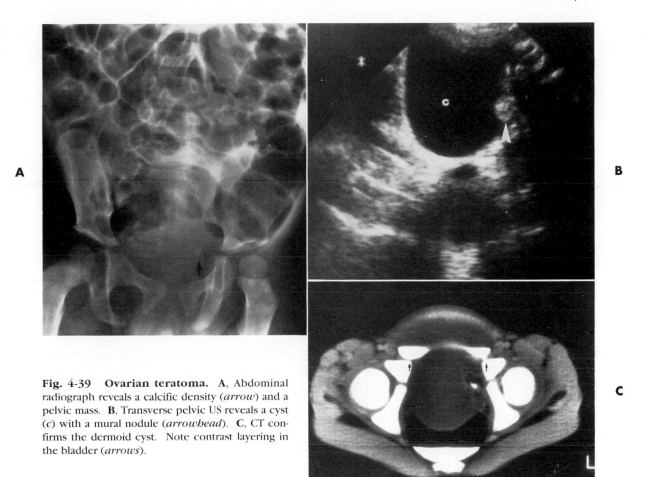

Fig. 4-39   Ovarian teratoma.   A, Abdominal radiograph reveals a calcific density (*arrow*) and a pelvic mass. **B,** Transverse pelvic US reveals a cyst (*c*) with a mural nodule (*arrowhead*). **C,** CT confirms the dermoid cyst. Note contrast layering in the bladder (*arrows*).

Dermoids contain mesoderm and ectoderm. The average age of presentation is 6 to 11 years. The average diameter of these tumors is 10 cm, and they are bilateral in 10% to 20% of patients. The most common presenting symptom is a mass, and 50% of children complain of pain. US demonstrates that two thirds of the tumors are complex masses with both echogenic and cystic components. A mural nodule is characteristic and occurs in two thirds of cases. Fat-fluid levels may also be noted. CT and MRI may reveal calcification of teeth or bone, hair, debris, or fat and again may show a mural nodule. Abdominal radiographs reveal calcification in 50% of these girls (Fig. 4-39).

Malignant ovarian tumors, although rare, comprise 35% of ovarian tumors in girls. They consist of (1) the germ cell variety (85%; immature teratomas and dysgerminoma); (2) the stromal cell variety (10%; granulosa cell tumor, Sertoli-Leydig cell tumor); or (3) the epithelial cell variety (5%; cystadenocarcinoma). They usually come to clinical presentation in the postpubertal age group and are often large (>10 cm in diameter) and mostly solid, although they may contain cystic areas as a result of necrosis. Abdominal or pelvic pain is common.

US is the initial imaging modality to determine the origin, size, and characteristics of the mass. Staging is accomplished better by MRI or CT.

Metastatic involvement of the ovaries is rare; lymphoma/leukemia and neuroblastoma have been reported.

Male Genitalia

Penile urethra   The penile urethra and its abnormalities usually are assessed on a VCUG and include posterior urethral valves, strictures, and anterior diverticula. Strictures are postinflammatory or iatrogenic (postinstrumentation) in origin.

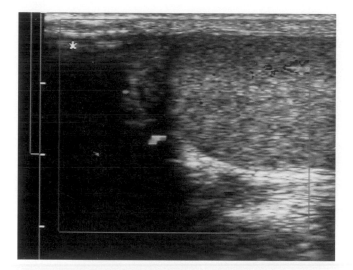

Fig. 4-40   Normal testicular echogenicity and flow (see Color Plate 1).

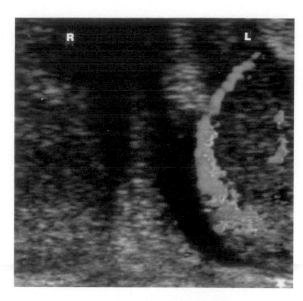

Fig. 4-41   Color-flow Doppler US demonstrating increased flow in the epididymis consistent with epididymitis (see Color Plate 2).

Scrotum   The scrotal content consists of two testicles in 96% of all full-term male infants. Descent of testicles is related to birth weight, and only two thirds of premature infants have completed testicular descent at birth. Cryptorchidism (occurring in 10% of boys at age 1 year) is a failure of descent, not a mechanical obstruction. Intraabdominal location is uncommon, and most (85%) lie within the inguinal canal. During the first year of life, 80% of cryptorchid testes in full-term neonates and 95% of premature cryptorchid testes descend spontaneously to a normal scrotal position. In a boy with cryptorchid testes, histologic changes can be expected to occur by 2 years of age, and he is 10 to 40 times more likely to develop malignant degeneration, with seminoma the most common entity. To preserve fertility, some surgeons consider orchiopexy of the undescended testicle around the age of 2 years.

Total absence of one testis (1:5000) is four times as common as testicular absence and usually occurs on the left side.

An imaging search for the undescended testicle usually involves US (90% specific and accurate) and MRI (>90% sensitive and specific).

US evaluation reveals the normal testis as an oval organ of uniform echogenicity. The echogenic, linear mediastinum testis should be identified. Posteromedially the epididymis is characterized as an echogenic structure adjacent to the testis. Measurements vary with the boy's age and vary from 2 cm^3 until age 11 years to 3 to 10 cm^3 at ages 12 to 14 and to an average 13 cm^3 after that (Fig. 4-40).

Scrotal masses   The imaging approach to scrotal pathology can be divided into two tiers: (1) a painful scrotal mass and (2) a painless scrotal mass. Testicular nuclear scans will evaluate for torsion in a boy with a painful scrotal mass by demonstrating decreased flow to the affected testicle. Color-flow Doppler US can reliably exclude torsion by demonstrating the increase in flow of epididymitis (Fig. 4-41). US is the imaging modality of choice to differentiate cystic from solid lesions in a boy with a painless scrotal mass.

Causes for a *painless* scrotal mass include hydrocele, with or without a hernia, or a varicocele (dilation of the pampiniform plexus of veins in the scrotum). Doppler US examination may show a venous flow pattern in boys with the latter condition. Rarely cysts of the spermatic chord or neoplasms occur. Testicular carcinoma is rare, particularly in African American and Asian boys.

Painful scrotal masses should be treated as torsion until proved otherwise. Torsion accounts for 20% of acute scrotal abnormalities. It is most common in boys 12 to 16 years old and occurs on the right side more commonly than on the left. On physical examination the scrotum is tender and swollen and does not transilluminate.

Epididymitis, the main differential point, is almost as common as torsion and often is caused by *S. aureus* or *E. coli.* Other infectious causes such as mumps and coxsackievirus are also common and can be associated with scrotal fluid, a reactive hydrocele. US findings vary and are often indistinguishable from those of trauma.

On US imaging, the spermatic cord and testis should have demonstrable arterial flow with Doppler imaging; the epididymis will not. Venous flow is sporadically seen in the testicle (see Figs. 4-40 and 4-41).

Findings on color-flow Doppler imaging of an acute condition in the scrotum are summarized in the box.

Findings on Color-Flow Doppler Imaging

Acute torsion: no flow in testis; no peripheral
  hyperemia
Epididymoorchitis: increased flow in testis and
  epididymis
Chronic torsion: no flow in testis; increased peripheral
  hyperemia
Tumor: enlarged testis; increased flow *to* mass

Overall US accuracy approaches 100%.

Since epididymitis and orchitis can be associated with urinary tract abnormalities such as ectopic ureters and can lead to abscess formation, further evaluation of the entire urinary tract is needed with a VCUG and an excretory urogram.

Neoplasms   Approximately 80% of all testicular tumors in boys are malignant. Clinically, they appear as a painless, slowly enlarging testicular mass. Approximately 25% of these masses have an associated hydrocele. Two thirds are of the germ cell variety, with half of them embryonal adenocarcinomas.

Embryonal adenocarcinomas (yolk-sac tumor or endodermal sinus tumor) are associated with high levels of serum α-fetoprotein (90%). After 3 years of age, the occurrence of embryonal carcinoma and teratocarcinoma is rare. Non-germ cell (Leydig's cell) tumors appear in boys near 4 years of age and occur more commonly in African-American boys. Metastatic disease to the testis is seen in boys with leukemia or lymphoma, neuroblastoma, and Ewing's sarcoma. US examination is sensitive but not specific because it can show a variety of patterns, changing from a diffuse decrease in echogenicity to an inhomogeneous parenchymal pattern.

SUGGESTED READING
Text

Kirks DR, editor: *Practical Pediatric Imaging*, Boston 1992, Little, Brown and Co., pp 916-1056.

Siegal MJ, editor: *Pediatric sonography*, New York 1991, Raven Press, pp 257-368.

Silverman FM, Kuhn JP, editors: *Caffey's pediatric X-Ray Diagnosis*, ed 9, vol 1, St Louis, 1992, Mosby, ed 9, vol 2, pp 1201-1442, 2101-2147.

Slovis TL, Sty JR, Haller JO: *Imaging of the Pediatric Urinary Tract*, Philadelphia, 1989, WB Saunders, pp 69-162.

Sty JR, Wells RG: Imaging of neuroblastoma. In *Neuroblastoma Tumor Biology and Therapy*, 1990, CRC Press, pp 147-160.

Sty JR, Wells RG, Starshak FJ et al: *Diagnostic Imaging of Infants and Children*, vol 1, Gaithersburg, 1992, Aspen Publishers, pp 1-138.

Swischuk LE: *Imaging of the Newborn, Infant and Young Child*, ed 3, Baltimore, 1989, Williams & Wilkins, pp 589-705.

Taybi TL, Lachman RS: *Radiology of Syndromes, Metabolic Disorders and Skeletal Dysplasias*, ed 3, St Louis, 1990, Mosby, pp326-328.

Teele RL, Share JC: *Ultrasonography of Infants and Children*, Philadelphia, 1991, WB Saunders, pp 137-213, 462-490.

Articles

Beckwith JB, Kiviat NB, Bonadio JF: Nephrogenic rests, nephroblastomatosis, and the pathogenesis of Wilms tumor, *Pediatri Pathol* 10:1, 1990.

Blickman, JG: *Pediatric urinary tract infection: imaging techniques with special reference to voiding cystourethrography*, thesis, Rotterdam, 1991, Pasmans Publishers.

Brown T, Mandell J, Lebowitz RL: Neonatal hydronephrosis in the era of sonography, *AJR* 148:959, 1987.

Cohen HL, Eisenberg P, Mandel F et al: Ovarian cysts are common in premenarchal girls: a sonographic study of 101 children 2 12 years old, *AJR* 159:89, 1992.

Kaariainen H, Jaaskelainen J, Kivisaari L et al: Dominant and recessive polycystic kidney disease in children: classification by intravenous pyelography, ultrasound, and computed tomography, *Pediatr Radiol* 18:45, 1988.

Kier R, McCarthy S, Rosenfield AT et al: Non-palpable testes in young boys: evaluation with MR imaging, *Radiology* 169:429, 1988.

Krensky AM, Reddish JM, Teele RL: Causes of increased renal echogenicity in pediatric patients, *Pediatrics* 72:840, 1983.

Lebowitz RL, Avni FE: Misleading appearances in pediatric uroradiology, *Pediatr Radiol* 10:15, 1980.

Lebowitz RL, Mandell J: Urinary tract infection in children: putting radiology in its place, *Radiology* 165:1, 1987.

Patriquin H, Robitaille P: Renal calcium deposition in children: sonographic demonstration of Anderson-Carr progression, *AJR* 146:1253, 1986.

Stalker HP, Kaufman RA, Stedje K: The significance of hematuria in children after blunt abdominal trauma, *AJR* 154:569, 1990.

Strife JL, Souza AS, Kirks DR et al: Multicystic dysplastic kidney in children: US follow-up, *Radiology* 186:785, 1993.

CHAPTER 5

Skeletal System

IMAGING TECHNIQUES

Conventional radiographs
Computed tomography
Magnetic resonance imaging
Ultrasonography
Radionuclide scintigraphy
Arthrography

Conventional radiographs

Conventional radiographs depict the bony density of the skeletal system adequately and remain the mainstay in the evaluation of musculoskeletal disease. Adequate evaluation by means of conventional radiographs must include imaging in at least two perpendicular directions. Oblique projections are useful in certain instances, whereas comparison views need be obtained only if confusion between a suspected abnormality with a possible normal variant occurs.

Computed tomography

Computed tomography (and conventional tomography in limited instances) is indicated in certain anatomic regions (e.g., sternoclavicular joint) to delineate the extent of a bony lesion (e.g., stress fracture, metastatic and primary bone lesions) better and in preoperative and postoperative imaging. The three-dimensional-reconstruction capability and the superior visualization of casted skeletal structures are the most useful attributes of CT imaging.

Magnetic resonance imaging

Magnetic resonance imaging (MRI) has established itself as an excellent modality for directly imaging the bone marrow, joints, cartilaginous structures, and soft tissues. Tumor extent, its architecture, the degree of

vascular compromise, and intraosseous medullary involvement of bone lesions are depicted best by this modality.

Ultrasonography

Ultrasonography (US) and the skeletal system interact in the evaluation of the neonatal hip and, with its Doppler capability, in the evaluation of soft tissues, vascular anatomy, and complications of osteomyelitis.

Radionuclide scintigraphy

Radionuclide scintigraphy remains the primary modality in the detection of osteomyelitis, metastatic bone lesions, and any disorder that may affect different portions of the skeleton (e.g., nonaccidental trauma). Agents used are technetium 99^m methylene diphosphate (MDP) and, increasingly, iridium 111-labeled white blood cells and gallium 67 citrate.

Arthrography

Arthrography of the double- or single-contrast variety has been replaced by MRI in most situations.

NORMAL DEVELOPMENT AND VARIANTS

Normal Development
   Ossification centers: upper extremities
   Ossification centers: lower extremities
   Accessory ossification centers, sesamoids
Normal Variants
   "Normal" periosteal new bone
   "Physiologic" sclerosis
   "Irregular" ossification
   "Ivory" epiphyses
   "Air vacuum" phenomenon
   "Lucent" anatomic areas
   Metaphyseal cortical irregularities

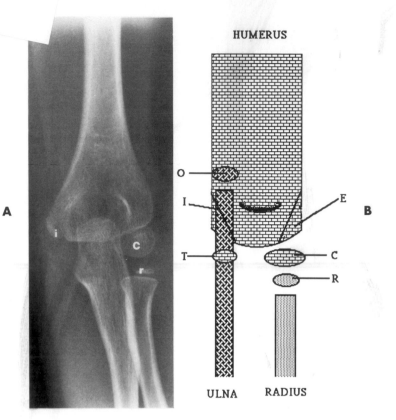

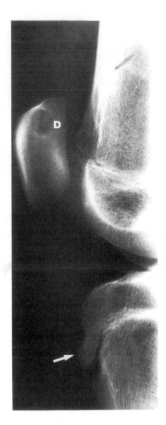

Fig. 5-1 **A**, AP radiograph of the elbow of a 5-year-old girl. (*C*, Capitellum; *r*, radius; *i*, medial epicondyle). **B**, CRITOE mnemonic.

Fig. 5-2 Lateral radiograph of the knee demonstrates a dorsal defect of the patella (*D*). Note the teardrop of the anterior tibial tubercle (*arrow*).

Normal Development

Ossification centers: upper extremities In upper extremities the proximal humeral primary growth (ossification) center ossifies between 38 and 42 weeks gestational age. The secondary growth center is radiographically visible in an infant around 1 year of age.

The multiple secondary ossification centers of the elbow can create confusion and may be difficult to differentiate from fractures in the setting of trauma. The sequential ossification of these centers—*c*apitellum, *r*adial head, *i*nternal or medial epicondyle, *t*rochlea, *o*lecranon, and *e*xternal (or lateral) epicondyle (CRITOE)—in boys occurs sequentially at approximately 1, 3, 5, 7, and 9 years of age and occurs 6 to 9 months earlier in girls (Fig. 5-1). Therefore in a trauma setting a bony structure at or near any of these sites at an earlier stage than expected most likely represents an (avulsion) fracture.

The distal radial epiphysis (growth or ossification) usually appears near the age of 2 years and the distal ulnar epiphysis around 6 years of age. An *apo*physis does not contribute to linear growth; an *epi*physis is located near or at a joint and does contibute to linear growth. The last epiphysis to close is the medial clavicle.

Ossification centers: lower extremities The earliest epiphysis to ossify in almost all children is the distal femur (at birth). The head of the femur contains an ossification center at approximately 4 months of life. This ossification center may ossify in an irregular fashion and before fusing with the metaphysis, may flatten somewhat. The ossification centers for the proximal fibula and the patella often do not ossify until the child is 5 years of age. The most striking epiphysis or physis is that of the proximal tibia. The anterior tibial tubercle "teardrop" reflects differential growth of the main proximal tibial ossification center and the tubercle and may be very irregular in appearance (Fig. 5-2). The dorsal defect of the patella is an anomaly of ossification that usually is noted incidentally. It is almost always located on the superolateral aspect of its dorsal surface and is seen as a well-defined, round lucency, with intact overlying articular cartilage. The differential diagnosis includes fibrous cortical defect, osteochondritis dissecans, osteomyelitis, chondroblastoma, Langerhans cell histiocytosis (LCH), and osteomyelitis.

Secondary ossification centers, especially the lesser trochanter, ischium, and base of the fifth metatarsal, occasionally are confused with fractures. If fractured and nondisplaced, this is often a clinical diagnosis accompanied by soft tissue swelling and pain. The apophysis of the fifth metatarsal is parallel to it, with a base of the fifth metatarsal fracture perpendicular to it. The apophysis of the acromion and the coracoid processes of the scapula are evident within 6 months of birth and fuse during adolescence. Their well-ossified edges usually differentiate them from avulsion fractures. The last apophysis in the body to close is the iliac crest, which closes in the early twenties; it appears at approximately 12 to 14 years of age.

The ossification center that appears earliest often fuses last; and skeletal maturation generally occurs proximal to distal. The relative contributions to bone length reveal that the wrist and proximal humerus grow the fastest, the elbow the slowest. In the lower extremity the knee, including the distal femur and the proximal tibia, grows most rapidly.

Accessory ossification centers Most commonly surrounding the ankle, accessory ossification centers can be difficult to differentiate from previous trauma if no soft tissue swelling is present. The os subtibiale and the os subfibulare are examples of accessory ossification centers.

Accessory (false) ossification centers may be seen in the proximal aspect of the metacarpals (and metatarsals) II through V and in the distal aspect of the first metacarpal (and metatarsal). They contribute little or nothing to the bone length and they are seen commonly in children with cleidocranial dysostosis and hypothyroidism.

The function of sesamoid bones is to ameliorate the tension on tendons. The largest sesamoid bone in the body, the patella, and other sesamoids may be bipartite or tripartite, an appearance that occurs bilaterally in 50% of patients. Sesamoid bones are more common around the first and second rays of the feet and hands. Sesamoid bones around the knee, in addition to the patella, include a fabella (in the lateral head of the gastrocnemius muscle) and a cyamella (in the head of the popliteal muscle).

Normal variants

"Normal" periosteal new bone The "normal" periosteal new bone of the newborn is seen in approximately 50% of all infants less than age 6 months. It is characterized by a thin, smooth layer of new bone paralleling the diaphysis of the humerus, radius, and femur and is caused by relatively rapid growth during this time (Fig. 5-3). The bone itself is often dense and appears sclerotic as a result of a combination of cortical

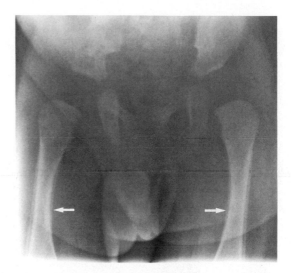

Fig. 5-3 "Normal" newborn periosteal new bone of both femora.

thickening, a narrow medullary canal, and dense spongy bone. These findings may disappear (normalize) in the first weeks to months of life. The differential diagnosis of this normal variant includes osteomyelitis, hypervitaminosis A, and metastatic leukemia or neuroblastoma, although the medullary canal often is not normal, in fact moth-eaten, in the later two instances.

"Physiologic" sclerosis In children less than 6 years of age "physiologic" sclerosis often is present at the zones of proximal calcifications of the metaphyses. This band frequently is difficult to distinguish from one caused by heavy metal (lead) intoxication or syphilis. "Lead" bands, caused by inhibition of osteoclasts in the zone of provisional calcification, have broader dense bands that also involve the proximal fibulae to distinguish them from the physiologic sclerosis (Fig. 5-4).

Irregular ossification Irregular ossification is seen often in the lateral epicondyle of the humerus and the trochlea and at the medial and lateral edges of the medial and lateral condyles of the femur. A similar appearance may be noted on the medial aspect of the distal femoral or proximal tibial epiphysis (See Fig. 5-4, *B*). These findings must be differentiated from those of osteochondritis dissecans (Fig. 5-5), which are located in areas in the line of weight-bearing.

"Ivory" epiphyses "Ivory" epiphyses are sclerotic-appearing epiphyseal variants seen most commonly in the distal phalanges, occasionally the middle ones. They may be accompanied by symmetric vertical fissures of the secondary ossification centers in proximal epiphyses, especially of the hallux (big toe) that must not be mistaken for fractures. This complex of lucent lines and increased density is often noted in the calcaneal apophysis, which appears in a child near 7 years

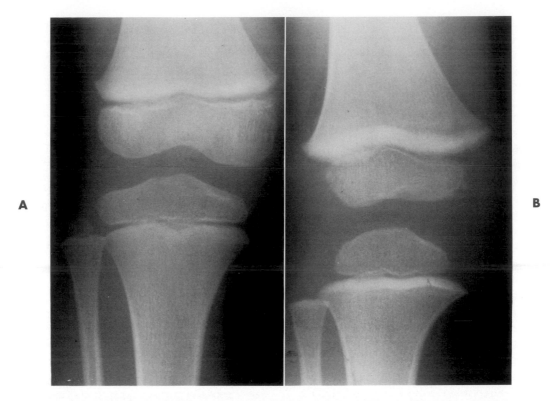

Fig. 5-4 A, Normal "physiologic" sclerosis. **B**, "Lead" bands. Note dense fibular metaphysis. There is irregular ossification of the medial distal femoral epiphysis, a normal variant.

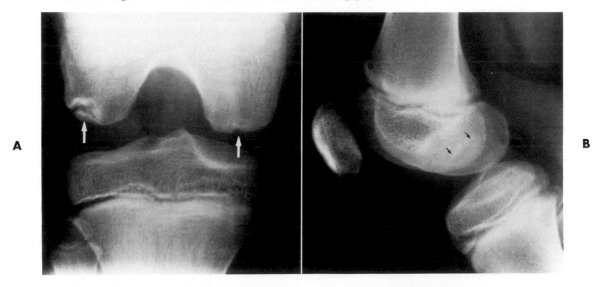

Fig. 5-5 Irregular ossification. A, Tunnel view demonstrates pseudoosteochondritis dissecans of both femoral condyles (*arrows*) in a **B**, posterior, non-weight bearing location (*arrows*).

of age. It is the result of multiple ossification centers that coalesce in an irregular fashion to fuse during the midteenage years. The fused apophysis then becomes the same density as the remainder of the calcaneus.

"Air vacuum" phenomenon In an immobilized patient, even when gentle traction is applied to the elbow, wrist, hip, knees, or ankles, an "air vacuum" phenomenon may occur. Negative intraarticular pressure allows nitrogen gas to come out of solution to become free within the joint space. The inability to elicit this crescent of air has been used to exclude the presence of joint effusions. This sign is not very specific.

"Lucent" anatomic areas Several "lucent" anatomic areas that are normal can be seen, especially in the greater tuberosity of the humerus, the bicipital tuberosity of the radius and the body of the calcaneus. These "cysts" are caused by an area of bone that is relatively thin when compared with the normal trabeculae around it. Benign fibrous cortical defects (nonossifying fibroma) are also commonly seen in the distal femur or proximal tibia and occur in children 2 to 6 years old. They occur at tendinous insertions (of the adductor muscle group most commonly) and may be related to avulsive cortical irregularities.

The metaphysis may develop a lucent metaphyseal band caused by "stress" of prematurity, cyanotic congenital heart disease (CHD), or any systemic illness. It is thought that blood flow to the zone of provisional calcification is "diverted" to other parts of the body with resultant retardation of ossification. When this stress is relieved, bone growth resumes, as evidenced by the growth "recovery" (or "arrest") line of Parks (Fig. 5-6).

Metaphyseal cortical irregularities Metaphyseal cortical irregularities are relatively common and must be differentiated from the classic findings of the "bucket handle" fracture seen with child abuse. These cortical irregularities are seen particularly frequently on the dorsal and medial aspects of the distal femur and the medial aspect of the distal fibula and are seen proximally and distally in the humerus and in the distal radius. An interruption of the cortex with slight spiculation, these irregularities disappear with growth and probably represent a fenestration in the metaphyseal cortex.

CONGENITAL ABNORMALITIES

Skeletal Dysplasias
  Short-limbed dwarfism
    Rhizomelic dwarfism
    Mesomelic shortening
    Acromelic shortening
    Asymmetric short stature
    Nonspecific short-limb dwarfism
  Short-trunk dwarfism
  Proportionate dwarfism
  Asymmetric dwarfism
    Multiple enchondromatosis
    Multiple hereditary cartilaginous exostoses
    (osteochondromas)
Focal Bony Deficiencies
  Hypoplasia or aplasia
  Hyperplasia
  Congenital amputations
Defects of Ossification
  Cleidocranial dysostosis
  Sclerosing bone dysplasias
    Osteoclerosis
    Hyperostosis

Skeletal Dysplasias

Skeletal dysplasias are congenital disturbances of bone growth and structure. Shortening of the limbs or

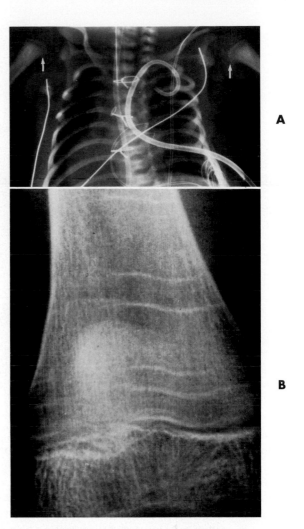

Fig. 5-6 **A,** "Stress" lacunar metaphyseal bands (*arrows*) in an infant S/P surgery for CHD. **B,** Growth recovery lines (of Parks) in a child with cystic fibrosis and repeated bouts of pulmonary infection.

spine below the third percentile for a normal newborn constitutes congenital dwarfism. The tubular bones are affected symmetrically, and these short-limbed infants can be categorized according to the portion of the extremity that is maximally shortened. The majority of *symmetric* short-statured infants can be divided into short-limbed dwarfs, short-trunk dwarfs, and proportionate dwarfs.

Short-limbed Dwarfism

Rhizomelic dwarfism Noted at birth, thanatophoric dwarfism is a fatal condition whose clinical and radiologic features differ from those of achondroplasia only in their severity. The limb shortening affects the proximal segment of the extremities predominantly. Autosomal dominant inheritance is noted in both conditions.

In a surviving short-limbed dwarf, achondroplasia is the most common abnormality. The clinical features

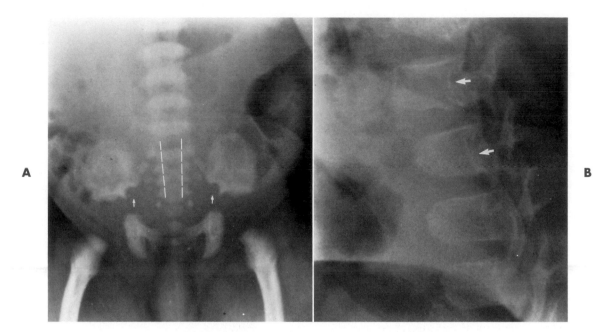

Fig. 5-7   Achondroplasia. A, Frontal radiograph demonstrates tapering interpedicular distances, small sacroiliac notches (*arrows*), and wide acetabula. **B,** Lateral radiograph of the lumbar spine shows posterior scalloping (*arrows*).

include shortening and bowing of the extremities, with profound lumbar lordosis and an enlarged cranium with frontal bossing, a sunken nasal root, and prognathism. Knee pain is a frequent complaint. Key imaging findings are located in the spine and pelvis and consist of narrow interpedicular distances, posterior vertebral body scalloping, decreased vertebral body height, and short pedicles, resulting in a narrow spinal canal and thoracolumbar kyphosis. Characteristic findings in the pelvis include hypoplastic, "square" iliac bones, the "champagne glass" pelvic inlet resulting from small sacroiliac notches, and wide triradiate cartilages (Fig. 5-7).

A milder form of rhizomelic dwarfism manifests in late childhood and reveals the more subtle findings of achondroplasia: hypochondroplasia. Clinically, the characteristic facies of achondroplasia often are not seen; radiographically, the features of achondroplasia are present in a milder form.

Mesomelic shortening Mesomelic shortening affects the middle portions (i.e., radius, ulna, tibia, and fibula) of the extremities. The fatal form consists of camptomelic ("bent limbs") dwarfism, which probably has an autosomal recessive mode of inheritance. Clinically, there is striking symmetric anterior bowing of the lower extremities, with pretibial dimples. It is characterized further by an enlarged cranium, micrognathia, cleft palate, and low-set ears. Radiographically, tibial bowing, hypoplastic scapulae, and absent thoracic pedicles are diagnostic. The vertebral bodies are normal. Dislocated hips, kyphoscoliosis, and 11 pairs of ribs often are seen in addition. Another form of mesomelic dysplasia is normal at birth, limb shortening becoming evident at age 2 years, and is known as dyschondrosteosis, including the Nievergelt and Langer types. They are autosomal dominant entities occurring in girls and are characterized by bilateral Madelung deformities. This deformity consists of growth retardation of the medial portion of the distal radial growth plate with resultant shortening and ulnar deviation of the radius, causing ulnar deformity and occasional synostosis (Fig. 5-8). This deformity also may occur after trauma or infection of the radius and occasionally as a result of multiple cartilaginous exostoses.

Acromelic shortening Acromelic shortening affects the distal segments of the extremities. Is is exemplified best by asphyxiating thoracic dystrophy (Jeune syndrome). This is a form of short-limb dwarfism that is usually fatal and is inherited as an autosomal recessive condition. Clinically, the infants present with respiratory distress (short ribs resulting in a narrow, tubular chest), with short hands and feet and polydactyly in up to one third of patients. Radiographic findings feature the long and narrow chest, flattened acetabular angles, and osseous spurs projecting inferiorly from the medial and lateral aspects of the acetabula. Similar findings in surviving acromelic infants are known as *chondroectodermal dysplasia* (Ellis-van Creveld syndrome), a triad of dwarfism, ectodermal dysplasia, and polydactyly. This syndrome has an autosomal recessive mode of

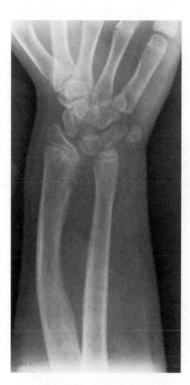

Fig. 5-8 Madelung deformity. There is shortening and ulnar deviation of the radius causing mild ulnar deformity (bowing). Carpal bones have wedged into the resulting V of radius and ulna.

Common Causes of Limb Shortening

RHIZOMELIC SHORTENING (AD)

Thanatophoric dwarf*
Achondroplasia
Hydrochondroplasia
Chondrodyplasia punctata

MESOMELIC SHORTENING (AR)

Camptomelic dwarf*
Dyschondrosteoses

ACROMELIC SHORTENING (AR)

Asphyxiating thoracic dystrophy*
Chondroectodermal dysplasia
Pyknodysostosis

NONSPECIFIC SHORTENING (AR/AD)

Osteogenesis imperfecta
Congenita ⎫
          ⎬ Types 1-4
Tarda   ⎭

*AR, Autosomal recessive inheritance; AD, autosomal dominant inheritance.

inheritance, and an infant with this condition clinically presents with hypoplastic nails; thin, sparse hair, eyebrows and eyelashes; and polydactyly on the ulnar aspect of the hands. There is associated CHD, most commonly an atrial septal defect (ASD) or ventricular septal defect (VSD), in two thirds of patients.

Another acromelic variant is pyknodysostosis, characterized by generalized osteosclerosis, acromelic short-limb dwarfism, typical craniofacial changes, and repeated fractures. It is inherited as an autosomal recessive condition. Clinically, there may be delayed closure of the anterior fontanelle, a large cranium, bulging eyes, a "parrotlike" nose, and a receding chin. Radiographically, there is striking generalized osteosclerosis, with multiple fractures of varying age. Multiple wormian bones and hypoplastic facial bones also may be seen. Short phalanges of the fingers and toes, with hypoplastic terminal phalanges, are common. (Toulouse-Lautrec is said to have suffered from this variant).

The most common limb-shortening syndromes are summarized in the box.

Asymmetric short stature Asymmetric short stature is seen most commonly in children with chondrodysplasia punctata (stippled epiphyses), which is a rare X-linked dominant anomaly fatal in boys. There are two forms: an autosomal recessive rhizomelic and an autosomal dominant (Conradi disease) variety. Facial features resembling those of achondroplasia are the clinical hallmarks, along with contractures of the extremities, cataracts, and long delicate fingers. Transient calcifications in the skeletal and respiratory cartilage are the imaging hallmarks. Stippled epiphyses may also be seen in infants with cretinism, fetal warfarin syndrome, and trisomy 18.

Nonspecific short-limb dwarfism Nonspecific short-limb dwarfism is illustrated best by osteogenesis imperfecta (OI). This condition classically was divided into an autosomal recessive (AR) (congenita, lethal) form and an autosomal dominant (AD) (tarda; late) form. The former was characterized by thickened tubular bones caused by multiple healing fractures, whereas the latter was characterized by thin tubular bones. Currently, gene probes have elucidated mutations in genes that regulate collagen formation, resulting in defective conversion of reticulum fibers into adult collagen fibers.

Currently four types of OI are recognized:
- Type 1: appears in late teen years with deafness (otosclerosis), and blue sclera; autosomal dominant inheritance. This, the former tarda form, is characterized by repeated fractures that heal, with resultant skeletal deformities beginning in infancy or early childhood. Other clinical hallmarks are blue sclerae, a small triangular face, and a bulging skull. Deafness caused by otosclerosis may develop but is uncommon. Radiographically, progressive kyphoscoliosis,

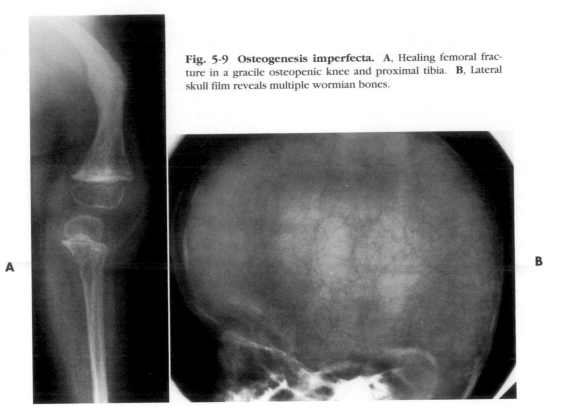

Fig. 5-9 Osteogenesis imperfecta. A, Healing femoral fracture in a gracile osteopenic knee and proximal tibia. **B**, Lateral skull film reveals multiple wormian bones.

wormian bones, and multiple fracture are seen along with an osteopenic skeleton (Fig. 5-9).

- Type 2: lethal, former congenita form that can be recognized on prenatal US by multiple fractures, demineralized calvaria, and a femur length more than 3 SD below the mean for gestational age. Most infants are born prematurely; many are stillborn; blue sclerae are always present; and the condition is AR inherited.
- Type 3: characterized by normal sclerae and progressive deformity of the limbs, with only occasional fractures.
- Type 4: characterized by osteoporosis, without fractures, and the presence of discolored teeth.

Short-trunk dwarfism Short-trunk dwarfism is represented by achondrogenesis. Four types associated with decreasing levels of severity are inherited as autosomal recessive conditions. They clinically are seen in infants with severe micromelia and a large head and are associated with neonatal death. Absence of ossification on conventional radiographs if the infant survives and a reduction in limb length on prenatal US can be diagnostic. Rarer forms of short-trunk dwarfism are the KNIEST syndrome and spondylometaphyseal dysplasia, both with autosomal dominant inheritance and spinal and metaphyseal abnormalities. Platyspondyly frequently is associated with coronal clefts and anterior wedging and has characteristic vertebral anomalies often associated with kyphosis and/or scoliosis.

Children with mucopolysaccharidoses have skeletal findings that develop later in childhood termed *dysostosis multiplex*. The abnormality of mucopolysaccharide or glycoprotein metabolism (incomplete degradation and resultant abnormal storage) is manifested radiographically by osteopenia, an enlarged cranium with a thick calvaria, anteroinferiorly beaked oval vertebral bodies (Fig. 5-10), dysplastic capital femoral epiphyses and short and wide metacarpals and phalanges. These metacarpals and phalanges tend to taper proximally and may result in a clawlike hand deformity. Clinically, knowledge of the patient's age, intelligence level, and the presence of urinary acid mucopolysaccherides is paramount for accurate diagnosis. Hurler syndrome (mucopolysaccharidosis I; AR) is the most common form and serves as a variant prototype both clinically and radiographically. A milder form very similar to Hurler syndrome is Hunter syndrome (mucopolysaccharidosis II; X linked). A characteristic gargoyle face with a broad, flat nasal bridge, wide-spaced eyes, puffy cheeks, and thick lips surrounding an open mouth with a prominent tongue may be evident. Hepatosplenomegaly, hernias, and stiff joints are present in addition to psychomotor retardation. Mucopolysacharidosis III (Sanfilippo syndrome; AR) represents an even milder form of dysostosis multiplex. Morquio syndrome (mucopolysaccharidosis IV) is characterized by short stature (<4 feet tall), lax joints, and a short neck.

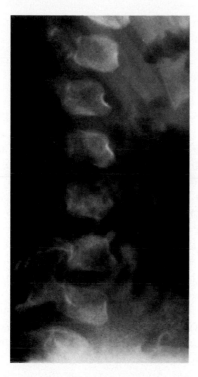

Fig. 5-10 Dysostosis multiplex. Characteristic anteroinferiorly beaked oval vertebral bodies.

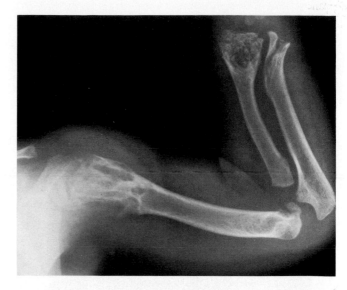

Fig. 5-11 Enchondromatosis. Characteristic metaphyseal lesions with popcorn calcification that have resulted in radial and ulnar deformities and contour abnormalities of the proximal humerus.

Hypoplastic and beaked vertebral bodies are characteristic imaging findings.

These children often die before age 10 years, are deaf, and have CHD (murmurs from varying causes). The mucolipidoses types (I, II, III) are clinically and radiographically identical to the mucopolysaccharidoses and sphingolipidoses, but these children do not excrete mucopolysaccharides in their urine.

Proportionate dwarfism Proportionate dwarfism is noted in patients with short stature. However, skeletal dysplasias are not the most common cause. These children are more likely to have pituitary, renal, nutritional, or chromosomal abnormalities resulting in short stature. Proportionate short stature can also be normal, for 2% of all children measure below the third percentile of the growth chart.

Asymmetric dwarfism The most common entities causing asymmetric dwarfism are multiple enchondromatosis and diaphyseal aclasis (multiple exostoses).

Multiple enchondromatosis A child with multiple enchondromatosis has cartilaginous masses infiltrating the metaphyses of the long and short tubular bones and the flat bones. Enchondral bones are not affected. It is a nonhereditary disorder. There are six types, of which three are common types: if the multiple enchondromas are purely unilateral or if they are unevenly distributed throughout the metaphyses of the long bones,

sparing the cranium and spine, it is called *Ollier disease*; if the condition is associated with multiple cutaneous hemagiomas, it is called *Maffucci syndrome*; and if it is symmetrically distributed throughout the body with involvement of the cranium and hands and feet, it is known as *generalized enchondromatosis*. The former two are more common in boys (2:1). Less frequent variants include metachondromatosis, affecting the short tubular bones of the hands and feet; spondyloenchondroplasia, in which the enchondromas are associated with platyspondyly; and enchondromas with irregular vertebral lesions.

Radiographically, multiple lucent metaphyseal lesions that often contain punctate ("popcorn") calcifications are characteristic. Eventually these lesions may result in angular limb deformities (Fig. 5-11). Chondrosarcomas reportedly can occur with both Maffucci syndrome and Ollier disease, usually in adults; 5% of patients with chondrosarcomas have Ollier disease. Symptoms such as pain may indicate a pathologic fracture. CT or MR are rarely indicated. The differential diagnosis includes polyostotic fibrous dysplasia and diaphyseal aclasis.

Multiple hereditary cartilaginous exostoses (osteochondromas) Among the most common bone dysplasias, osteochondromas are characterized by multiple cartilaginous exostoses arising from the metaphyses of, in particular, the tubular bones (i.e., distal femur, proximal tibia) and ribs (80%) and the pelvis and scapulae (10%) (bones preformed in cartilage) (Fig. 5-12). If the resultant pain or deformity created by these lesions interferes with the patient's life-style, the osteochondromas can be removed to improve appearance and function, but if they cause pain by compressing nerves and/or vessels, sarcomatous degeneration should be suspected. This occurs in approximately 5% of patients. Osteochondromas are more common in boys (AD). Approximately 50% of these patients have affected parents. Radiographically, CT may image a cartilaginous cap that should be thin and sharply demarcated. A thick cap (>2 to 3 cm) raises the possibility of malig-

nant degeneration. MRI is more specific than CT in identifying this cartilaginous cap.

Focal Bony Deficiencies

Hypoplasia or aplasia Along with hypoplasia, aplasias constitute the most common congenital malformations. Unilateral absence of the fibula is most common, occurring more commonly than bilateral absence. Clinically, there is pitting of the skin over the apex of a bowed, shorter lower leg. Following, in order, is absence of the radius, femur, ulna, and humerus. Radial deviation of the hand is usually seen in a child with *radial* ray shortening, which may occur in children with Holt-Oram syndrome, VACTERL, Fanconi anemia, or the trisomy 13 and 18 syndromes. The *femur* may be hypoplastic to absent, a set of anomalies grouped together as proximal femoral focal deficiency (PFFD) (Fig. 5-13). Most cases are unilateral and may be associated with aplasia or hypoplasia elsewhere in the same limb. In addition, these anomalies may occur as part of the caudal regression syndrome.

Hyperplasia Hyperplasia may include hemihypertrophy and an excessive number of structures (e.g., *polydactyly*). Of the autosomal recessive inherited short-rib–polydactyly syndromes, Ellis-van Creveld is the most common. Known as chondroectodermal dysplasia, these dwarfs have short ribs, hypoplastic or aplastic nails, sparse hair, and polydactyly. *Synostoses*, most commonly affecting the carpal or tarsal bones, are failures of segmentation. Of them, tarsal coalition (fusion) is the most common and is the most frequent cause for foot pain in an adolescent. It often results in

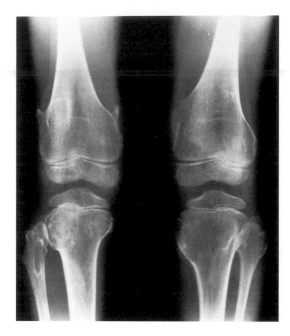

Fig. 5-12 Exostoses. Multiple bony excrescences arising in the distal femurs, proximal tibiae, and fibulae.

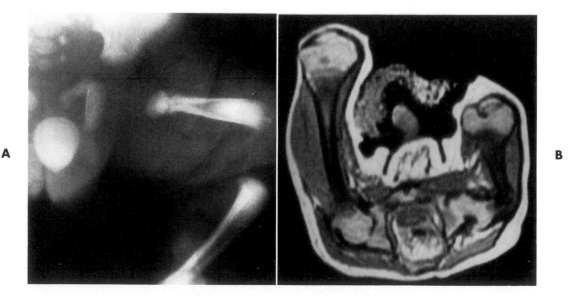

Fig. 5-13 Proximal femoral focal deficiency. A, Conventional radiograph demonstrates deformed shortened proximal left femur. **B,** MRI representation of same.

a spastic flatfoot (pes planus) deformity. The talonavicular variety is most common (60%), and a calcaneonavicular coalition is present in 30% of these patients. CT imaging is the modality of choice for detection and evaluation of the (bony) bridging tissue.

Congenital amputations Constricting amniotic bands can result in stumps or focal soft tissue constrictions of limbs (Streeter bands), fused digits, or club foot deformity (Fig. 5-14). These findings are grouped together in the amniotic deformity, adhesion, mutilation (ADAM) complex. Disruption of the amniotic membrane from the chorion is thought to lead to adhesions that trap parts of the developing fetus. Alternatively, a vascular anomaly or focal vascular dysplasia may be the underlying cause.

Defects of Ossification

Cleidocranial dysostosis An autosomal dominant disorder of mesenchymal skeletal development (30% are spontaneous mutations), cleidocranial dysostosis is characterized by a triad of cranial, clavicular, and pelvic abnormalities. Clinically, the patients have a soft cranium and delayed closure of the fontanelles, resulting in a brachycephalic skull with a small face; eventually, drooping shoulders, short stature, and an abnormal gait develop. Radiographically, wormian bones are common in widely patent sutures, and hypoplastic facial bones and widely placed orbits are seen. Clavicles are totally absent in 10% to 15% of patients and are partially absent in most. There is delayed ossification of the symphysis pubis, and this abnormality creates the *appearance* of widening of the symphysis pubis (Fig. 5-15). These patients have normal maturation and can expect a normal life span.

Sclerosing bone dysplasias Increased bone density and abnormalities of tubularization are the characteristic radiographic findings in patients with sclerosing bone dysplasias. There are two groups of dysplasias: increased mineralization causing osteosclerosis and active overgrowth causing hyperostosis.

Osteosclerosis Osteoclerosis can manifest as osteopetrosis, osteopoikilosis, or osteopathia striata.

In patients with osteopetrosis, osteoblast dysfunction (carbonic anhydrase II deficiency) causes a failure of resorption of cartilage and bone matrix (primary

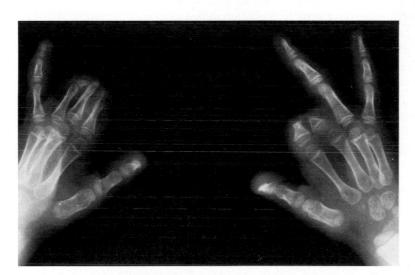

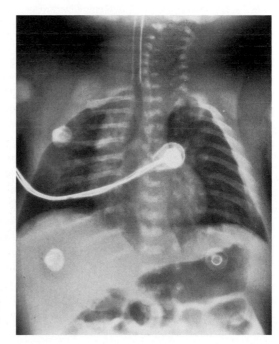

Fig. 5-14 Amniotic bands. Amputations of multiple phalanges of both hands.

Fig. 5-15 Cleidocranial dysostosis. Delayed ossification of the posterior neural arches, absent clavicles, and short ribs are demonstrated on a chest radiograph.

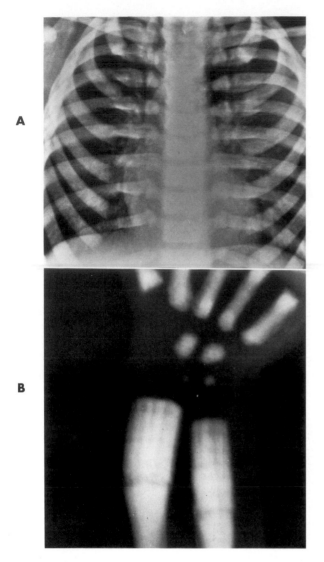

A

B

Fig. 5-16 Osteopetrosis. A, Generalized osteosclerosis of all bony structures. **B,** Fine, longitudinal striations in flared metaphyses.

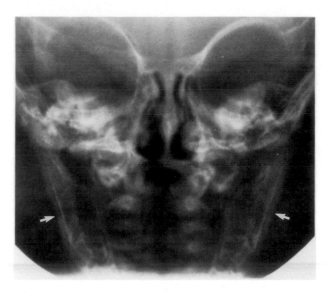

Fig. 5-17 Caffey disease. Periosteal new bone formation is seen along both mandibles.

spongiosa). Dense bones are present as a result of marrow underdevelopment (marble bones). The condition can be of a congenital infantile (Albers-Schönberg disease) or adult (tarda) type. In the former (AR) there is an increase in the density of all the bones, with club-shaped metaphyses and bone-within-bone appearance of the vertebral bodies. The base of the calvaria is thickened. This can lead to deafness or optic atrophy, and there may be longitudinal striations in the distal long bone shafts. The latter variant is usually noted incidentally in childhood or adolescence and is an autosomal dominant condition. Transverse lucent bands in the phalanges, arcuate bands in the iliac bones, and bone-within-bone appearance of vertebral bodies are manifestations of the temporal fluctuations of this affliction. Bone pain and a propensity for fractures are the common presenting symptoms clinically (Fig. 5-16).

In children with *osteopoikilosis* multiple small, rounded foci of osteosclerosis affect the end of large and small tubular bones, including the epiphyses. It is a symptomless autosomal dominant dysplasia that can be regarded as an incidental finding.

Osteopathia striata is characterized by fine linear striations in the metaphyses of long bones and may represent a stage in the osteosclerosis conditions. It is very rare.

Hyperostosis Hyperostosis, or bone hypertrophy, can take the form of Caffey disease, melorheostosis, or diaphyseal dysplasia.

The cause of Caffey disease (infantile cortical hyperostosis) is unknown. It occurs during the first few months of life (average age of onset, 9 weeks), often in clusters of patients and locales. Clinically, the child is irritable, has an elevated temperature, and has soft tissue swelling around affected areas: the mandible, clavicle, and tubular bones. The erythrocyte sedimentation rate (ESR) is elevated. Prostaglandin E, a virus, and a familial tendency have been implicated as causes. It is a self-limited disease.

Imaging reveals periosteal new bone in relation to the mandible, ribs, clavicle, and ulna in decreasing order of frequency (Fig. 5-17).

Melorheostosis is an uncommon disorder and appears in children as asymmetry of the limbs with no pain. It is characterized radiographically by usually unilateral extracortical and endosteal hyperostotic "waves" resembling molten wax flowing down the side of a candle.

Diaphyseal dysplasia (Camurati-Englemann disease) manifests as a waddling gait in a malnourished child and is very rare. Radiographically, there is endosteal and periosteal thickening of the diaphyses of the tubular bones.

In the differential diagnosis of these sclerosing bone dysplasias, only children with melorheostosis and Caffey disease reveal abnormal uptake on a radionuclide bone scan.

SYSTEMIC AND GENERALIZED SKELETAL DISORDERS

Metabolic Disorders
  Rickets
  Hyperparathyroidism
  Renal osteodystrophy
  Hypothyroidism
  Scurvy
  Hypervitaminosis A
  Heavy metal poisoning
Anemias
  Hemophilia
  Sickle cell disease
  Thalassemia
Neurofibromatosis
Langerhans Cell Histiocytosis
  Letterer-Siwe disease
  Hand-Schüller-Christian disease
  Eosinophilic granuloma
Fibrous Dysplasia

Metabolic Disorders

Rickets Rickets, a relative or absolute deficiency in vitamin D or its derivatives, causes failure of normal mineralization of the growing cartilage into bone and ground substance of bone. There are several causes of rickets: *nutritional causes* as a result of deficient vitamin D in the diet or lack of sunlight (ultraviolet rays); *malabsorption* as a result of hepatobiliary disease (lack of bile) or small bowel malabsorptive disease; or *a defect in synthesis* such as in a child with renal glomerular failure, vitamin D-resistant rickets, or inherited renal tubular acidosis (RTA). Rarely it is caused by *familial* vitamin D-resistant rickets or hypophosphatemia. Rickets almost always is diagnosed in an infant before age 2 years and is seen radiographically before it is clinically evident in up to one third of patients. The classic radiographic appearances occur after 4 to 6 weeks of vitamin D deficiency, especially in the most rapidly growing ends of bones. There is widening of the physis and cupping, fraying, and irregularity of the metaphyseal region, the zone of provisional calcification in particular, accompanied by generalized osteopenia (Fig. 5-18). The most rapidly growing areas of the infant skeleton, namely the wrist, knees, and proximal humeri, are the most affected. The bone age may be delayed. The classic "rachitic rosary" at the anterior rib ends and transverse radiolucent bands in the diaphyses ("umbauzonen") are rarely seen today.

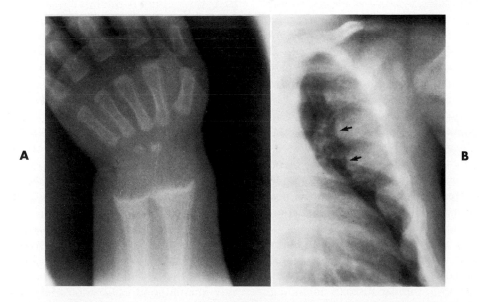

Fig. 5-18 Rickets. A, Widening of the physis; cupping, fraying and irregularity of the zone of provisional calcification. **B,** Rachitic rosary (*arrows*).

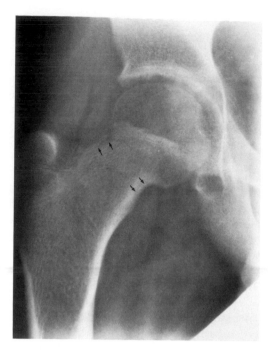

Fig. 5-19   Secondary hypoparathyroidism (renal rickets). Osteopenia and subperiosteal resorption of the femoral neck (*arrows*).

Rickets and Ricketslike Conditions

RICKETS

Nutritional

Premature infant (receiving hyperalimentation)
Prolonged breast-feeding
Unusual diet
Lack of sunlight

Malabsorption

Bile deficiency: secondary to biliary obstructive or
   liver disease
(Regional) enteritis
Pancreatic dysfunction (cystic fibrosis)

RICKETSLIKE CHANGES

Renal Osteodystrophy

Tubular disorders
Congenital: renal tubular acidosis
Aquired: nephrotic syndrome, vitamin D deficiency

Glomerular Disorders:

Glomerulonephritis, polycystic disease, chronic
   pyelonephritis

Hyperparathyroidism   *Primary* hyperparathyroidism is due to a parathyroid adenoma's secreting increased levels of parathormone. In children this is a rare, often hereditary condition. *Tertiary* hyperparathyroidism occurs after the prolonged presence of secondary hyperparathyroidism. Escape of the parathyroid glands from the regulatory effects of serum calcium levels is the underlying mechanism. *Secondary* hyperparathyroidism ("renal rickets") is due to chronic hypocalcemia. The radiographic changes are seen most commonly in children with renal failure who are treated by peritoneal dialysis or those suffering from intestinal malabsorption. Growth retardation may accompany this renal osteodystrophy. Radiographic changes include generalized osteopenia with areas of subperiosteal resorption, which are most prominent along the radial margins of the middle phalanges. The distal clavicles and inner aspects of the femoral necks likewise are frequently involved (Fig. 5-19). Soft tissue calcification may occur. Intraosseous localized fibrous tissue accumulation (osteoclastomas) are known as "brown" tumors that may be diagnostic in conjunction with the rachitic changes already described.

Renal osteodystrophy   Renal osteodystrophy refers to changes that occur in children with chronic renal insufficiency. These conditions can be thought of as belonging to two groups: tubular disease, including congenital (e.g., RTA) or acquired (e.g., nephrotic syndrome, vitamin D deficiency) variants; or *glomerular*

disease (chronic pyelonephritis, glomerulonephritis, polycystic disease). Both result in ricketslike changes in the metabolically inactive bones of these children (see box). In children with renal osteodystrophy, if growth failure is severe, the radiographic alterations of hyperparathyroidism predominate. With skeletal growth, the changes of rickets appear.

Hypothyroidism   Cretinism, the congenital form of hypothyroidism, is the most common metabolic abnormality found during routine laboratory testing of newborns. Thyroid hormone is necessary for bone growth and maturation and for development of the central nervous system. Hypothyroidism slows skeletal growth and maturation. It is usually due to congenital absence of hypoplasia of the thyroid gland. Congenital hypothyroidism is usually sporadic but occasionally is autosomal recessive. It occurs three times more frequently in girls than boys. Radiographically, the bone age is usually more than 2 SD below the mean. The epiphyseal ossification centers are irregular and fragmented, and there is delay in closure of the cranial sutures, with wormian bones frequently present.

Associated abnormalities in which hypothyroidism is common include Down syndrome, autoimmune endocrine abnormalities, and congenital heart disease.

Hyperthyroidism is extremely rare in neonates and is rare in childhood. (Pre)adolescent females may have a toxic goiter, but skeletal maturation is usually normal.

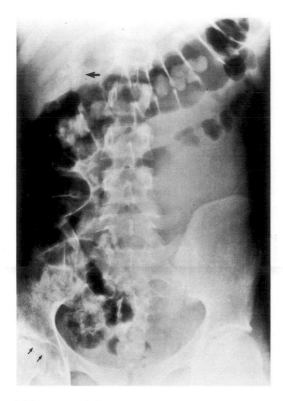

Fig. 5-22 Hemophilia. Abdominal radiograph demonstrates gallstones (*arrow*), destructive arthritis of the right hip joint (*arrows*), and a soft tissue mass in the left lower quadrant (hemophilic pseudotumor).

radiographs or US and other cross-sectional imaging modalities in the *acute* phase. *Chronic* hemophilic arthropathy is characterized by thickening of the synovium, premature ossification of epiphyses, epiphyseal overgrowth, and resultant premature fusion of the growth plates. All these changes are caused by increased blood flow to this region. Avascular necrosis also may occur secondary to occlusion of epiphyseal vessels by the hemarthrosis. Cartilage destruction results in joint space narrowing, subchondral cyst formation, and eburnation of the articular cortex. In the knee the classic findings are epiphyseal overgrowth and widening of the intercondylar notch (differential diagnosis includes juvenile rheumatoid arthritis, tuberculous arthritis), and there may be squaring of the inferior aspect of the patella. Pseudotumor formation occurs in approximately 1% of severe hemophiliacs. The majority of these pseudotumors occur in the femur and pelvis and present as a painless, slowly expanding mass. There may be calcification within the "tumor" and associated bone erosion and periosteal new bone formation. Conventional radiographs and CT are the primary diagnostic modalities (Fig. 5-22). Marrow recruitment and resultant hyperplasia is demonstrated

on MR marrow imaging (T1). Because there is more red marrow to compensate, there is a retardation of normal conversion process of red marrow into yellow (high T1 signal) marrow.

Sickle cell disease Hemoglobin S is the most common hemoglobin variant resulting from substitution of valine for glutamic acid on the sixth position of the beta chain. When hemoglobin S is the predominant hemoglobin, it indicates homozygosity (Hb SS; 1:650 African-Americans), but hemoglobin SA and other variants (e.g., Hb S Thal) also can result in sickle cell disease (sickle trait is present in 10% of African-Americans).

The presence of hemoglobin F (fetal hemoglobin) causes symptoms in the first years of life. Toward the end of the second year of life, swollen fingers or toes ("hand-foot" syndrome) are the usual first clinical signs of sickle cell disease.

Abdominal pain, bone infarction, and joint pain become more frequent presentations through childhood. Skeletal abnormalities in children with sickle cell disease are due to three factors: bone infarction, bone infection, and marrow hyperplasia.

On conventional radiographs the "hand-foot" syndrome is characterized by soft tissue swelling, periosteal new bone formation along the phalangeal shafts, and mild expansion. This syndrome may be difficult to distinguish from osteomyelitis. The skull may reveal diploic space widening, with vertical striations causing the "hair-on-end" pattern, although this finding is seen much less frequently than in children with thalassemia. Infarction is uncommon in the skull. In the spine, however, on the lateral view the end plates reveal central cupping, resulting in the vertebral body's resembling the letter H (also known as *Lincoln log*) (Fig. 5-23). These findings are caused by the infarction secondary to rouleau-x-formation of red blood cells in the smaller vessels supplying the central portion of the end plates. The larger vessels supplying the epiphyseal rings or the vertebral bodies remain patent. These changes may also be seen on the anteroposterior view of the vertebral body.

Infarction of the long bones, most commonly the femur, occurs at the junction of the metaphysis and diaphysis because the epiphyses and metaphyses are individually supplied by collateral circulation. Infarction of the marrow may heal with fibrosis, which can calcify, or it may be complicated by osteomyelitis, often caused by *Salmonella*. Scintigraphy has been used in the acute phase of suspected marrow infection, but because patients with sickle cell disease often have had previous infarctions, findings on bone scintigraphy are unreliable. Combining bone and marrow imaging has been helpful in differentiating osteomyelitis from infarction immediately after the occurrence of an

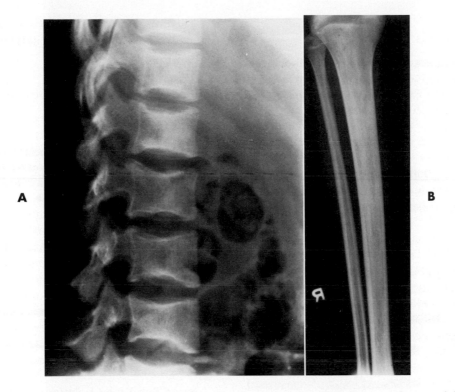

Fig. 5-23 Sickle cell disease. **A**, End-plate infarction resulting in "Lincoln log" deformity of the thoracolumbar spine. **B**, Diffuse areas of increased density throughout the tibia, representing the sequelae of bone infarcts.

infarct. Avascular necrosis of the epiphyseal portion of the long bone usually occurs after closure of the growth plate. The hip is the most common site for this to occur, and it is seen in approximately one third of patients with sickle cell disease, usually adults. MRI is the imaging modality of choice to detect avascular necrosis in its earliest phase.

Thalassemia Cooley anemia is the major (homozygous) form of thalassemia, a severe childhood anemia (often leading to death by age 12 years); thalassemia minor is a milder (heterogeneous) form. Both occur more frequently in patients of Eastern Mediterranean descent. The polypeptide chain involved determines further characterization of the variants, with the beta chain involved most commonly. Radiographic changes are mainly the result of marrow hyperplasia. In particular, the hands and feet show widened medullary cavities with coarse trabecular patterns and squaring of the bone (Fig. 5-24). During adolescence, these peripheral findings involute and sclerose as a result of hematopoietic marrow-to-fat conversion. In the calvaria, diploic widening with "hair-on-end" appearance may be seen, and there may be progressive obliteration of the paranasal sinuses. In the axial skeleton osteopenia and expansion of the shafts occur. Extramedullary hematopoiesis may also be evident in the paraspinal region (usually unilaterally) and is identified best by CT or MRI.

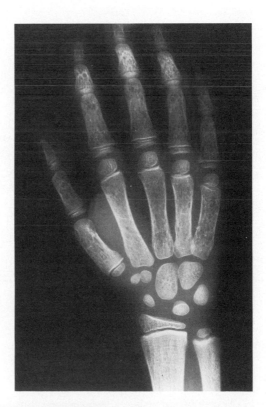

Fig. 5-24 Thalassemia. Widened medullary cavities with coarse trabecular markings of the metacarpals and phalanges.

Neurofibromatosis

Inherited as an autosomal dominant condition with variable penetrance and an almost 50% mutation rate, neurofibromatosis (NF) is a hereditary hamartomatous disorder with potential for involvement of any organ system of the body. Von Recklinghausen first described it as one of the most devastating, destructive, and debilitating diseases known to man. There is an incidence of one in 3000 live births, and the classic clinical symptoms include café au lait spots, neurofibromas of the skin or peripheral nerves, and Lisch spots in the iris. One half of the patients has a family history, and approximately one half has scoliosis, indistinguishable from idiopathic scoliosis. More than five café au lait spots, each .5 cm or larger in diameter, are considered the hallmark of neurofibromatosis. Characteristic skeletal radiographic findings in children with neurofibromatosis include "erosive" cortical defects, probably related to adjacent nerve enlargement caused by neurofibromatosis, and the "empty orbit" sign. The most commonly associated skeletal lesion is congenital pseudarthrosis of the tibia. This lesion is characterized by bowing in an area of fibrosis in the tibial midshaft (Fig. 5-25).

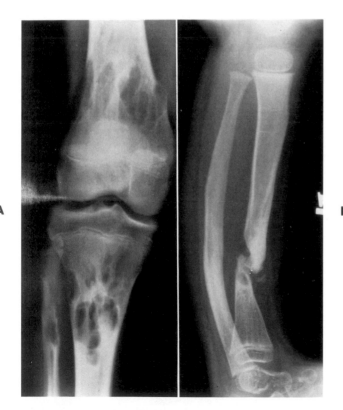

Fig. 5-25 Neurofibromatosis. A, Erosive cortical defects of the distal femur, proximal tibia, and fibula. **B,** Congenital pseudarthrosis of the tibia.

The erosion of adjacent bony structures is seen best on conventional radiographs, although MRI occasionally is useful.

Langerhans Cell Histiocytosis

LCH is a disease complex of unknown cause (? defect in immunoregulation) characterized by proliferation of a distinct histiocyte called a *Langerhans cell* and includes Letterer-Siwe disease (<10%), Hand-Schüller-Christian disease (10% to 20%), and eosinophilic granuloma (75%). There is considerable overlap between these groups, and up to 50% of patients are not clearly "groupable." It is a self-limiting disease in most cases. Age at diagnosis (<2 years) and severity of liver, lungs, or bone marrow involvement are important prognostic factors.

Letterer-Siwe disease Letterer-Siwe disease is the acute disseminated form of LCH seen in infants less than 6 months of age. These infants initially have hepatosplenomegaly, lymphadenopathy, purpura, and anemia. The prognosis is poor. Skeletal lesions are rare.

Hand-Schüller-Christian disease Hand-Schüller-Christian disease is a more slowly progressive form of disseminated LCH seen in children between the ages of 3 and 6 years. The children often have polyuria (diabetes insipidus), and bone pain. Lymphadenopathy, hepatosplenomegaly, and exophthalmos also are frequent presentations. The classic triad of exophthalmos, diabetes insipidus, and cranial lytic lesions occurs in 10% to 15% of patients. Skeletal lesions are present in 85% of these children. Prognosis is related to the degree of organ involvement.

Eosinophilic granuloma Eosinophilic granuloma is a form of LCH limited to bone and occurs in children 6 to 10 years of age and young adults. It is most often monostotic, and the male to female incidence ratio is 2:1. Prognosis is excellent, and skeletal involvement is common.

This skeletal involvement (Fig. 5-26) is most common in the skull (25%), ribs (14%), femur (14%), and pelvis (10%), followed by the spine, mandible, and humerus (each approximately 8%). Thus approximately 70% affect the flat bones and 30% the long bones. The lesions characteristically are punched out and destructive, with well-defined but not sclerotic, although often beveled, margins. In the vertebral column an almost pathognomonic finding is uniformly flattened vertebra plana. Affected vertebral bodies may return to normal or at least half their normal height over years. CT and MRI exquisitely define the extent of the lesion into the surrounding tissues.

Bone scintigraphy is less reliable because not all lesions (only 60%) take up the isotope, for the uptake depends on active skeletal response.

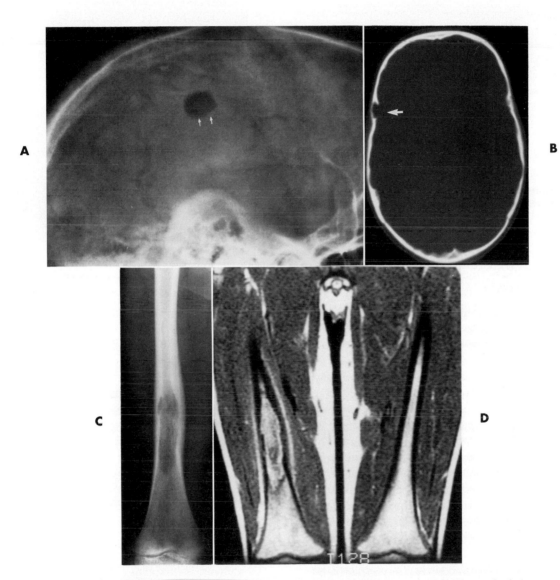

Fig. 5-26 Langerhans cell histiocytosis. A, B, Lateral skull radiograph and CT reveal a lytic lesion with beveled edges (*arrows*). **C,** Destructive central lesion of the distal diaphysis is well defined and slightly expansile. **D,** MRI better delineates marrow extent, degree of expansion of the lesion, and extent of the soft tissue involved.

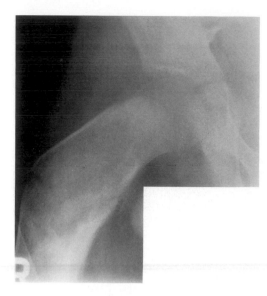

Fig. 5-27 Fibrous dysplasia. Radiograph of proximal femur reveals a mildly expansile ground-glass lesion with a pathologic fracture (shepherd's crook deformity).

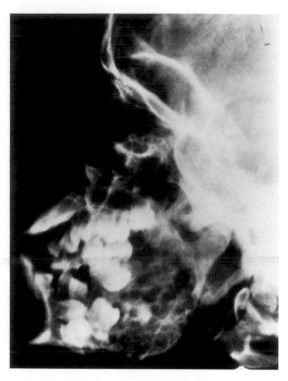

Fig. 5-28 Cherubism. Extensive multilocular lesions of the mandible in a patient presenting with swelling of the jaw.

Fibrous Dysplasia

Fibrous dysplasia, a nonhereditary, common disorder involving replacement of bone by fibrous tissue, occurs in a monostotic (70%) and a polyostotic form.

Approximately one third of patients will have the polyostotic form, and one third to one fifth will have cutaneous café au lait spots of the "coast of Maine" variety. Males and females are affected equally. The association between precocious puberty in girls, café au lait spots, and polyostotic (typically unilateral) fibrous dysplasia is known as McCune-Albright syndrome and is characterized by advanced bone age and sexual precocity. This syndrome occurs in approximately one third of girls with fibrous dysplasia. Radiographically, expansile lytic lesions occupy the medullary canal, may thin the cortex, and involve the diaphysis but may extend into the metaphysis (Fig. 5-27). A ground-glass appearance may result from a preponderance of dysplastic trabeculae replacing marrow with fibrous tissue. The proximal femur (35%), tibia (20%), face, and ribs (15%) are the most common sites of involvement. Bowing deformities such as the "shepherd's crook" deformity of the proximal femur occur, probably as a result of the biomechanical forces, in a third of patients. Involvement of the facial bones and skull base is often sclerotic and may result in asymmetric thickening called *leontiasis ossea* ("resembling a lion's face"). CT is the most useful modality for imaging the facial region and the remaining skeleton to define extent of involvement; radionuclide bone scanning shows the distribution of lesions most reliably in the polyostotic form by usually producing intense uptake. Use of MRI is adjunctive.

Cherubism presents as bilateral swelling in the jaw, with expansile, multilobular lesions. It is considered a hereditary form of fibrous dysplasia, most often occurring in children less than 4 years of age (Fig. 5-28).

INFECTION

Osteomyelitis
  Acute osteomyelitis
  Subacute osteomyelitis
  Chronic osteomyelitis
Unique Forms of Inflammation
  Septic Arthritis
  Toxic synovitis
  Syphilis
  Rubella

Osteomyelitis

Bones and joints can become infected through three routes: from the bloodstream (most common), from a contiguous site of infection, or by infected foreign material penetrating into these structures.

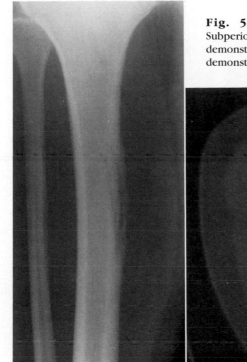
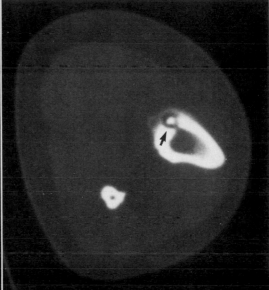

A

B

Fig. 5-29   Acute osteomyelitis.   A, Subperiosteal resorption and periosteal elevation demonstrated in the tibial metadiaphysis. **B,** CT demonstrates a sequestrum (*arrow*).

Osteomyelitis is primarily a disease of infants and children. Its origin is hematogenous seeding, and it may develop from a transient, asymptomatic bacteremia. Spread from adjacent structures or puncture wounds constitutes other routes of infection. There are three classic forms of osteomyelitis: acute, subacute, and chronic.

Acute osteomyelitis   Acute hematogenous osteomyelitis affects primarily the metaphyses. Blood-borne organisms flourish in the large venous sinusoids (terminal capillary loops) within the intramedullary portion of the metaphysis. Spread may occur through the transphyseal vessels to the physis, epiphysis, and joints. However, since transphyseal vessels disappear after 18 months of age, transphyseal spread is unlikely in children more than 18 months of age. The inflammatory response, exudate, and resultant increased intraosseous pressure cause stasis of blood flow and thrombosis that then may develop in bone necrosis and bone resorption. A *sequestrum* is a piece of necrotic bone within the inflammatory process, whereas periosteal new bone formation around dead bone constitutes the *involucrum*, which may contain an exit to the skin, a *cloaca*. Today an involucrum and/or sequestrum is seldom seen with proper use of antibiotic therapy. More than three fourths of cases of osteomyelitis involve the long bones, with the faster growing and largest metaphyses (wrist, humerus, knee) usually affected first. Flat bones (e.g., ilium, vertebrae, calcaneus) are involved in 25%. One third of all cases of osteomyelitis occur in the first 2 years of life, more commonly in boys than girls (2:1). The most common organism is *Staphylococcus aureus* (85%), followed by group B β-hemolytic streptococcus. The ESR is always elevated, whereas the white blood count (WBC) and blood culture results are positive in only 50%. Conventional radiographic findings should never be used to exclude acute osteomyelitis in a patient with fewer than 10 days of symptoms.

Deep soft tissue swelling may be seen within days after onset of infection. Destructive bone changes do not occur until 10 to 14 days after the onset of infection and consist of subperiosteal resorption, creating radiolucencies within cortical bone, which may progress to irregular destruction with periosteal new bone formation (Fig. 5-29). This process is caused by the bony trabeculae withstanding the soft tissue swelling from infection. The increased intraosseous pressure is then relieved through the haversian canals of the cortex and exits to the subperiosteal space. During the first 2 to 3 days of symptoms, radionuclide imaging is particularly useful in showing this well-defined focus of increased radioactivity on the dynamic perfusion, with early blood pool and delayed images

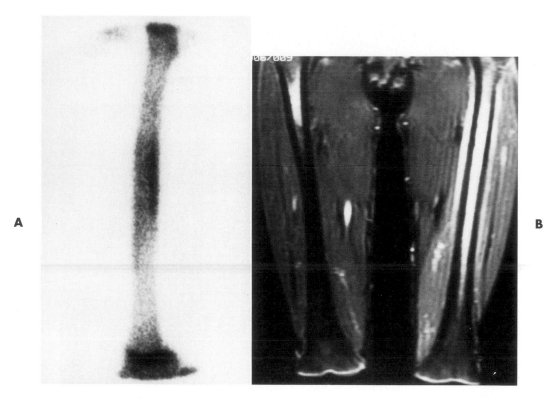

Fig. 5-30 Acute osteomyelitis. A, Radionuclide imaging demonstrates area of increased uptake in left femoral diaphysis. **B**, MRI better illustrates extent of marrow involvement and soft tissue edema.

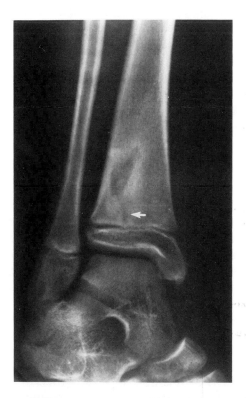

Fig. 5-31 Subacute osteomyelitis. Brodie abscess extending to the growth plate (*arrow*) of the distal tibia.

corresponding to the area of hyperemia. Over 90% sensitivity and specificity can be expected, although experience in pediatric bone scanning is mandatory. On occasion, the use of gallium citrate (Ga 67) or indium-111 labeled leukocyte scans increases the sensitivity and specificity. Cross-sectional imaging modalities such as US may confirm periosteal elevation in the first few days; MRI and to a lesser degree CT can detect marrow (T2) and cortex alterations caused by edema and destruction after 10 days (Fig. 5-30). A sequestration is shown well by CT (see Fig. 5-29).

The differential diagnosis, as in subacute osteomyelitis, may include Ewing sarcoma, metastatic neuroblastoma, leukemia, and EG.

Subacute osteomyelitis Subacute osteomyelitis is more insidious in presentation (2 weeks of symptoms) and more classic on conventional radiographs: single or laminated periosteal new bone formation or a Brodie abscess in the metaphysis abutting the growth plate, with well-defined dense margins seen most commonly in the tibia and femur (Fig. 5-31). CT and MRI may delineate the extent of these findings exquisitely but are not really necessary.

Chronic osteomyelitis Chronic osteomyelitis, a continuous infection of a low-grade type or of a recurrent type, is characterized by predominantly bony scle-

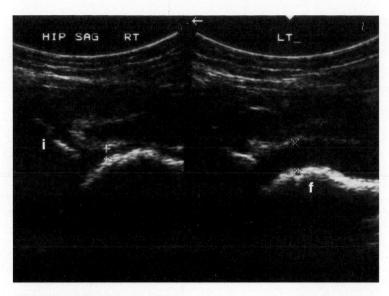

Fig. 5-32 Hip effusion (*markers*) demonstrated on coronal US on the left side (i, iliac wing; f, femoral neck).

rosis, periosteal new bone formation, and the presence of a few sequestra and/or draining sinuses. It is very uncommon in children. CT or MRI defines the extent better than conventional radiographs. If the new bone formation is considerable and mimics an osteoid osteoma, the imaging findings are known as *Garré sclerosing osteomyelitis*, which is caused by multiple small foci of repeated infarction, resulting in new bone formation.

Unique Forms of Inflammation

Septic arthritis Septic arthritis frequently is encountered in the neonate, often in the intensive care unit, and is caused by secondary joint involvement through vascular channels that cross the growth plate. It most often is seen in the shoulder or hips, followed by the knee, elbow, and ankle. Multifocal involvement is common, with the hip the most frequent site (60%). *Haemophilus influenzae* is the most likely causative organism in children less than age 2 years; after that age *S. aureus* is the most common organism. Imaging findings may include joint effusion and apparent dislocation. In the hip avascular necrosis may occur as a result of increased joint pressure compressing the vascular supply to the femoral head. Demineralization, destruction, and subsequent remodeling are rare late sequellae.

Toxic synovitis Toxic (transient) synovitis (irritable hip) consists of pain, a limp, and/or spasm in children less than age 10 years, with a male predominance. Although increased joint fluid is present, a causative organism is seldom if ever found. A recent viral illness often is noted.

Radiographs of the hips are usually normal. Any effusion (e.g., inflammatory, hemarthrosis, or juvenile rheumatoid arthritis) can increase the teardrop-femoral head distance. A difference of more than 1 mm from side to side is considered significant to indicate the presence of an effusion. US is much more sensitive for imaging joint effusions (Fig. 5-32). Radionuclide imaging may show increased periarticular activity or if vascular compression has occurred, a photopenic femoral head area. Neither imaging modality is specific for synovitis.

Syphilis Caused by transplacental spread of *Treponema pallidum* in the second or third trimester, syphilis can cause a skin rash, anemia, hepatosplenomegaly, ascites, and nephrotic syndrome in the infected infant. Because the skeletal manifestations (eventually present in 80% of patients) may take up to 2 months to manifest themselves, diagnosis may be delayed. It is rare today. A metaphyseal lucent band (metaphysitis) is directly subjacent to a dense band in the subphyseal region. Focal areas of lytic destruction may occur in the diaphyses (Fig. 5-33). If the bilateral proximal and medial metaphyseal destruction is present, it is known as the (other) *Wimberger* sign (see "scurvy"). This destructive lesion is also seen in infants with bacterial osteomyelitis and hyperparathyroidism. There may be pathologic fractures and abundant periosteal new bone formation, and in the cranium and flat bones lytic lesions may occur. With specific therapy, most lesions heal.

Rubella Maternal infection with rubella during the first half of pregnancy results in intrauterine growth retardation, cataracts, deafness, hepatosplenomegaly, cardiovascular lesions, and skeletal changes in approxi-

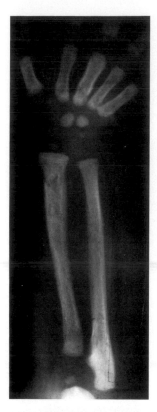

Fig. 5-33 Syphilis. Destructive metadiaphysitis in an infant's radius and metacarpals.

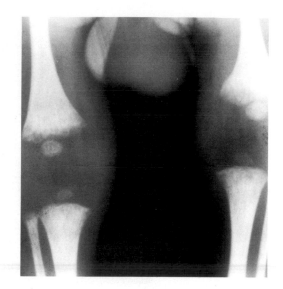

Fig. 5-34 Rubella. Celery-stalk appearance of distal femoral and proximal tibial metaphyses.

mately half of the infants born to these women. Conventional radiographs may demonstrate abnormal metaphyses and show the classic "celery stalk" appearance of the metaphyses of long bones, particularly around the knee (Fig. 5-34). All the (toxoplasmosis, rubella, cytomegalovirus, herpes, and syphilis (TORCHS) entities should be included in the differential possibilities. Periosteal new bone formation is rare except in patients with syphilis. Most changes are trophic and heal by 3 to 6 months of life. Skeletal maturation often is delayed.

AGGRESSIVE BONE LESIONS

Osteosarcoma
Ewing Sarcoma
Primitive Neuroectodermal Tumor
Chondrosarcoma
Metastatic Lesions
    Leukemia
    Lymphoma
        Non-Hodgkin lymphoma
        Hodgkin lymphoma
    Rhabdomyosarcoma

Osteosarcoma

Osteosarcoma is the most common primary malignant neoplasm of bone that occurs in children and young adults and accounts for 60% of malignant bone lesions in the first two decades of life. Boys outnumber girls. The lesion appears in children 10 to 25 years of age and usually is located in the metaphysis of a long bone (80%), especially around the knee joint (65%). There are three subgroups of osteosarcoma: osteoid producers (50%); chondroblastic (25%); and fibroblastic (25%). Pain and swelling of the affected area are the common clinical findings. Conventional radiographic findings include an aggressive mixed lytic and sclerotic, and eccentric metaphyseal lesion that penetrates the cortex and is accompanied by "sunburst" periosteal new bone formation that may be flocculent. A Codman triangle may be present. Multicentric or metachronous (skip) lesions occur in up to 10% of these children. MRI defines bone marrow and soft tissue extent exquisitely both before and after therapy (Fig. 5-35). Metastatic lesions are noted most commonly in the lung on CT and may ossify; they are present in 10% to 20% of patients at presentation. Radionuclide scintigraphy has a diminished role in the presence of CT and MRI and does not reliably detect skip lesions. Treatment includes preoperative and/or postoperative chemotherapy, resection, and allograft replacement. Overall, the probability of 5 years' survival is 70% with absence of metastatic disease.

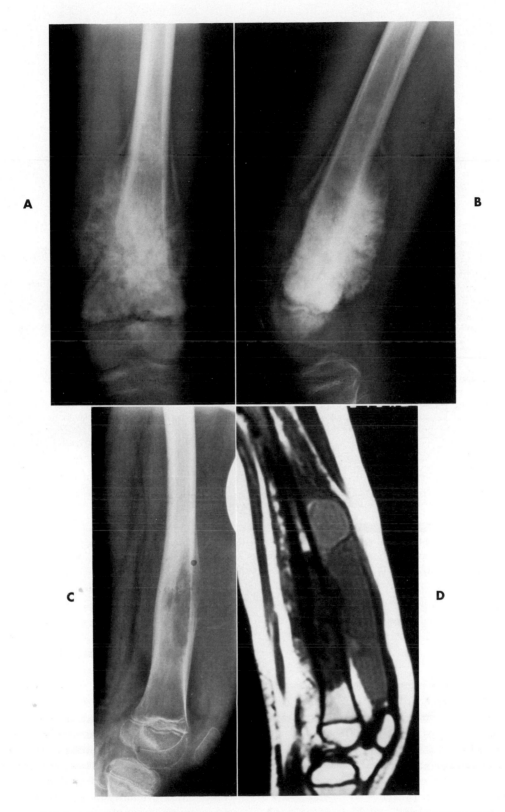

Fig. 5-35 Osteosarcoma (OSA). A, B, Conventional radiographs of a classic bone-forming tumor with sunburst periosteal new bone formation and elevation of the femur. **C,** Conventional radiograph of a lytic OSA of the distal femur. **D,** MRI exquisitely delineates the marrow and soft tissue extent.

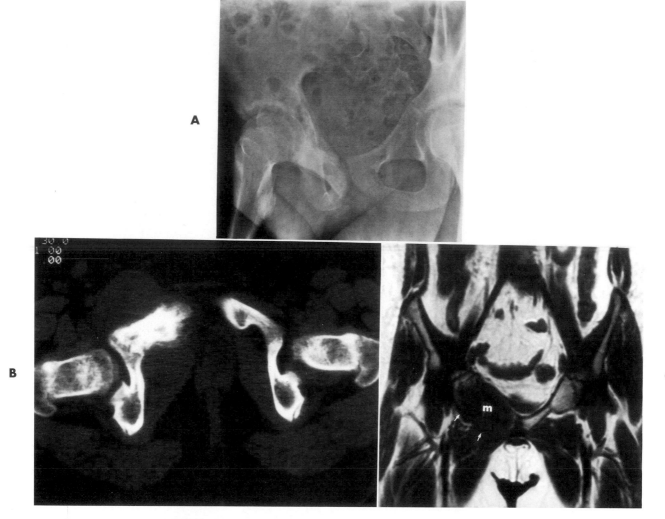

Fig. 5-36 **Ewing sarcoma.** **A,** Conventional pelvic radiograph demonstrates an inhomogeneous, sclerotic, and slightly expansile lesion of the acetabulum with periosteal new bone formation. **B,** CT demonstrates the bony involvement and soft tissue extent in the axial plane. **C,** T1 MRI in the axial plane confirms the CT findings (*m,* mass; *arrows*).

Ewing Sarcoma

Ewing sarcoma affects a somewhat younger age group than osteosarcoma and is more common in males (2:1). The tumor is rare in African-American and Asian populations and in patients over 30 years old. It is the most common bone lesion in the first decade and second to osteosarcoma in the second decade and rarely occurs before 5 years of age. Peak incidence is at 15 years of age. The patient presents with pain, fever, and leukocytosis. Long bones (femur) are primarily affected, followed by the spine and ribs, and 25% occur in the pelvis. On conventional radiographs this diaphyseal lesion is characteristically permeative, with poorly defined margins. There may be periosteal new bone formation with an "onion skin" appearance. CT and MRI clearly delineate the often very large soft tissue component, especially in the more commonly sclerotic lesions in the flat bones of the pelvis and thoracic cage (Fig. 5-36). Bone scintigraphy is useful for the early detection of the bone metastases common in children with Ewing sarcoma. Metastatic lesions are seen in the lungs, skeletal system, and lymph nodes and are present in 15% to 25% of children at presentation. Treatment is primarily by radiotherapy and chemotherapy, sometimes combined with resection. The 5-year survival rate approaches 50%.

Differential diagnosis includes eosinophilic granuloma, non-Hodgkin lymphoma, leukemia, and osteomyelitism (see box).

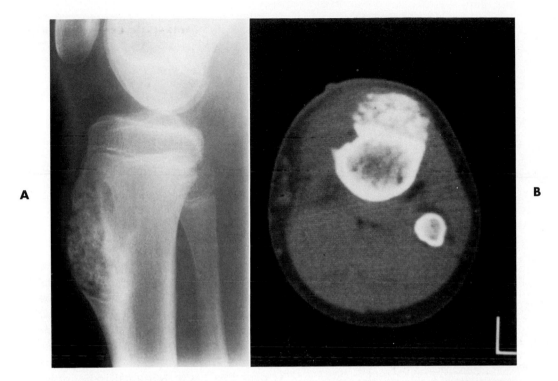

Fig. 5-37 Chondrosarcoma. **A**, Lateral radiograph of proximal tibia reveals an expansile lesion with popcorn calcification in the region of the tibial tubercle. **B**, CT confirms extent and popcornlike calcification.

Primitive Neuroectodermal Tumor

Clinically similar to Ewing sarcoma, primitive neuroectodermal tumors (PNETs) are small round cell tumors likely neural in origin. A highly malignant tumor, a PNET is located most often in the thoracopulmonary region and has been called an *Askin tumor*. In the thorax there is often an associated pleural effusion and a rapidly enlarging soft tissue mass (see Fig. 2-13). CT defines its extent well. If there is no tumor spread at the time of diagnosis, the survival rate is approximately 50%.

Chondrosarcoma

Extremely rare in the pediatric age group, chondrosarcoma, a tumor of cartilaginous origin, is characterized by slow growth and progression, and it may present initially as a very large lesion. If primary (central), its location might be metaphyseal in the femur, ribs, and humerus and in the pelvis, but the lesion more commonly is diaphyseal. Secondary (peripheral) chondrosarcoma in a preexisting benign cartilaginous lesion, especially multiple enchondromatosis or osteochondromatosis, and after radiation therapy more commonly occurs in flat bones. The clinical presentation often is that of pain and interval growth and swelling of

<table>
<tr><td>**Differential Diagnosis of Irregular Metaphyseal Lucency**</td></tr>
<tr><td>Leukemia/lymphoma
Metastatic neuroblastoma
Trauma/stress
Eosinophilic granuloma
Syphilis
Ewing sarcoma (PNET)</td></tr>
</table>

the lesion. Conventional radiographs may show the typical "popcorn" or "cumulus cloud" type of calcification, again seen better on CT or MRI with better delineation of the extent (Fig. 5-37). These lesions are radioresistant, and treatment consists of wide excision.

Metastatic Lesions (see box on p.176)

Leukemia Leukemia is the most common childhood cancer, with 80% the acute lymphoblastic type (ALL). The peak age incidence is 2 to 5 years. Bone and joint pain is a common clinical finding, and there may be tenderness and swelling of the extremities. More than half of patients have skeletal findings classically consisting of metaphyseal lucent bands, osteolytic lesions, and periosteal new bone formation in association with gen-

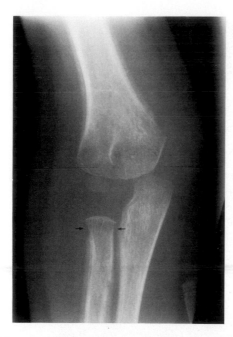

Fig. 5-38 Acute lymphocytic leukemia. AP radiograph of elbow demonstrates the metaphyseal lucent band as part of moth-eaten appearance of the proximal radius (*arrows*). There is periosteal new bone formation of all the visualized bones.

eralized demineralization (Fig. 5-38). MRI exquisitely delineates the low-signal cellular infiltrate of leukemia/lymphoma (or metastatic neuroblastoma) contrasting with the high signal of the normal fatty marrow on T1-weighted images. The definite diagnosis is made by bone marrow aspiration. A chloroma is an extramedullary manifestation of leukemia in which leukemic cell aggregates are noted in the soft tissue, such as the prevertebral region in the neck.

Lymphoma There is no distinct skeletal appearance of lymphoma.

Non-Hodgkin lymphoma A child with non-Hodgkin lymphoma rarely has bone lesions as the only manifestation. As such, the lesions are not characteristic and may mimic those of leukemia, neuroblastoma, eosinophilic granuloma, and Ewing sarcoma. Permeative lesions are usually seen, vertebra plana may occur, and periosteal new bone formation, if present, is minimal.

Hodgkin lymphoma Radiographic findings in a child with Hodgkin disease do not differ significantly from those with non-Hodgkin lymphoma. Vertebral involvement usually, as in adults, manifests as an ivory vertebra; skeletal lesions may be secondary to adjacent nodal enlargement.

Rhabdomyosarcoma Rhabdomyosarcoma is the most common soft tissue sarcoma in children, with one third occurring in the head and neck, one third in the

genitourinary tract, and one third in the bony skeleton. There are two types. The *embryonal* type is the most common, and the *alveolar* type shows slightly more mature muscle cells and more often involves the extremities. Cytologic classification seems to have more bearing on prognosis: anaplastic, monomorphous round cell, and mixed types have been described. Conventional radiographs may show an indistinct soft tissue mass with adjacent bone erosion, which is seen better on CT and MRI. Metastatic disease occurs primarily to the lung and regional lymph nodes (15%).

Metastatic Lesions to Bone
Lymphoma/leukemia
Neuroblastoma
Wilms tumor
Retinoblastoma
Medulloblastoma
Ewing sarcoma or multicentric (metachronous) osteosarcoma
Rhabdomyosarcoma

Imaging: Bone scintigraphy is more sensitive than MRI, which is more sensitive than conventional radiography.

BENIGN AND CYSTIC BONE LESIONS

Solitary, Unicameral, or Simple Bone Cysts
Aneurysmal Bone Cyst
Benign Fibrous Cortical Defect
Chondroblastoma
Chondromyxoid Fibroma
Desmoplastic Fibroma
Osteoid Osteoma
Hemangioma
Giant Cell Tumor

Solitary, Unicameral, or Simple Bone Cysts

Solitary, unicameral, or simple bone cysts, relatively common bone lesions, usually are found in the proximal metaphysis of the humerus and femur (80%) and contain clear, yellow fluid. They occur most commonly in patients 2 to 20 years old, with boys outnumbering girls 3:1. Radiographically (Fig. 5-39), they appear as well-demarcated, central lucent lesions that may be mildly expansile or contain septae, and they occasionally are complicated by a pathologic fracture. Like fibrous cortical defects, they gradually disappear and are seldom seen in adulthood. As a result of a pathologic fracture, a "fallen fragment" may be noted and will

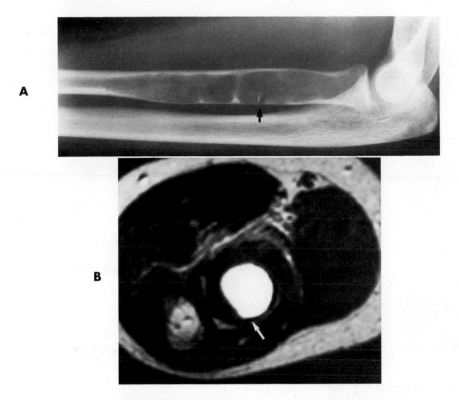

Fig. 5-39 Unicameral bone cyst. Mildly expansile lytic lesion of the proximal radius (**A**) with a fallen fragment (*arrow*). **B**, MRI confirms cystic nature and the fluid-fluid level (*arrow*).

be located in the most dependent portion of the lesion. CT findings are comparable; MRI demonstrates the cyst contents with a uniformly high T2 signal. If for mechanical reasons treatment is necessary, it consists of curettage and packing with bone chips. Intracavitary steroid or methylmethacrylate injection has also had success, but in such cases there is a 20% recurrence rate of the cyst.

Aneurysmal Bone Cysts

Although once considered a giant cell variant, aneurysmal bone cysts (ABCs) are cavernous, blood-filled spaces most often seen in the metaphyses of tubular bones and in the posterior elements of the vertebral column. Eighty percent of them occur in patients younger than 20 years of age. They are located eccentrically, are expansile, and are considered posttraumatic or reactive lesions. Expansion may break through the cortex, with reactive periosteal new bone formation suggesting an aggressive lesion. In one third of these patients CT and MRI reveal a fluid-fluid level, which is highly suggestive but not diagnostic of an aneurysmal bone cyst (Fig. 5-40). It is the only bone tumor named after its radiographic appearance and is slightly more common in girls than boys. Treatment is resection or curettage.

Benign Fibrous Cortical Defect (Nonossifying Fibroma)

Benign, asymptomatic lesions, fibromas, derive from fibrous tissue and are metaphyseal or diaphyseal in location in the major long bones. Boys outnumber girls (1.6:1) with this lesion. The differentiation between these lesions primarily is based on age and size of lesion, but pathologically they are identical. Fibrous cortical defects are usually less than 2 cm and are well-defined, rounded lesions in the cortex that disappear during the teenage years. Nonossifying fibromas are larger than 2 cm, are most often seen in the distal tibia, and may present with a pathologic fracture. They do not grow or spread, and they regress spontaneously with age. Multiple nonossifying fibromas may be found in association with NF (see Fig. 5-25).

Chondroblastoma

Uncommon, chondroblastoma (Codman tumor) is usually seen in teenagers, with boys outnumbering girls (1.7:1). The proximal humerus, tibia, and distal femur are commonly involved; 50% are located around the knee. Conventional radiographs show a well-defined lytic, rounded lesion located in an epiphysis, sesamoid bone, or an apophysis (Fig. 5-41). There may be carti-

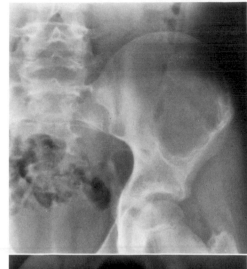

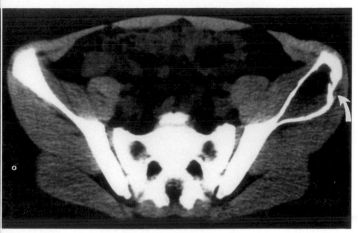

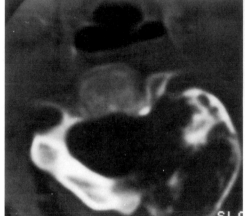

Fig. 5-40 **A,** Frontal radiograph of pelvis demonstrates a lucent, well-demarcated left iliac lesion with minimal internal architecture. **B,** Axial CT demonstrates both a fluid-fluid level within the expansile left iliac lesion and the pathologic fracture (*arrow*). **C,** Axial CT demonstrates an aneurysmal bone cyst of the posterior elements of C5.

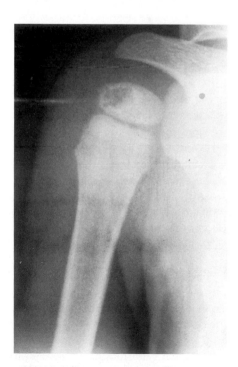

Fig. 5-41 **Chondroblastoma.** Well-demarcated, lytic, round epiphyseal lesion.

laginous calcification within it, which often is seen better with CT. The differential diagnosis includes osteomyelitis (especially TB), eosinophilic granuloma, and fibrous dysplasia.

Chondromyxoid Fibroma

This least common benign cartilaginous tumor, chondromyxoid fibroma is most often seen in the metaphyseal region of long bones, with approximately one half in the proximal tibia. It occurs in the teenage years. The scalloped, oval, and lytic eccentric lesions with chondroid flecks of calcification are seen best on CT. MRI defines the extent of the lesion and its chondromyxoid contents (Fig. 5-42). Malignant transformation has been described.

Desmoplastic Fibroma

Desmoplastic fibroma is a member of the family of fibromatosis lesions that are all rare, purely lytic lesions without matrix, causing pain and swelling in the second decade with equal frequency in boys and girls. It may be locally aggressive, and wide resection is necessary for cure (Fig. 5-43).

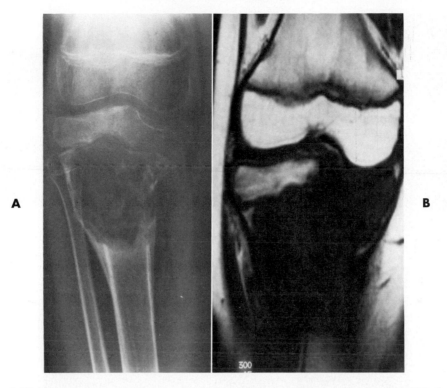

Fig. 5-42 Chondromyxoid fibroma. A, Slightly expansile metaphyseal lesion with chondroid flecks and scalloping. **B**, MRI reveals epiphyseal extension of the lesion.

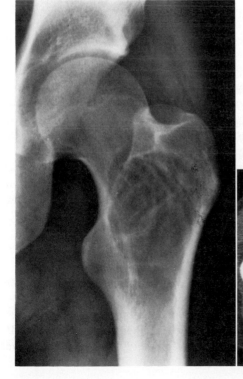

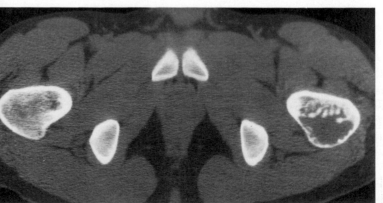

Fig. 5-43 Desmoplastic fibroma. A, Conventional radiographic appearance of an intertrochanteric well-defined lytic lesion. **B**, CT confirms no bony breakthrough or soft tissue extension.

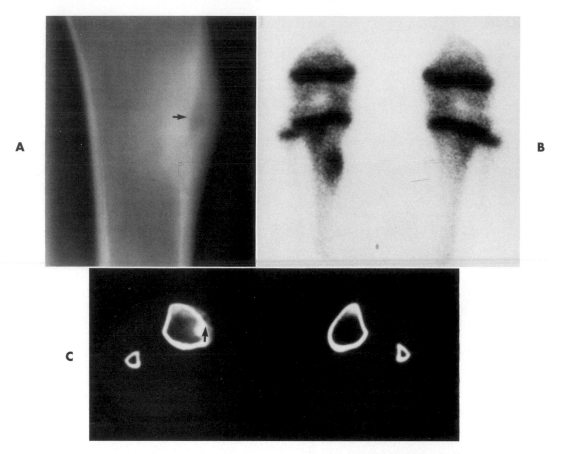

Fig. 5-44 Osteoid osteoma. A, Conventional tomography demonstrates cortical thickening and a lucent nidus (*arrow*). **B,** Radionuclide bone scan confirms increased uptake. **C,** Axial CT delineates the nidus as well in the right proximal tibia (*arrow*).

Osteoid Osteoma

Osteoid osteoma, a common bone-forming lesion occurs in children over age 3 years (mainly 10 to 20 years of age) and occurs twice as often in boys as in girls. The classic clinical presentation consists of pain, characteristically worse at night and relieved by aspirin in three fourths of patients. The majority of lesions are seen in the femur and tibia and the posterior elements of the vertebral column. The nidus is usually less than 1 cm, is usually lucent but may calcify, and is surrounded by an exuberant zone of reactive sclerosis. This dense sclerosis may obscure the nidus, best demonstrated on CT; MRI is less useful. Radionuclide scintigraphy shows a well-circumscribed area of intense uptake (Fig. 5-44). The differential diagnosis includes a healing stress fracture or chronic osteomyelitis. Surgery is the treatment of choice, with confirmative imaging of the excised specimen a necessity.

Much less common but with the same age and gender incidence, as well as microscopic and radiographic appearance, is the giant osteoid osteoma, or osteoblastoma. There are less reactive sclerosis and more expansion of the lesion, and the nidus is larger than 2 cm.

Hemangioma

Hemangiomas are the most common benign tumors in infancy and children and occur commonly in the skin and subcutaneous tissues. The two main forms include cavernous hemangiomas (conventional radiographs may show calcified phleboliths) and capillary hemangiomas, masses of capillaries that, as opposed to cavernous hemangiomas, have a connection to the systemic circulation. These lesions may also be categorized according to the site of origin: cutaneous, intramuscular, and synovial. They may be summarized as venous or arteriovenous hemangiomas and angiomatoses. This diffuse involvement in a neonate with hemangiomatosis characteristically involves one extremity that often is enlarged because of hyperemia. The Klippel-Trenaunay syndrome is characterized by limb hypertrophy with subcutaneous hemangiomas; Kasabach-Merritt syndrome is the association of cavernous hemangiomas and disseminated intravascular coagulation (DIC). Intraosseous hemangiomas are rare and more commonly are found in the spine and skull. Prominent bony trabeculation, represented in vertebral bodies by vertical, prominent, dense trabeculation with mild expansion, is the typical radiographic finding. Malignant entities include (lymph) angiosarcoma and an intermediate variant, hemangioendothelioma.

Capillary hemangiomas range from the juvenile form (strawberry nevus in 1:22 live births) to deep skeletal involvement, most commonly found in the lower extremity.

The synovial variant is rare, most often occurring in the knee. US with color-flow Doppler imaging may be useful. MRI usually has distinctive flow features.

Giant Cell Tumor

Giant cell tumors (osteoclastomas) are very rarely seen before closure of the growth plate. Only 2% of giant cell tumors occur in patients less than age 15 years. Radiographically, they resemble aneurysmal bone cysts and seldom cause symptoms. There is an equal gender incidence, and the lesion is rare in African-Americans. Osteoclastic overactivity resulting in essentially fibrous lesions is considered its cause. Treatment consists of curettage and packing with methylmethacrylate cement. There is a 10% to 15% recurrence rate. A pathologic fracture occurs in up to one third of patients.

TRAUMA

Pediatric Fractures
    Growth plate fractures
    Upper-extremity fractures
        Clavicle
        Humerus
        Elbow
    Lower-extremity fractures
        Slipped capital femoral epiphysis
        Toddler's fracture
        Stress fracture
Osteochondroses
    Osteochondritis dissecans
    Legg-Calvé-Perthes disease
Nonaccidental Trauma (Trauma X; Child Abuse)
Birth Trauma

Pediatric Fractures

The *pattern* of fractures in the pediatric population depends on the age of the child, the stage of the child's development, and the knowledge that both dislocations and ligamentous injuries are uncommon in children. There are also age-related differences in the composition of the bones and soft tissues, including a relatively stronger and thicker periosteum and stronger but slightly more lax ligaments. In addition, in children the

haversian canals comprise more of the cortical bone than in adults; thus children have more incomplete fractures than adults because the forces can be absorbed more easily. The weakest point in the bony structure is the physis, or growth plate. Finally, the type of fracture often is influenced by the kind of activity in which the child of a certain age is engaged (e.g., toddler's fractures seldom occur after age 2 years; shoulder dislocation and/or clavicular fracture are characteristic of birth trauma).

The degree of *fracture healing* is also an important adjunct in the correct evaluation of pediatric fractures. There are three stages: the *inflammatory* stage, with an acute hematoma; the *callus* formation stage; and finally the *reparative* stage when mature bone replaces the fibrocartilage and immature bone bridging the fracture site. The callus formation stage can be radiographically identified by 10 to 14 days after the fracture; by 6 weeks, well-organized bone is usually present. The amount of callus formation depends on the fracture site, the degree of displacement, and on the degree of immobilization during healing. These same factors also directly affect the amount of remodeling that can be achieved in the healing process. The younger the child, the greater is the potential for remodeling. Internal fixation is rarely necessary, for nonunion seldom occurs. Thus the most important complications of pediatric fractures are caused by growth disturbances that can result when the fracture involves the growth plate. Resultant bony bridging of the growth plate is exquisitely delineated on MRI and has influenced therapy positively.

Depending on the child's age, different *fracture mechanisms* are identified in children. In infants and toddlers incomplete fractures can result in a *bowing* (plastic) type, with no obvious break in the cortex; a *greenstick* fracture, which is a fracture on the convex side of the cortex but not on the concave side; or a *buckle* fracture, which can occur on the opposite side of the greenstick fracture. This buckling is also known as a torus (little hill) fracture (Fig. 5-45).

Growth plate fractures Fractures involving the growth plate reflect the relative weakness of the growth plate cartilage, the greater laxity and strength of the ligaments, and the tight attachment of the periosteum. There are four zones to the growth plate: aligned from the epiphysis to the metaphysis is the germinal zone; the proliferating zone; the hypertrophic zone; and the zone of provisional calcification. The relative abundance of collagen matrix in the germinal and proliferating zones and the calcium deposition in the zone of provisional calcification result in the hypertrophic zone's being the relative weakest zone. It is here that fractures occur. The Salter-Harris classification of epiphyseal complex fractures recognizes at least

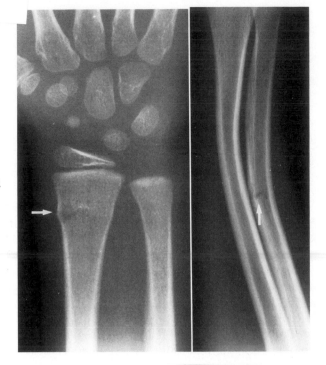

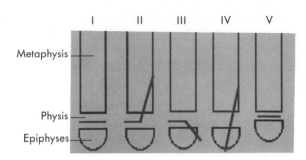

Fig. 5-46 Schematic diagram of the Salter-Harris classification.

B

Fig. 5-45 A, Torus fracture resembling a "little hill" (*arrow*). **B,** Bowing fracture of the radius and greenstick fracture of the ulna (*arrow*).

five types, I through V. In type I the fracture passes through the growth plate only, and it is more common in children less than 5 years old. In type II the fracture line exits through the metaphysis. Salter II fractures account for approximately 70% of all fractures involving the growth plate and is most commonly seen in the distal radius and tibia. In type III (10%) the fracture line extends through the epiphysis, is thus intraarticular, and most often affects the ankle and knee and the medial epicondyle of the humerus. Type IV (10%) occurs when the fracture extends through both the metaphysis and the epiphysis and most often affects the lateral condyle of the humerus. Type V, rare (1%), involves a crush of the growth plate and may lead to premature fusion. Salter types I and II have an excellent result if properly treated as does type III if properly reduced. Types IV and V may result in growth deformity and often need open reduction and/or internal fixation (Fig. 5-46).

Unique apophysis fractures include Osgood-Schlatter disease and Sinding-Larson-Johansson disease.

Osgood-Schlatter "disease" In a teenager with Osgood-Schlatter disease, clinically characterized by tenderness over the tibial tubercle, overuse and repeated trauma to the infrapatellar tendon insertion site may lead to tearing of the infrapatellar tendon fibers without evidence of inflammation, avascular necrosis, or osteochondritis. The incidence in teenage boys outnumbers

that in girls (3:1), and 30% are bilaterally affected. Conventional radiographs support the diagnosis if there is obliteration of the posterior aspect of the infrapatellar tendon bordering Hoffa's infrapatellar fat-pad as a result of edema. Fragmentation and/or swelling of the anterior tibial tubercle alone is not sufficient for the radiographic diagnosis (Fig. 5-47). Rest, physiotherapy, and antiinflammatory medications usually comprise the treatment of choice. The differential diagnostic possibilities are infection, chondrosarcoma (rare), and stress fractures.

Sinding-Larson-Johansson "disease" Similar fragmentation changes at the lower margin of the patella are seen at the tendinous insertion site. A similar avulsive mechanism is involved, usually in active children, and therapy is identical to that for Osgood-Schlatter disease.

Upper-extremity fractures Two thirds of fractures of the *clavicle* occur in children less than age 10 years. The most common involve the middle third; acromioclavicular separations are rare. The surgical neck of the *humerus* is the site of the second most common injury, and the appearance of the growth plate at two "levels," due to the "peaked" orientation of the proximal humeral physis, a normal variant, should not be mistaken for a fracture. Midshaft fractures are unusual, but they put the radial nerve and brachial artery at risk. The *elbow* is one of the more common sites of injury and the most difficult area in which to interpret the imaging findings. An effusion most likely indicates a fracture, even if one is not found after a diligent search. The quintessential finding on the lateral view is known as the *fat-pad sign.* Normally, there is fat visible in the anterior, coracoid fossa, whereas the fat in the posterior olecranon fossa is deeply buried and not visible. An effusion will elevate these fat-pads, deforming the anterior fat-pad and allowing visualization of the posterior fat-pad. In younger children a nondisplaced distal humeral (supracondylar) fracture is most common, whereas in older children an occult radial head fracture is more likely (Fig. 5-48).

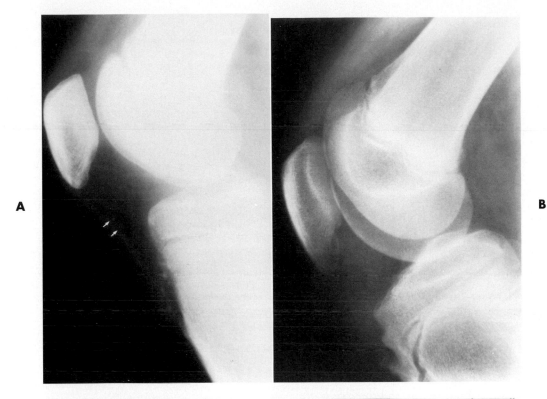

Fig. 5-47 Osgood-Schlatter disease. A, Normal infrapatellar tendon (*arrows*) and normally "fragmented" anterior tibial tubercle. **B,** Obliteration of the infrapatellar tendon—Hoffa's fat-pad interface.

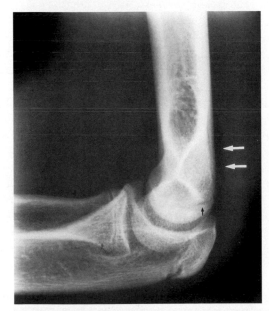

Fig. 5-48 Positive fat-pad sign (*arrows*) indicates the posterior fat-pad in a patient with a nondisplaced distal humeral fracture (*small arrow*).

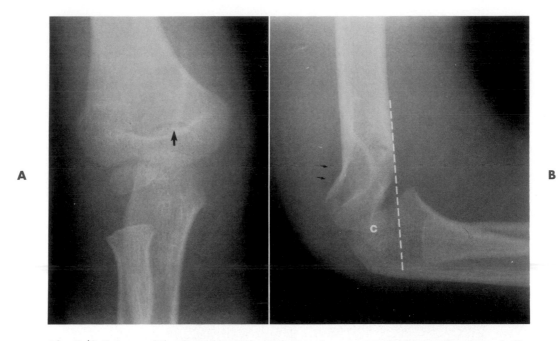

Fig. 5-49 Intracondylar fracture. A, Anterior view demonstrates the fracture line (*arrow*). B, Lateral view demonstrates degree of dislocation. Note location of the capitellum (*c*) posterior to the anterior humeral line (*interrupted line*). A positive fat-pad sign is present also (*arrows*).

More than half of the fractures around the elbow are of the supracondylar variety. To assess the degree of dislocation and determine the subsequent mode of treatment, the *anterior humeral line* is used. A line drawn down the anterior aspect of the shaft of the humerus on a lateral projection should pass through the middle of the ossification center of the capitellum. A line through the center of the radius should do the same. The degree of dislocation—a spectrum from mild avulsion to fractures with posterior dislocation of the elbow—will dictate open or closed reduction (Fig. 5-49).

Avulsion fractures of the medial epicondyle are seen in up to 15% of elbow injuries in children. This fracture is known as a "little leaguer's elbow" because it occurs when the flexor carpi ulnaris tendon pulls off the medial epicondyle. This classically is associated with the snapping of the wrist and/or elbow when throwing a curveball. There is usually significant soft tissue swelling in association (Fig. 5-50). The bony fragment, often still attached to the tendon, may be trapped within the elbow joint, causing pain and/or locking. Internal fixation by pinning the fragment is the treatment of choice.

Traumatic dislocation of the elbow joint is virtually always in a posterior direction. Avulsion of the medial epicondyle is often associated.

In infants the "nursemaid's elbow" results from an adult's pulling the infant's arm. The radial head slips out of its figure-eight ligament and usually is reduced

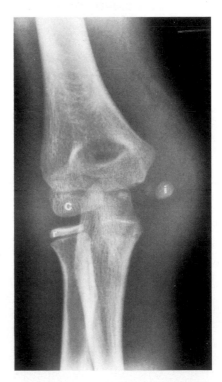

Fig. 5-50 Little leaguer's elbow. Avulsion fracture of the medial epicondyle (*t*) with marked soft tissue swelling (*c*, capitellum).

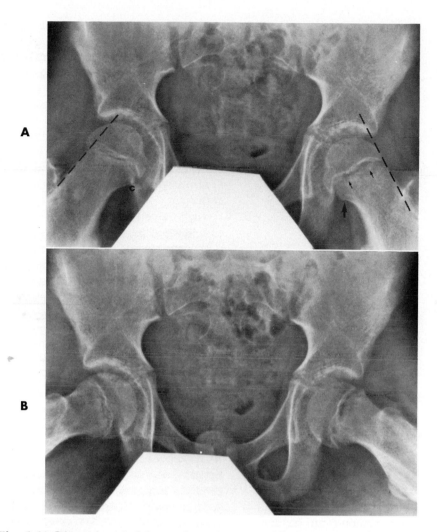

Fig. 5-51 Slipped capital femoral epiphysis. A, AP radiograph reveals a widened physis (*small arrows*) and decreased height of the epiphysis on the left. In addition, there is loss (*large arrow*) of the Capener triangle (*c,* normal double density of the medial metaphysis superimposed on the posterior acetabular rim on right) and an abnormal lateral femoral neck line (normal on right). **B,** Frog lateral view confirms the inferomedial position of the slipped capital femoral epiphysis.

by supination of the forearm and flexion of the elbow. When positioning the child for a radiograph, the radiographer often accomplishes this reduction, thus explaining why radiographs frequently are noncontributory except for an occasional avulsion fracture.

Lower-extremity fractures Common fractures in the lower extremity mostly occur in the hip and the ankle.

Slipped capital femoral epiphysis In children slipped capital femoral epiphysis (SCFE) is a type of Salter I fracture of the proximal femoral growth plate that is relatively common in adolescents who are obese, more likely boys, and African-American. It may be hereditary. Both mechanical and endocrine factors have been implicated as causes. SCFE has also been associated with hypothyroidism, as well as avascular necrosis and chondrolysis. The fracture occurs between the proliferative and hypertrophic zones of

the metaphysis, as opposed to a classic Salter I. As a result of normal muscular forces, the femoral neck moves anteriorly and slightly superolaterally, resulting in rotation of the epiphysis posteriorly and inferomedially (retroversion). Conventional radiographs can show (1) a subtle difference in joint and femoral head symmetry, with the frontal view revealing loss of height of the affected epiphysis; (2) widening of the affected growth plate; and (3) loss of the intersection of the lateral femoral neck line. On the frog lateral view, the widened growth plate and displacement of the femoral head are delineated better. Obtaining both views is mandatory in all cases (Fig. 5-51). Contralateral SCFE occurs in 10% to 15% of patients. Treatment consists of pinning the epiphysis in its normal position, usually after reduction of the ensuing fracture. Controversy exists about whether the contralateral femoral head should be pinned prophylactically.

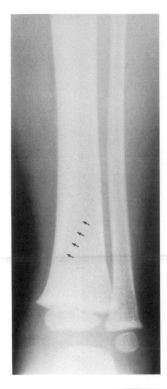

Fig. 5-52 Toddler's fracture. Spiral fracture (*arrows*) of the tibia.

Fractures around the knee are not common, but those of the Salter II variety do occur. Fractures of the patella are uncommon and are transverse or stellate in configuration. A bipartite patella should not be confused with a fracture.

Toddler's fracture   A toddler's fracture is a spiral fracture of the tibia in a child who is starting to walk, thus between the ages of 1 and 2 years. It consists of an undisplaced fracture of the middle to distal tibial shaft (Fig. 5-52). Oblique radiographs may be needed for confirmation. The child usually has a limp and is afebrile, as opposed to a child with toxic synovitis.

Stress fracture   Stress fractures result from subjecting normal bone to abnormal chronic or repetitive stresses. Excessive osteoclastic activity results and has been implicated in explaining the imaging findings. It is seen most commonly in the teenage years. The proximal tibial shaft is the most common location, but the fibula, femur, and the metatarsals are also often involved. The use of a radionuclide bone scan assists the diagnostic process and may increase overall sensitivity. Periosteal elevation can be detected on US.

Osteochondroses

Osteochondritis dissecans   Osteochondritis dissecans most likely has a traumatic origin and predominantly affects teenagers and young adults. Males out-

number females (3:1), and the condition most commonly occurs in the lateral aspect of the medial condyle of the femur, followed by the talus and the elbow. Bilaterality occurs in 25% of cases. The fragment of articular cartilage, with or without some underlying bone, may be floating free in the joint space, causing pain and/or locking. Conventional radiographs are often diagnostic (Fig. 5-53). Whether the covering cartilage is intact can be assessed by arthrography and MRI. If the cartilage covering is intact, surgical intervention is not deemed necessary, and treatment is expectant.

Legg-Calvé-Perthes disease   Legg-Calvé-Perthes disease, idiopathic avascular necrosis of the femoral head, is the most common cause of hip pain in the young child (age 4 to 8 years), but it may cause a limp or knee pain. Bilateral but not symmetric or simultaneous involvement is seen in less than 20% of these children. There may be delayed maturation (<2 SD). Boys outnumber girls (5:1), and the cause is deemed ischemic, although the exact cause is unclear. Classic radiographic findings initially include subchondral fractures, the extent of which can be appreciated better on the frog lateral view. These (micro) fractures then can progress to fragmentation, flattening of the femoral head, and joint space widening (Fig. 5-54). The increase in the joint space medially, often the initial finding, is caused by swelling of the legamentum teres, hypertrophy of the articular cartilage (nourished by synovial fluid), and/or continued growth of unossified cartilage. In approximately 75% of these patients there is slight lateral displacement of the femoral head.

MRI can reveal avascular necrosis, whereas conventional radiographs still appear normal; thus MRI is a much better-suited modality for treatment planning than CT. Bilateral avascular necrosis of the femoral heads is seen in children with multiple epiphyseal dysplasia, Gaucher disease, and sickle cell disease; unilaterally occurring SCFE and chronic dislocation of the hips should be considered as well. The patient's age and pertinent clinical findings are essential components when considering this differential diagnosis.

Nonaccidental Trauma (Trauma X; Child Abuse)

Child abuse traverses all social lines. It is estimated that 1 1/2 million children per year in the United States are abused or neglected and approximately 1000 children die annually as a result of trauma X. Boys and girls are affected equally, and almost all are less than 2 years of age. Imaging plays an important role in determining physical abuse since approximately two thirds of these patients have positive findings, although other types of abuse (i.e., sexual, psychologic) do occur and occasion-

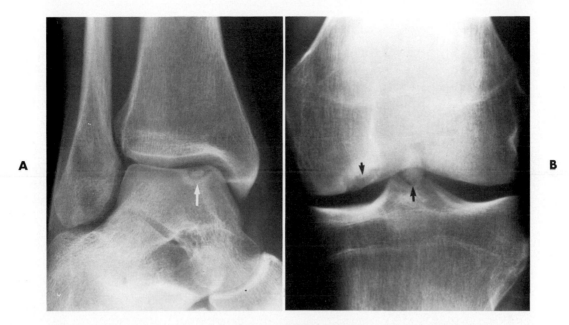

Fig. 5-53 Osteochondritis dissecans. A, Lytic talar dome lesion with a sclerotic margin and a sclerotic nidus (*arrow*). B, Loose, bony fragment in the joint space and the donor site (small *arrow*).

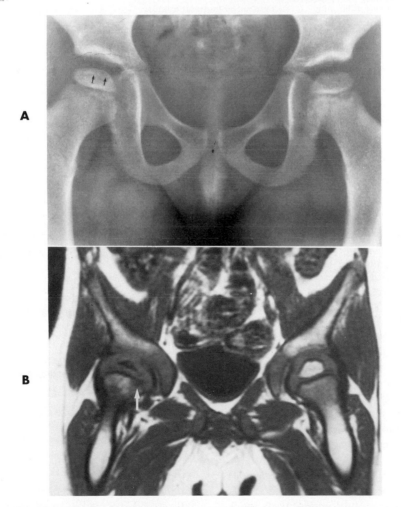

Fig. 5-54 Legg-Calvé-Perthes disease. A, Conventional radiograph demonstrates increased sclerosis of the right femoral epiphysis with a subchondral lucent line (*arrows*). B, MRI shows signal void in the right femoral epiphysis and synovial hypertrophy.

A   **B**   **C**

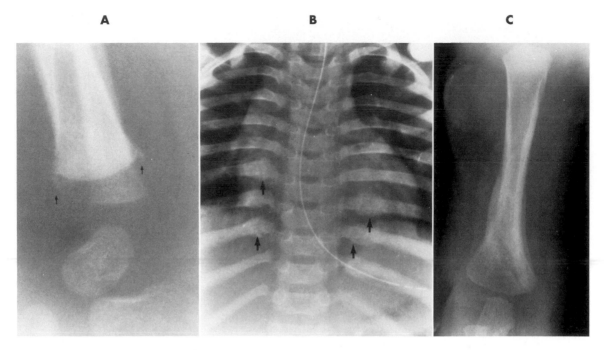

Fig. 5-55 **Nonaccidental trauma.** **A**, Metaphyseal corner fractures (*arrows*). **B**, Posterior rib fractures (*arrows*) bilaterally. **C**, Healing spiral humeral fracture.

ally require pediatric imaging in an adjunctive role. It is the radiologists' legal obligation to report findings compatible with child abuse. For the child less than age 5 years, because it often is difficult to obtain a satisfactory history from the child, a skeletal survey is the screening modality of choice; for an infant less than 2 years old it is mandatory. In the child older than 5 years a skeletal series is of little diagnostic value, and a bone scan is considered the initial study in these circumstances. CT and MRI, particularly in the neuraxis, play complementary imaging roles.

Highly suggestive imaging findings in children with nonaccidental trauma (Fig. 5-55) include the following:

- Metaphyseal corner fractures; "bucket handle" distal femur, proximal and distal humerus fractures
- Fractures in different stages of healing
- Spiral fractures of the femur, humerus, and tibia in infants and toddlers
- Multiple fractures, especially in different stages of healing, and those occurring in "unusual" locations and containing abundant callus as a result of poor immobilization.

In long bones of young children, the bucket handle, or "corner," fracture is considered pathognomonic of child abuse. Periosteal avulsion with microfractures of the growing bone at its metaphyseal insertion that occurs when the child is shaken is considered the causative mechanism. Posterior rib fractures and avulsion fracture of the spinous processes are highly suggestive of abuse, particularly in children less than age 5 years. The same holds true for spiral fractures of long bones in infants less than age 1 year. Metacarpal and metatarsal fractures, fractures of the lateral end of the clavicle, or sternal fractures are similarly rare and should be viewed with suspicion. Cranial CT classically reveals a parietooccipital subdural hematoma, often associated with parenchymal injury (shaken-baby syndrome). The differential diagnosis of the skeletal findings includes OI, congenital syphilis, leukemia, multifocal osteomyelitis, and meningococcemia, but scurvy, Caffey disease, hypervitaminosis A, and prostaglandin therapy in infants should also be considered.

Birth Trauma

Birth trauma occurs in approximately five of every 1000 live births. Skeletal manifestations include clavicular fracture, humeral or femoral fractures, and hip dislocation. Soft tissue deformity of the cranium is a frequent occurrence during the birthing process. The generalized form of cranial deformity caused by subcutaneous edema and possible hematomas is called *caput succedaneum*, which will resorb within a couple of weeks. A localized form is called a *cephalohematoma*, a subperiosteal hematoma that does not cross suture lines because of its containment by the periosteum. It may ossify and result in asymmetry of the skull that may persist for months (see Fig. 6-6). Subgaleal hematomas do cross suture lines and are rare but may also be present. Associated skull fractures are rare, although molding of the skull tables can resemble a depressed fracture.

MISCELLANEOUS CONDITIONS

Developmental Dysplasia of the Hip
Blount Disease
Joints
    Chronic arthritis
    Ankylosing spondylitis

Developmental Dysplasia of the Hip

The femoral head and the acetabulum depend on intimate contact between the two to develop normally. Lack of these normal stress forces can lead to deficient development of the cartilage and/or the bone, resulting in developmental dysplasia of the hip, or congenital dislocation of the hip. Dislocation of the femoral head may be caused by intrauterine forces, the most common one of which is breech presentation. The incidence is 1:200 live births; the dislocation is rare in African-Americans and Chinese. The condition occurs bilaterally in up to 30% of patients. Ligamentous laxity is also a contributing factor, with the laxity increased because of endogenous estrogens in the female infant. This partially explains the female-to-male incidence ratio of 9:1. Ossification of the femoral head usually is apparent by 2 months in girls and by 3 months in boys. Asymmetric ossification of the femoral head may be an indication of subluxation but may also be a normal variant.

US is currently the screening modality of choice to confirm normal anatomy. The depth of the acetabulum and the coverage of the cartilaginous head are visualized better with US than on conventional radiographs, and dynamic evaluation can visualize suspected subluxation. The methods described by Graf and modified by Harcke both have merits; a hybrid of the two methods is favored. Operator dependency is great, and dynamic imaging is mandatory to clarify and identify any abnormality. US is 100% sensitive and highly specific for evaluating the position of the femoral head and the anatomy of the hip joint. The normal US appearance of the hip in the sagittal plane with the hip flexed should resemble a "lollipop," whereas the configuration on the transverse view in the flexed hip should resemble a "seagull" or "rising sun" (Fig. 5-56, A and B). Stress views can dynamically assess the stability of the joint. Correlation of these maneuvers with Barlow sign and Ortolani "click" is disappointing.

Conventional radiographs of the pelvis make use of several lines that assist in assessing whether the femoral heads are normally seated. On the anteroposterior pelvic view, the *horizontal line of Hilgenriner* connects the superior portions of the triradiate cartilage. A *perpendicular line of Perkin* is then drawn from the lateral margin of the ossified rim of the acetabular roof. The femoral head should normally project into the inferior medial quadrant created by these lines. The acetabular angle can then be computed and normally measures between 15 and 30 degrees, with the larger of these values pertaining to the younger neonate. Values greater than 30 degrees suggest dysplasia. The curved line along the under surface of the trocanter and the superior portion of the obturator foramen, Shenton's line, should be normally bilaterally smooth, interrupted on the dislocated side. The lines and measurements should be performed on the anteroposterior view, for the frog lateral view often reduces the dislocation and creates a false negative result (Fig. 5-56, C). Three to five sequential 3-mm thick CT images through the acetabulum are useful for postreduction evaluation of femoral head position, especially postoperatively. MRI is useful if the joint space cartilage needs further assessment.

Blount Disease

Blount disease, a developmental deformity of the proximal tibial epiphysis (osteochondrosis deformans tibiae), can be traumatic in origin and/or a sequella of physiologic bowing. The early onset (*infantile*) form develops in children between the ages of 1 and 3 years when the child begins ambulating. Therefore it is often (80%) bilateral and symmetric. It affects boys and girls equally but is more common in African-Americans. Disordered ossification of the medial portion of the proximal tibial growth plate results in tibia vara. The characteristic radiographic feature shows sloping and medial fragmentation of the epiphyseal center, widening and irregularity of the growth plate, and beaking of the metaphysis. If bridging of the growth plate occurs it may be seen well on MRI (Fig. 5-57). Physiologic bowing of the legs, OI, trauma, infections, and rickets are the main differential diagnostic possibilities.

In children between 7 and 14 years of age there may be sclerosis of the medial growth plate and narrowing, with accompanying widening of the lateral aspect of the growth plate. This condition has been called *late-onset (adolescent) Blount disease*, resulting in similar premature fusion of the medial growth plate and varus deformity.

Joints

Chronic arthritis Inflammation of the joints, or arthritis, is the most important chronic disease of children. When chronic polyarthritis coexists with splenomegaly and lymphadenopathy, it is known as *Still disease*. It is seen in children between 3 and 5 years of age with symptoms of pain and swelling of joints.

Sites of involvement for chronic polyarthritis are

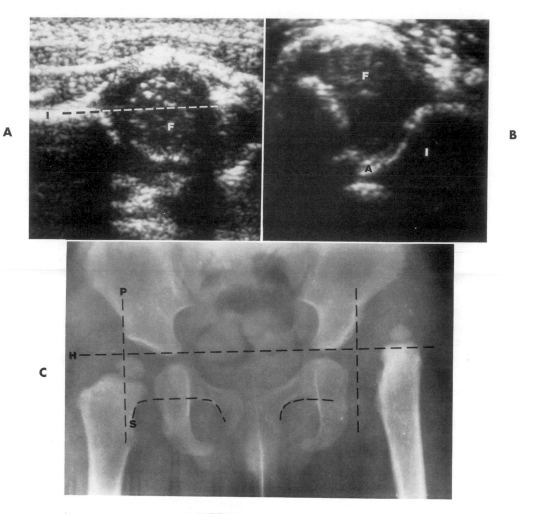

Fig. 5-56 Developmental dysplasia of the hip. Normal US: **A**, Lollipop view, with the iliac wing (*I*) bisecting the femoral head (*F*). **B**, Seagull or rising sun view: (*A*, acetabulum; *F*, femoral head; *I*, ischium). **C**, Conventional radiograph depicting Hilgenreiner (*H*), Perkin (*P*), Shenton's (*S*) lines, and a left hip dislocation.

hands (50%), wrist (70%), feet, and knees (90%). Cervical spine involvement is seen in 2% of both variants. Radiographic findings are identical to those of adult rheumatoid arthritis but lack the symmetric component. They include soft tissue swelling, accelerated bony maturation, periosteal new bone formation, and bony erosions (Fig. 5-58). Joint space narrowing, widening of the intercondylar notch, effusions, and ankylosis of the apophyseal joints may supervene. Skeletal scintigraphy is useful to monitor distribution and progression of the disease. MRI is superior for joint imaging, especially of cartilage depiction and the detection of hemosiderin.

The rheumatoid variants such as psoriatic arthritis, arthritis of inflammatory bowel disease, and Reiter syndrome are rare in children but may be considered in the differential diagnosis.

Ankylosing spondylitis Although the onset of spondylitis occurs in early adulthood, juvenile ankylosing spondylitis in children occurs in boys older than 8 years. Chronic inflammatory changes of the spine and sacroiliac joints resulting in ascending ankylosis and spine deformity are of unknown cause, which is partly genetic (positive result for HLA-B27 in 95% of patients). In the pediatric age group blurring and sclerosis with eventual fusion of the sacroiliac joint are the most common radiographic findings, but syndesmophytes are rare.

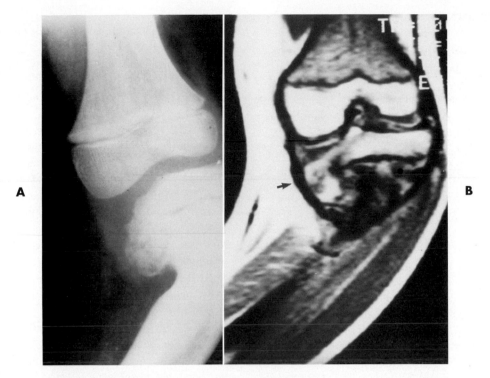

Fig. 5-57 Blount disease. **A,** Sloping and medial fragmentation of the proximal tibial epiphysis. **B,** MRI depicts bony bridge of the growth plate (*arrow*).

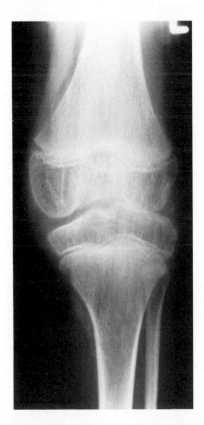

Fig. 5-58 Juvenile rheumatoid arthritis. Joint space narrowing, widening of the intracondylar notch, and epiphyseal overgrowth.

SUGGESTED READINGS
Texts

Kirks DR, editor: *Practical Pediatric Imaging*, Boston, 1991 Little, Brown and Co, pp 263-409.

Kleinman PK: *Diagnostic Imaging of Child Abuse*, Baltimore, 1987, Williams &4 Wilkins.

Ozonoff MB: *Pediatric Orthopedic Radiology*, Philadelphia, 1992, WB Saunders.

Reed MH, editor: *Pediatric Skeletal Radiology*, Baltimore, 1992, Williams & Wilkins.

Silverman FM, Kuhn JP, editors: *Caffey's Pediatric X-Ray diagnosis*, ed 9, vol 2, St Louis, 1992, Mosby, pp 1443-1966.

Sty JR, Wells RG, Starshak RJ et al: *Diagnostic Imaging of Infants and Children*, vol 3, 1992, Aspen Publisher, pp 233-404.

Swischuk LE: *Imaging of the Newborn, Infant and Young Child*, ed 3, Baltimore, 1989, Williams & Wilkins, pp 706-982.

Taybi H, Lachman RS: *Radiology of Syndromes, Metabolic Disorders and Skeletal Dysplasias*, ed 3, St Louis, 1990, Mosby.

Articles

Bickerstaff DR, Neal LM, Booth AJ et al: Ultrasound examination of the irritable hip, *J Bone Joint Surg* 72B:549, 1990.

Blickman JG, Wilkinson RH, Graef AW: The radiologic lead band revisited, *AJR* 146:245, 1986.

Burrows PE, Mulliken JB, Fellows KE et al: Childhood hemangiomas and vascular malformations: angiographic differentiation, *AJR* 141:483, 1983.

Caffey J: Infantile cortical hyperostosis, *J Pediatr* 29:541, 1946.

Colavita N, Orazii C, Danza SN et al: Premature epiphyseal fusion and extramedullary hematopoiesis in thalassemia, *Skeletal Radiol* 16:533, 1987.

Graff R: Fundamentals of sonography diagnosis of infant hip dysplasia, *J Pediatr Orthop* 4:735,1984.

Gupta NC, Prezio JA: Radionuclide imaging in osteomyelitis, *Semin Nucl Med* 18:287, 1988.

Harcke HT, Grissom LE: Performing dynamic sonography of the infant hip, *AJR* 155:837, 1990.

Hernandez RJ, Posnansky AK: CT evaluation of pediatric hip disorders, *Orthop Clin North Am* 16:513, 1985.

Jaramillo D, Hoffer FA: Cartilagenous epiphysis and growth plate: normal and abnormal MR imaging findings, *AJR* 158:1105, 1992.

Keller MS, Chawla HS, Weiss AA: Real time sonography of infant hip dislocation, *Radiographics* 6:447, 1986.

Marchal GJ, Van Holsbeeck MT, Raes M et al: Transient synovitis of the hip in children: the role of US, *Radiology* 162:825, 1987.

Moore SG, Bisset GS III et al: Pediatric Musculoskeletal MR Imaging, *Radiology* 179:345, 1991.

Park EA: The imprinting of nutritional disturbances on the growing bone, *Pediatrics* (Suppl) 33:815, 1964.

Reynolds J: Sickle cell disease: the skull and spine, *Semin Roentgenol* 22:168, 1987.

Rush VH, Bramson RT, Ogden JA: Legg-Calvé-Perthes disease: detection of cartilaginous and synovial changes with MR imaging, *Radiology* 167:473, 1988.

Schlesinger AE, Hernandez RJ: Diseases of the musculoskeletal system in children: imaging with CT, sonography, and MR, *AJR* 158:728, 1992.

Tredwell SJ, Davis LA: Prospective study of congenital dislocation of the hip, *J Pediatr Orthop* 9:386, 1989.

CHAPTER 6

Neuroimaging

WITH PATRICK D. BARNES

IMAGING TECHNIQUES

Conventional Radiography
Computed Tomography
Magnetic Resonance Imaging
Ultrasonography
Radionuclide Imaging
Other Modalities

Imaging techniques include conventional radiography, computed tomography (CT), magnetic resonance imaging (MRI), ultrasonography (US), and radionuclide imaging. These techniques generally have displaced or replaced more expensive and invasive modalities such as cerebral angiography, myelography, ventriculography, and cisternography.

Conventional Radiography

A skull series should include frontal views (i.e., those of Caldwell and Towne) and horizontal beam lateral views. The orbits, facial bones, and paranasal sinuses are evaluated with upright frontal Caldwell and Waters views and lateral projections. Conventional radiographs of the skull and sinuses are not used routinely, but occasionally they assist in evaluating trauma, infection, or craniofacial anomalies (e.g., craniosynostosis). Conventional radiographs of the spine routinely are used in the evaluation of any child with suspected dysraphism, scoliosis, torticollis, pain, and any neurologic symptoms or signs relating to the spine. Tomography is especially helpful in evaluating children with spine trauma or craniocervical anomalies.

Computed Tomography

CT imaging can be performed without contrast enhancement initially. Only if uncertainty persists should intravenous (IV) contrast medium be used. Superior bony resolution and sensitivity for hemorrhage make CT unsurpassed in the investigation of acute and subacute trauma. Whenever the use of a skull series is contemplated in the setting of trauma, CT should be considered first. CT evaluates the intracranial structures, the essence of clinical concern, yet readily assesses the orbits, facial bones, and cranium, and possesses the additional assets of direct coronal imaging and three-dimensional reconstruction. Additional indications for CT include hydrocephalus (macrocephaly), determining the sequelae of surgery, and detailed imaging of the orbits, sinuses, and temporal bones. Further evaluation for the presence of calcifications (e.g., tuberous sclerosis) and evaluation of localized spinal column abnormalities (e.g., spondylolysis) also are in the realm of CT.

Magnetic Resonance Imaging

MRI is the modality of choice for imaging the central nervous system (CNS; craniospinal neuraxis). It can also be performed to evaluate further the intracranial anatomy, the extent of CNS development, the degree of blood-brain barrier breakdown (with the addition of gadolinium), and vascular integrity (with magnetic resonance angiography [MRA]). The use of sedation is often necessary in infants and younger children (<6

The following illustrations are reprinted from Wolpert SM, Barnes PD: MRI in pediatric neuroradiology, St. Louis, 1992, Mosby: Figures 6-5; 6-9; 6-13; 6-43; 6-44; 6-52; 6-54; 6-55, B; 6-57; and 6-58.

years of age); and examination times may be long relative to those of CT or US and occasionally are accompanied by discomfort caused by claustrophobia.

MRI's ability to detect nonflowing water as a high intensity on proton-density images aids in distinguishing flowing cerebrospinal fluid (CSF)–containing structures or abnormalities (low intensity) from high-intensity lesions such as edema, inflammation, infarction, and tumor. Unexplained seizures, unexplained neuroendocrine disorders, and unexplained hydrocephalus are best approached by MRI, as are the neurocutaneous syndromes, migrational anomalies, neurodegenerative disease, encephalitis, hemorrhagic lesions, vascular anomalies, neoplasms, and any abnormalities of the spinal neuraxis.

Ultrasonography

Real-time US through the anterior fontanelle is noninvasive and provides rapid real-time and multiplanar imaging of brain anatomy in the fetus and the preterm or term infant. Standardized views allow rapid screening for intracranial hemorrhage, gross malformations such as with the Dandy-Walker complex or agenesis of the corpus callosum, ventricular size, atrophy, and large extracerebral fluid collections and cysts. Sedation usually is not needed.

US is useful in evaluating intracranial blood flow, for example, in patients undergoing extracorporeal membrane oxygenation (ECMO), in patients with a suspected vein of Galen aneurysm and other vascular malformations, or in the determination of brain death. In the screening of spinal dysraphism US gives exquisite delineation of the normal conus medullaris, which normally terminates above the L2-3 level. A tethered cord with thickened filum and tethering masses such as lipomas often are identified.

Radionuclide Imaging

There are a number of uses for radionuclide imaging, especially single photon emission computed tomography (SPECT) imaging, including the evaluation of children with epilepsy, the differentiation of tumor progression from treatment effects (e.g., radiation necrosis), and the determination of brain death. In the evaluation of bony spine disease (e.g., spondylolysis, spondylitis, or tumor) radionuclide imaging is useful for the detection and delineation of multifocal disease, especially when conventional radiographs are negative.

Other Modalities

Ventriculography, encephalography, and myelography are rarely used. Angiography is still important in evaluating vascular anomalies (e.g., aneurysm, arteriovenous malformation), arterial occlusive disease, and for neurointerventional therapy.

THE SKULL

Normal Development and Variants
    Convolutional markings
    Vascular markings
    Sutures
    Molding
Congenital and Developmental Abnormalities
    Craniosynostosis
    Cranioschisis and cranium bifidum
Systemic Diseases
Infections
Vascular Lesions
Trauma
    Perinatal trauma
    Fractures
Tumors

Normal Development and Variants

The cranial calvaria (frontal, parietal, squamous temporal, and occipital bones) are formed by membranous ossification from the dura mater. The cranial base (mendosal suture to the cranial portion of the ethmoid bone) is formed by enchondral ossification. The calvaria, or neurocranium, reflects the growth of the brain, whereas the facial structures and skull base follow the somatic growth curve. Craniofacial proportion can be estimated on lateral radiographs; normally in the newborn this ratio is approximately 3.5:1, at 2 years 3:1, and at 12 years 2:1, whereas in the adult the craniofacial ratio is normally 1.5:1 (Fig. 6-1).

Characteristic markings of the the pediatric skull with which to be familiar include the following.

Convolutional markings Convolutional markings are inner table indentations that conform to the cerebral surface of the growing brain. They are most prominent during the two periods of rapid brain growth: 2 to 3 years and 5 to 7 years. They become less prominent after approximately 8 years of age. These markings should be differentiated from the "lacunar skull" findings (lückenschädel) related to defective calvarial ossification and characterized by multiple oval lucencies of the inner table and diploic space (Fig. 6-2). Lacunar skull often is associated with myelomeningocele or encephalocele and is most prominent in the parietal and occipital bones. Occasionally this is a normal finding and disappears by 6 months of age. It is *not* related in any way to the increased intracranial pressure (ICP) of hydrocephalus, and lückenschädel

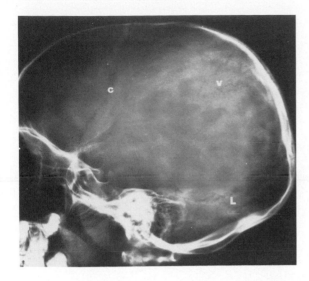

Fig. 6-1 Lateral skull radiograph illustrating the 3:1 craniofacial ratio of a 2-year-old child. Note also the coronal suture (*c*), lambdoid suture (*L*), venous channels (*v*), and convolutional markings.

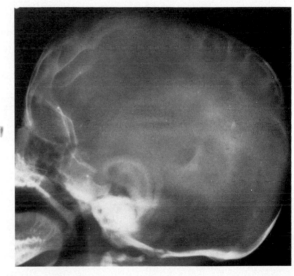

Fig. 6-2 **Lacunar skull.** Multiple oval lucencies of the inner table and diploic space.

should be differentiated from the accentuated convolutional markings of chronic increased ICP. The latter may also be manifested as macrocrania (increased craniofacial ratio), splitting of the sutures, or as demineralization, erosion, or enlargement of the sella turcica.

Vascular markings Vascular markings commonly seen as bony grooves in children after age 3 years are those of the middle meningeal arteries, the emissary veins, the parietal and frontal diploic veins, and the dural venous sinuses. The grooves are often serpiginous in appearance and conform to the distribution characteristic of a particular vessel. There is often marked variation in size (lakes) and configuration (stellate) of the diploic veins (see Fig. 6-1).

Sutures Sutures are the remnants of the original membranous cerebral capsule (dura mater), a structure identifiable in the fontanelles at the junctions of the major sutures. The sutures allow for ossification and spatial adjustment of the cranium during brain growth. The sutures have smooth edges in the neonate and remain so on the inner table, whereas on the outer table the sutures become interdigitated when the child reaches 1 year of age. The primary sutures include the sagittal, metopic, coronal, lambdoidal, mendosal, and the squamosal (Fig. 6-3). Other sutures take their names from bordering bony structures. The anterior fontanelle is diamond shaped and ossifies (closes) by approximately 1 year of age, whereas the posterior fontanelle, if present at birth, usually closes by 6 months of age. The sutures begin to obliterate by the second to third decades.

Diastasis, or splitting, of the sutures is normal during the periods of rapid brain growth. It also occurs in premature infants and those with osteogenesis imperfecta,

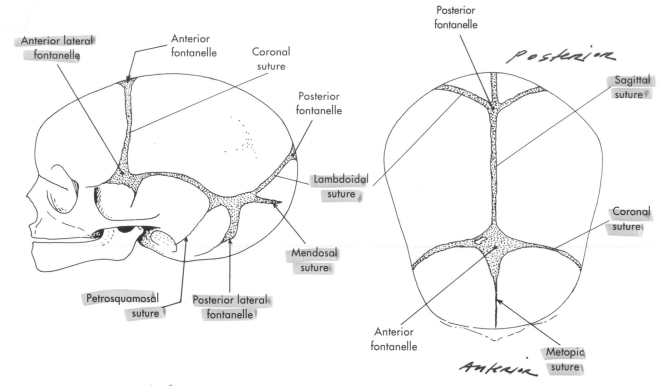

Fig. 6-3 Schematic depiction of the common landmarks and sutures of the skull.

hypothyroidism, hypophosphatasia, rickets, and cleidocranial dysostosis in which it represents a reflection of the underlying metabolic disturbance. Wormian bones (named after Dr. Olaus Worm, a Danish anatomist, who first described them in the 1600s) are intrasutural ossicles most commonly seen along the lambdoid sutures and are usually considered a normal variant. However, they may be excessive in children with osteogenesis imperfecta, cleidocranial dysostosis, hypothyroidism, pyknodysostosis, and healing rickets (Fig. 6-4).

Molding Molding of the skull with overlapping of the sutures is seen in an infant during the first few days after delivery. The remodeling that occurs in subsequent weeks of life will differentiate it from craniosynostosis. Bathrocephaly ("step-in-the-head") is a normal occipital bony variant of the mendosal sutures believed caused by a postural deformity resulting from a breech position. An "inca" bone (parietooccipital intrasutural ossicle) is common in this situation. This variant may remodel after a few months of life. Another skull variant is the parietal foramen (in 60% of normal infants), which occasionally is quite large and bilateral, often hereditary, but of no significance. Mastoid foramina may also be present.

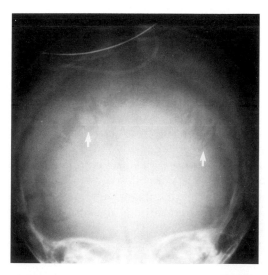

Fig. 6-4 Wormian bones in the lambdoid sutures (*arrows*).

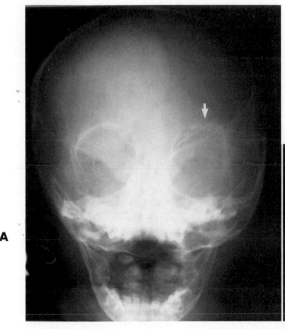

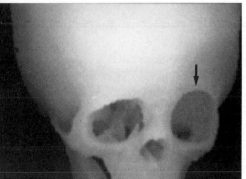

Fig. 6-5 Coronal synostosis. Frontal radiograph (**A**) and three-dimensional CT reconstruction (**B**) demonstrate the orbitocranial deformity (Harlequin eye) associated with unilateral coronal synostosis (*arrows*).

Congenital and Developmental Anomalies

Craniosynostosis   Craniosynostosis is the premature closure (bony fusion) of the sutures. It may be *primary* and possibly is related to faulty dural development or local injury (e.g., ischemia) or *secondary* to metabolic disease (e.g., rickets, hypophosphatasia), hematologic disorders (e.g., anemia), or decreased ICP (e.g., with shunted hydrocephalus or deficient brain growth). Craniofacial syndromes associated with multiple primary craniosynostoses include Apert syndrome (acrocephalosyndactyly), Carpenter syndrome (acrocephalopolysyndactyly), and Crouzon disease (craniofacial dysostosis). The synostosis occurs in utero or early infancy and the cranial deformity subsequently develops during active or rapid brain growth. There is a 3:1 male predominance, and the sagittal suture is involved in more than half the cases. Skull radiographs often reveal characteristic alterations of skull shape and specific changes along the involved suture. These changes include bony bridging of the suture (partial or complete), narrowing of the suture, or parasutural sclerosis. Three-dimensional CT is useful in planning surgical correction. Craniosynostosis of the sagittal suture is the most common type and produces *dolichocephaly* or *scaphocephaly.* Coronal synostosis is the second most common type and produces *plagiocephaly* when unilateral, resulting in a unilateral "harlequin eye" appearance (Fig. 6-5) and *brachycephaly*, when bilateral, resulting in a bilateral harlequin eye appearance. Metopic synostosis (associated with holoprosencephaly) and lambdoidal synostosis are less common types, the former resulting in the "quizzical eye" appearance (*trigonocephaly*) and the latter in severe flattening of the occipital region with plagiocephaly if unilateral and *brachycephaly* if bilateral. If all sutures have closed early (universal craniosynostosis), the "clover leaf" skull deformity (kleeblattschädel) results. It occurs in association with thanatophoric dwarfism in one third of patients.

Cranioschisis and cranium bifidum   Cranioschisis and cranium bifidum are characterized by calvarial defects located either anteriorly or posteriorly in the midline. In children with cranioschisis, herniation of meninges or brain tissues occurs through the bony defect, creating a meningocele or encephalocele, respectively. This does not occur with cranium bifidum. Cranioschisis is an uncommon defect of organogenesis and is seen more commonly in children with chromosomal anomalies (trisomy 13 or 18). The most frequent location is the posterior parietooccipital area, followed by the skull base (e.g., frontoethmoidal). Absence of the corpus callosum, Dandy-Walker complex, and the Chiari malformations are commonly associated cerebral anomalies. CT and MRI delineate the extent and location better than skull radiographs.

Systemic Diseases

Systemic diseases that can produce skull findings include the chronic hemolytic anemias such as thalassemia and sickle cell disease. Compensatory marrow hyperplasia can cause widening of the diploic space, the "hair-on-end" appearance. Eosinophilic granuloma, Langerhans cell histiocytosis (LCH), is characterized by histiocytic infiltration of the diploic space, resulting in well-circumscribed radiolucent lesions, classically with a "beveled" edge or "button" sequestrum, and occurring predominantly in the calvaria but also in the petrous bone. It is the most common lesion occurring in children with LCH (see Fig. 5-26). In the mandible such involvement produces a "floating teeth" appearance. Metabolic involvement consisting of frontal and parietal calvarial thickening classically is seen in children with vitamin D deficiency (rickets) and in those receiving long-term anticonvulsive therapy (e.g., phenytoin [Dilantin]).

Infections

Osteomyelitis caused by spread from sinusitis, mastoiditis, or trauma is uncommon. Osteomyelitis as a complication of a penetrating injury or compound fracture is also rare. *Streptococcus* and *Staphylococcus* are the most common bacterial agents in such an infection. In children with sickle cell disease *Salmonella* is the more likely offending agent. Primary tuberculosis, syphilis, and fungal involvement of the skull are very rare. Conventional radiographs or CT may reveal single or multiple lytic areas that, depending on the chronicity of the infection, may have sclerotic margins. Soft tissue swelling or thickening may also be a prominent feature. Radionuclide imaging may identify the site of infection in the first few days. CT is more reliable after 7 to 10 days.

Vascular Lesions

Vascular lesions of the diploic space of the skull may consist primarily of hemangiomas or vascular malformations (e.g., venous malformations). Lytic lesions with prominent trabeculations arranged in a radiating pattern without a sclerotic margin are seen on conventional radiographs.

Trauma

Perinatal trauma Perinatal trauma may result in hematomas of the subperiosteal compartment (cephalhematoma) or subgaleal compartment (caput succedaneum). A cephalhematoma usually does not cross suture lines because it is limited by the tight attachment of the periosteum along the sutures. Fractures are seldom associated with cephalhematomas. The lesion may calcify, and the skull deformity may persist for years (Fig. 6-6). Subgaleal collections, however, usually resolve in a matter of weeks.

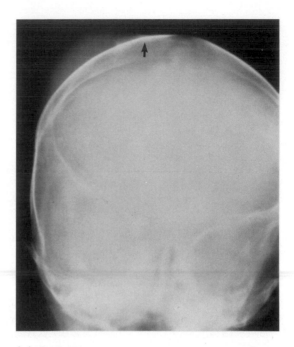

Fig. 6-6 Cephalohematoma characterized by soft tissue swelling limited by the periosteal attachment of the sutures (arrow).

Fractures Skull fractures rarely occur without a history of high-velocity impact (e.g., vehicular accidents or falls from a height). In the absence of such a history, child abuse should be considered, particularly if the fractures are multiple, bilateral, diastatic, or of differing ages. If there is overriding (depression) of the fracture fragments by more than the thickness of the calvaria, surgical elevation of the bony fragment may be indicated. Otherwise, most fractures heal with few or no sequelae (Fig. 6-7, *A*). Healing often occurs entirely in 3 to 6 months. If there has been an associated dural tear, pulsation of the CSF may impede the healing process and produce an enlarging bony defect ("growing fracture"). A complicating meningeal protrusion is known as a *leptomeningeal cyst* (Fig. 6-7, *B*). It occurs most frequently in patients less than age 3 years with diastatic or depressed fractures. Basal skull fractures may extend through the petrous bone or paranasal sinuses. CSF otorrhea or rhinorrhea may occur, and occasionally facial palsy or hearing loss does also. Meningitis, abscess, or vascular compromise (e.g., venous thrombosis, carotid-cavernous fistula) may occur. Skull films may show the fractures, whereas CT delineates associated findings (e.g., depression, hemorrhage, pneumocephalus). Imaging of a child with acute head trauma is best accomplished by CT, particularly in the presence of a depressed fracture (Fig. 6-8), impaired consciousness, or focal neurologic signs. The presence of a skull fracture does not necessarily indicate significant intracranial injury. Conversely, the

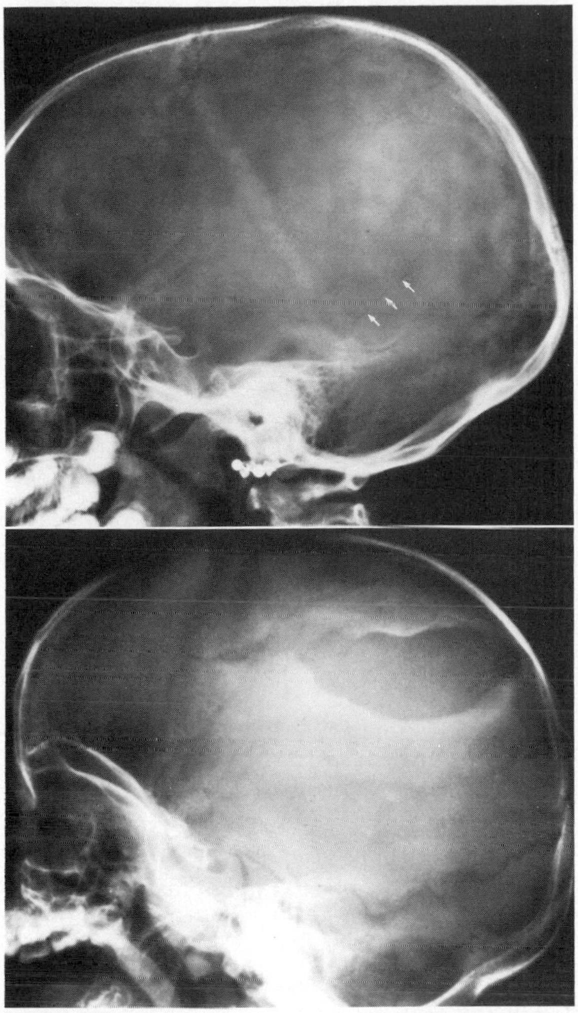

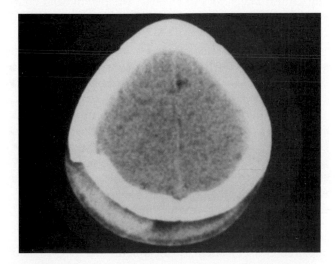

Fig. 6-7 **A**, Nondepressed linear skull fracture (arrows). **B**, "Growing fracture" caused by pulsation of the cerebrospinal fluid.

Fig. 6-8 Axial CT illustrating a depressed parietal fracture on the right with an acute subcutaneous hematoma.

absence of a skull fracture does not exclude serious neurologic injury.

Tumors

The common neoplastic lesions of the cranium include (epi)dermoid, hemangioma, and LCH. (See "Head and Neck Tumors," pp. 201-203.)

HEAD AND NECK

Orbit
Nasal Cavity and Paranasal sinuses
Petrous Temporal Bone
Tumors
  Benign malformative tumors
  Congenital lesions
  Inflammatory masses
  Neoplasms

Orbit

The orbits reach their adult size by 10 years of age and the globe by 7 years. The interorbital distance (IOD) ranges from 11 mm at birth to at least 22 mm in adults. *Hypertelorism* (increased IOD) occurs in children with cleidocranial dysostosis, Crouzon disease, Hunter or Hurler syndrome, encephaloceles, and thalassemia. *Hypotelorism* (decreased IOD) occurs in children with anomalies of orbit and brain development such as the holoprosencephalies or with sagittal or metopic synostosis.

The orbits share common walls with the paranasal sinuses that, if breached, expose the orbits to disease. They include the lamina papyracea (ethmoid air cells), the orbital floor (maxillary sinuses), and the orbital roof (frontal sinuses).

Orbital cellulitis occurs most often in children less than 3 years of age. Superficial or periorbital (preseptal) cellulitis is often of hematogenous origin (*Haemophilus influenzae*). Postseptal or intraorbital inflammation is usually related to spread of infection from the sinuses, especially the ethmoids (subperiosteal cellulitis or abscess). Periorbital swelling or exophthalmos often leads to CT evaluation. Intraorbital infection (orbital cellulitis or abscess) usually results in increased density of the orbital fat. Osseous inflammatory involvement (osteitis or osteomyelitis) may also occur. Differentiating orbital cellulitis from abscess is difficult except in the presence of air in the latter (Fig. 6-9).

Orbital pseudotumor is a lymphoid inflammatory process that characteristically responds to steroid therapy. It has a characteristic appearance, including

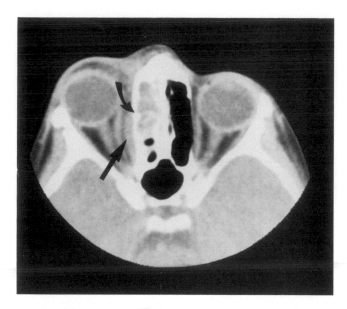

Fig. 6-9 Orbital cellulitis. Axial CT demonstrates ethmoid air cell opacification (*curved arrow*) plus an adjacent medial orbital collection displacing the medial rectus muscle (*straight arrow*) and consistent with ethmoid sinusitis plus orbital subperiosteal cellulitis.

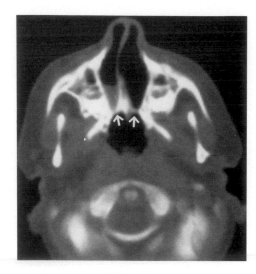

Fig. 6-10 Choanal atresia. Axial CT demonstrates bilateral membranous and bony atresia (*arrows*) with an air-fluid level on the right.

enhancing retroocular masses, enlarged extraocular muscles, and uveoscleral thickening.

Nasal Cavity and Paranasal Sinuses

The external nose consists of paired nasal bones composed of separate ossicles with a host of variably oriented sutures. They may be hypoplastic in children with Down syndrome or chondrodysplasia punctata.

Any horizontal lucent line (except for the frontonasal synchondrosis) should be considered a fracture. Often there is associated fracture of the anterior superior maxillary spine with resultant deformity. The vertical lines are venous channels.

Internally, the paired turbinates fuse dorsally with the choanae (posterior nares). Choanal atresia may be unilateral or bilateral and is more often bony (90%) than membranous (Fig. 6-10).

The paranasal sinuses are present in rudimentary form at birth. The maxillary, ethmoidal, frontal, and sphenoidal air cells develop sequentially. The maxillary antra and ethmoid air cells begin pneumatization before 6 months and are fully pneumatized by approximately 10 years. By 7 years of age, variable pneumatization of the frontal sinuses should be evident. The sphenoid sinus pneumatizes from anterior to posterior by 10 years of age. The size and shape of the pneumatized sinuses vary from individual to individual and with age. There is also wide variation in the appearance of soft tissues within the sinuses. In infants less than 2 years

of age normal mucosal development, engorgement caused by tearing, or enlarged adenoids may result in sinus opacification. For this reason, sinus radiographs in infants less than the age of 2 years are often not reliable for assessing sinusitis.

Inflammatory reaction to foreign material (e.g., allergies, viruses) often causes bilateral thickening of the mucosal membranes. However, a sinus air-fluid level in the absence of trauma suggests a bacterial infection. Chronic inflammatory changes of the mucosa may result in retention cysts, polyps, or mucoceles. Polyps are associated most often with cystic fibrosis and allergies. CT sets the standard for evaluating inflammation of the nasosinus structures for extension intracranially and intraorbitally, and to evaluate the ostiomeatal complex for planning of endoscopic paranasal sinus surgery (Fig. 6-11).

Of the benign nasal neoplasms, a nasal glioma represents sequestered brain tissue (heterotopia) at the nasal bridge (nasion). Differential diagnosis includes encephalocele or dermoid.

The most common aggressive lesion of the nasosinus structures is the juvenile angiofibroma. This is a benign but highly invasive fibrovascular tumor of adolescent males and arises from the posterolateral nasal cavity (sphenopalatine foramen). CT and MRI show an enhancing lesion (Fig. 6-12). Treatment usually necessitates angiography and preoperative embolization.

Petrous Temporal Bone

The *mastoid air cells* in the temporal bone become pneumatized and visible by 6 months of age but are

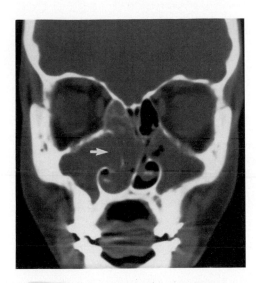

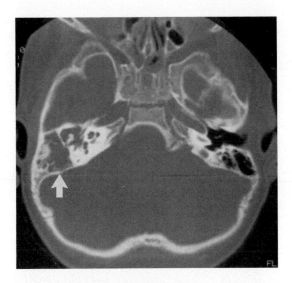

Fig. 6-11 Cystic fibrosis and nasosinus polyps. Direct coronal CT demonstrates bilateral opacification of the nasal cavities and sinuses with bony involvement (*arrow*) characteristic of cystic fibrosis with polyps and chronic sinusitis.

Fig. 6-13 Coalescent mastoiditis. Axial CT demonstrates middle ear and mastoid opacification with bony destructive changes (*arrow*) characteristic of mastoiditis.

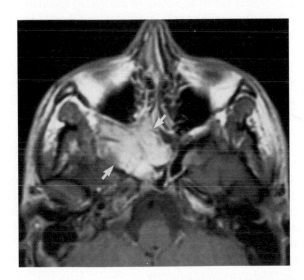

Fig. 6-12 Angiofibroma. Axial gadolinium-enhanced T1-weighted MRI demonstrates a markedly enhancing soft tissue mass involving the nasal cavity, nasopharynx, maxillary sinus, and sphenoid sinus (*arrows*).

quite variable in size, contour, and degree of aeration. They become progressively more pneumatized over the next 5 years. Common developmental anomalies associated with hearing loss include microtia and the Mondini spectrum of cochlear dysplasias. Extension of otitis media into the mastoid air cells is common. Mastoiditis implies an osteitis and occasionally is apparent on Towne views. CT is the definitive procedure for evaluating mastoiditis, chronic otitis media, and cholesteatoma. Findings include middle ear and mastoid opacification, bony demineralization or destruc-

tion, overlying soft tissue swelling, and occasionally sclerosis, especially if there is chronic inflammation (Fig. 6-13). Cholesteatomas can be acquired (secondary to chronic otitis media) or developmental (primary epidermoid). Neoplastic and pseudoneoplastic lesions, as discussed later, include histiocytosis, neuroblastoma, rhabdosarcoma, fibrous dysplasia, primitive neuroectodermal tumor (PNET), and leukemia. Multiplanar imaging is important in planning the surgical approach for definitive therapy of these lesions.

Tumors

Benign malformative tumors Along with inflammatory lesions, dysplastic lesions constitute the majority of head and neck masses in childhood (>80%), and they include dermoids, epidermoids, teratomas, and the vascular anomalies, which include hemangiomas. Hemangiomas are congenital lesions characterized by endothelial proliferation. Arterial and venous high flow is observed on Doppler US and MRI associated with a parenchymal component. Arteriovenous malformations (AVMs) are high-flow malformations without a parenchymal component. Lymphatic and venous malformations are low-flow anomalies with cystic spaces and an often fibrofatty stroma. Mixed lesions often occur and are identifiable on US and MRI.

A laryngocele is a developmental diverticular outpouching of the laryngeal ventricle and has a characteristic air-containing diverticulum adjacent to the larynx on conventional AP radiographs.

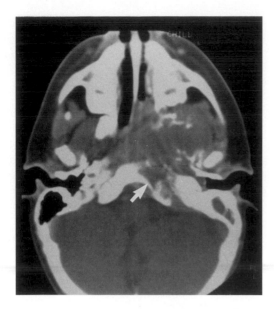

Fig. 6-14 Rhabdomyosarcoma. Axial CT demonstrates soft tissue mass with bony skull base destruction (*arrow*).

Other congenital lesions include cystic hygroma, branchial cleft cyst, and thyroglossal duct cyst.

The most common lesion, cystic hygroma, is a lymphatic malformation (see vascular anomalies on p. 201) presenting as a multilocular cystic mass that contains serous or chylous fluid and most often appears before age 3 years (50% at birth) as a lateral neck mass. There may be extension into the mediastinum (<10% of cases) (see Fig. 2-6).

Failure of obliteration of the cervical sinus, a structure originating from the second branchial arch, can result in a cystic mass and is the most common of the branchial arch anomalies. This branchial cleft cyst most commonly is located in the upper third of the neck anteriomedial to the sternocleidomastoid muscle.

A thyroglossal duct remnant is clinically apparent as a mass in the midline, localized anywhere from the tongue base to the region of the thyroid, and often complicated by recurrent infection. There may be a fistula, a cyst, or a sinus tract.

Inflammatory masses Inflammatory lesions are the most common cause of head and neck masses. Scalp infections are common but seldom involve bony or intracranial structures. Adenopathy is seen most often in the posterior occipital region. Neck masses include lymphadenitis, cellulitis, and abscess.

Adenopathy (see Chapter 2) is seen most commonly in the first 5 years of life. Differentiating cellulitis from abscess may be difficult on US, CT, or MRI.

Neoplasms Head and neck *neoplasia* may be of mesenchymal origin (osseous, chondroid, or reticuloendothelial tumors), of neural origin (neural crest, nerve sheath, and neuroectodermal neoplasms), or consist of benign malformative lesions (dermoid, cholesteatoma, and vascular anomalies). Imaging is accomplished best

by CT to evaluate bony involvement and calcification, whereas MRI is the modality of choice to evaluate neuroanatomic involvement, vascular involvement, and lesion extent. US may confirm a cystic component and provide guidance for needle aspiration or biopsy.

Mesenchymal tumors most commonly are located in the skull base and are rare. Chondrosarcomas of the sphenoid and osteochondromas associated with Ollier's disease are most common. Osteosarcomas and fibrosarcomas are rare. Chordomas arise from intraosseous notochordal remnants, usually near the sphenooccipital synchondrosis.

Rhabdomyosarcoma is the most common malignant soft tissue tumor of the head and neck region in children, followed by neuroblastoma, PNET, histiocytosis, and leukemia/lymphoma. Rhabdomyosarcoma is an aggressive and invasive neoplasm that may involve the orbit, sinus, otomastoid, or nasopharynx (Fig. 6-14). Non-Hodgkin lymphoma is more common than Hodgkin lymphoma, presenting with noncontiguous nodal spread, whereas with Hodgkin lymphoma, cervical lymphadenopathy frequently is present. They both may be associated with acquired immunodeficiency syndrome (AIDS).

Salivary gland tumors are rare in childhood and include the benign pleomorphic adenoma (40%) and hemangioma. Angiofibromas are discussed on p. 200.

Neuroblastoma is the most common neural tumor, followed by retinoblastoma, PNET, and rarely esthesioneuroblastoma. All of them have similar appearances on CT and MRI. Nerve sheath tumors, including schwannomas and neurofibromas, may be large enough to erode bone, but calcification is unusual. Paragangliomas primarily occur in adults. Retinoblastoma is the most common intraocular neoplasm of childhood. It

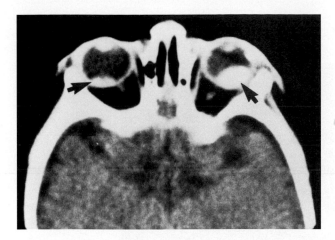

Fig. 6-15 Retinoblastoma. Axial CT demonstrates bilateral intraocular calcific high densities characteristic of retinoblastoma (*arrows*).

often is bilateral and occasionally familial. It almost always is calcified and may spread by direct extension along the optic nerve. Children with these tumors usually have leukocoria (white pupillary reflex) or strabismus (Fig. 6-15).

THE BRAIN

Myelination
Developmental Abnormalities
    Disorders of dorsal induction
        Cranioschisis
        Cephaloceles
        Chiari malformations
    Disorders of ventral induction
        Holoprosencephaly
        Septooptic dysplasia
        Dandy-Walker complex
    Disorders of neuronal proliferation and differentiation
        Micrencephaly
        Megalencephaly
        Hydranencephaly
    Disorders of histogenesis
        Neurofibromatosis
        Tuberous sclerosis
        Sturge-Weber syndrome
        von Hippel-Lindau disease
        Others
    Disorders of sulcation and migration
        Schizencephaly
        Neuronal heteropias
        Agyria
        Pachygyria
        Polymicrogyria
        Agenesis or dysgenesis of corpus callosum
    Arachnoid cysts

Metabolic and Degenerative Disorders
Infections and Inflammatory Processes
    Bacterial infections
    Viral infections
        Herpes simplex encephalitis
        Toxoplasmosis
        Leukoencephalitis
    Subacute and chronic infections
    Parasitic infections
Vascular Disease, Hemorrhage, and Trauma
    Hemorrhage
        Germinal matrix hemorrhage
        Intracerebral hemorrhage
        Epidural hemorrhage
        Subdural hemorrhage
        Benign extracerebral collections of infancy
        Contusions and shear injury
    Ischemia
        Hypoxic-ischemic brain injury
        Periventricular leukomalacia
        Ischemic cerebral cortical and subcortical injury
    Vascular occlusive diseases
    Vascular anomalies, malformations, and aneurysms
Neoplasms
    Cerebral hemispheric tumors
        Neuroepithelial tumors
    Tumors near the third ventricle
        Craniopharyngioma
        Optic or hypothalamic glioma
        Dermoid or epidermoid tumors
        Germ cell and pineal cell tumors
    Posterior fossa tumors
        Cerebellar astrocytoma
        Medulloblastoma
        Ependymoma
        Brain stem tumors

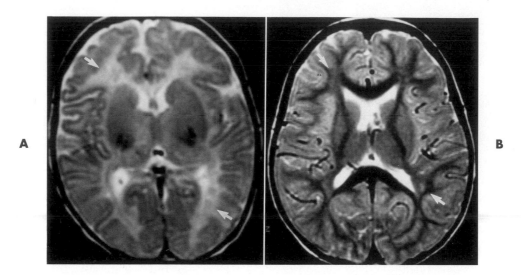

Fig. 6-16 MRI and myelination. Axial T2-weighted MRI in a 2-month-old infant (**A**) demonstrates the watery hyperintensity of the unmyelinated cerebral white matter (*arrows*) as contrasted with the axial T2-weighted MRI of a 2-year-old child (**B**) demonstrating hypointensities of the myelinated cerebral white matter (*arrows*).

Table 6-1 Classification of disorders of CNS formation by gestational age

Embrologic event	Gestational timing	Anomaly
Dorsal induction Primary neurulation	3-4 wk	Cranioschisis Cephaloceles (Myelo)meningocele } Primary Chiari malformations } neurulation Hydrosyringomyelia
Secondary neurulation	4 wk to postnatal	Diastematomyelia Tethered cord Neurenteric anamolies
Ventral induction	5-10 wk	Holoprosencephaly Dandy-Walker complex Absence of the septum pellucidum
Neural proliferation, differentiation, histogenesis	2-6 mo	Brain size anomalies Neurocutaneous syndromes Tumors, vascular anomalies
Sulcation, migration	2-5 mo	Lissencephaly Gyral anomalies Schizencephaly
Other		Arachnoid cyst

Modified from Vander Knaap MS, Valk J: *AJNR* 9:315, 1988.

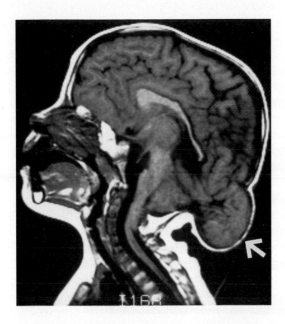

Fig. 6-17 Encephalocele. Sagittal T1-weighted MRI demonstrates an occipital encephalocele (*arrow*) and associated Chiari III malformation.

Myelination

Myelination is exquisitely displayed by MRI. During the myelination process, surface membrane glycolipids, proteins, and cholesterol increase as the water content of white matter decreases. Progression of myelination (T2 hypointensity of white matter) coincides with the development of neurologic function. At birth, the thalamus, cerebellar peduncles, and median longitudinal fasciculus are myelinated. By 3 months of age, the cerebellar white matter is myelinated, along with the posterior limb of the internal capsule and the paraventricular and paracentral white matter. By 6 months, the optic radiation and splenium are myelinated, and by 1 year of age the anterior limbs of the internal capsule and genu of the corpus callosum are myelinated. Cerebral lobar myelination progresses during the second year, and an adult pattern is reached between 18 and 24 months of age (Fig. 6-16).

Developmental Abnormalities

A classification of disorders of CNS formation according to gestation appears in Table 6-1.

Disorders of dorsal induction The formation and dorsal closure of the neural tube (neurulation) to form the brain and spinal cord originate with notochordal induction of the neuroectoderm (dorsal induction). Cephalic disorders of primary neurulation (craniospinal neural tube closure to the upper lumbar level) include cranioschisis, cephaloceles, and the Chiari malformations. Spinal defects resulting from disorders of primary and secondary neurulation (caudal spinal neural tube closure) are discussed in the section "The Spine."

Cranioschisis If the neural tube fails to close in utero, dorsal protrusions of the meninges and/or brain may occur (cranioschisis). Complete failure of closure at the cranial level results in anencephaly, which is incompatible with life. The mildest form of closure anomaly is represented by a small meningocele or sinus tract.

Cephaloceles Cephaloceles are protrusions of brain tissue, meninges, or both through a cranial defect. They most commonly occur in the midline. The *occipital* or *cervicooccipital* cephalocele is the most common (70%) and is associated with a Chiari malformation or the Dandy-Walker complex (Fig. 6-17). *Ethmoidal* cephaloceles may result in a nasal mass and hypertelorism. *Sphenoidal* cephaloceles frequently are seen as a nasopharyngeal mass and may be associated with facial anomalies.

Chiari Malformations There are four types of Chiari malformations.

Type I malformation represents "herniation" of or "low position" of the cerebellar tonsils, inferior vermis, or cervicomedullary junction below the foramen magnum. Now frequently noted on MRI, this "herniation" below the foramen magnum may be as much as 5 mm without downward placement of the brain stem. However, often there is associated hydrosyringomyelia (60%) or hydrocephalus (25%) and an association with the Klippel-Feil anomaly (e.g., C2-3 fusion).

Type II (Arnold-Chiari) malformation is almost always associated with a myelomeningocele. The frequently associated ventriculomegaly often worsens to frank hydrocephalus after the myelomeningocele is repaired. There is downward placement of the malformed hindbrain, with "beaking" of the tectum, a small fourth ventricle, and a small posterior fossa (Fig. 6-18). Aqueductal stenosis is common. Corpus callosal dysgenesis or agenesis (in 80%) is a common association along with other cerebral malformations. Conventional radiographs and CT findings may include a lückenschädel (lacunar) skull, a scalloped clivus, and an enlarged foramen magnum.

The very rare Chiari III malformation represents pronounced descent and dysplasia of the cerebellum and brain stem associated with a cervicooccipital encephalocele often containing hindbrain or occipital cerebral tissue. The Chiari IV malformation is an even rarer and more severe form of cerebellar and brain stem hypoplasia with caudal malposition and may not be related to the other three forms. Chiari III and IV are also commonly associated with heterotopias, agenesis of the corpus callosum, and hydrosyringomyelia.

Disorders of Ventral Induction Ventral induction is the process by which the primitive notochord induces the ventral neuroectoderm to form the primitive brain and facial structures. This results in the formation of the prosencephalon (forebrain), mesencephalon (midbrain), and rhombencephalon (hindbrain). The prosencephalon divides to form the telencephalon, the primitive cerebral hemispheres, and the diencephalon, the primitive thalamus and hypothala-

mus. The optic vesicles also develop as an outpouching of the diencephalon. The rhombencephalon becomes the pons, medulla, and cerebellum. US or CT is often adequate for screening children for these disorders.

Holoprosencephalies. The holoprosencephalies are the most severe of the ventral induction anomalies and occur when the forebrain fails to divide into two hemispheres. The optic and olfactory nerves are usually absent or hypoplastic. Holoprosencephaly commonly is associated with trisomy D (13 to 15) or trisomy E (16 to 18) and callosal agenesis.

The *alobar* type of holoprosencephaly, that is, complete failure of separation, presents in the fetus or infant as microcephaly and facial anomalies (e.g., hypotelarism). The prognosis is dismal. CT, US (Fig. 6-19), or MRI demonstrate the undivided cerebrum, an absent falx, a horseshoe-shaped monoventricle, fused basal ganglia, and fused thalami. The corpus callosum is always absent, but the posterior fossa may be normal.

The *semilobar* type shows mild separation of the two hemispheres and lateral ventricles by a dural fold, and a falx may be partially present. The brain is small, and the olfactory apparatus is lacking. Mental retardation and mild facial anomalies such as a median cleft lip may also be present.

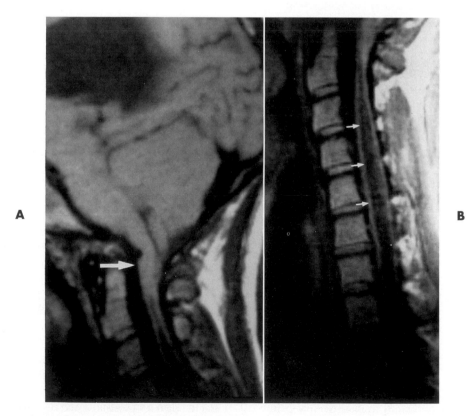

Fig. 6-18 Chiari II malformation and hydromyelia. Sagittal T1-weighted MRI demonstrates Chiari II malformation of the hindbrain (**A**, *arrow*) and associated hydrosyringomyelia (**B**, *arrows*).

The *lobar* type, the mildest form, may be evident only as an absent septum pellucidum and squared frontal horns. The cerebrum is normal in size but lacks hemispheric cleavage at the level of the frontal lobes.

Septooptic dysplasia (de Morsier syndrome) is considered a milder form of holoprosencephaly, with absence of the septum pellucidum and optic hypoplasia. Pituitary-hypothalamic dysfunction is often present. Hypotonia and blindness are evident in the first few days of life. Maternal diabetes, alcohol and drug abuse, and cytomegalovirus (CMV) infection have been implicated as risk factors. CT or MRI may reveal absence of one or both leaflets of the septum pellucidum, callosal dysgenesis, or schizencephaly (50%).

Dandy-Walker complex   Classically, Dandy-Walker complex (DWC) is characterized by hypoplasia or absence of the inferior cerebellar vermis and cystic dilation of the fourth ventricle. There is high position of the dural sinuses ("torcular Lambdoid inversion") with a large posterior fossa and absent falx cerebelli. Hydrocephalus is often present. Agenesis of the corpus callosum and encephaloceles are commonly associated findings (25%) (Fig. 6-20). The Dandy-Walker variant, mega cisterna magna, and Blake's pouch cyst may be considered as part of the Dandy-Walker spectrum.

These are to be distinguished from vermian hypoplasia (Joubert syndrome), the Chiari malformations, and cerebellar atrophy.

Disorders of neuronal proliferation and differentiation

Micrencephaly   Micrencephaly, an abnormally small brain, reflects an early intrauterine insult usually of

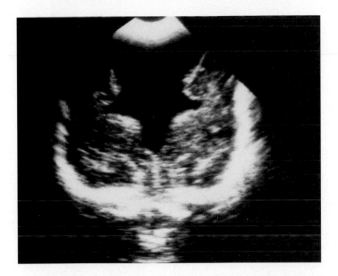

Fig. 6-19 Alobar holoprosencephaly demonstrated on coronal US as a monoventricle and an absent corpus callosum with fused basal ganglia and fused thalami.

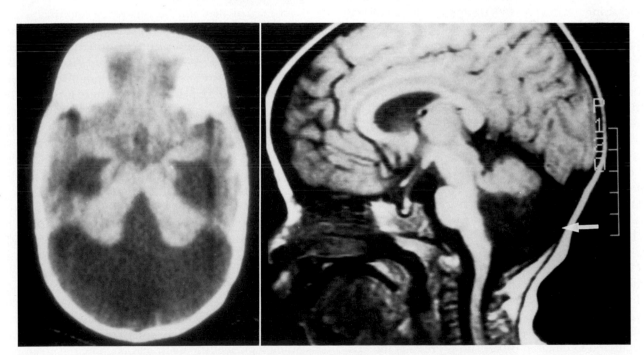

Fig. 6-20 Dandy-Walker complex. **A**, Axial CT and, **B**, sagittal T1-weighted MRI demonstrate absence of the inferior cerebellar vermis and wide communication between the fourth ventricle and retrocerebellar cystic space (*arrow*) consistent with Dandy-Walker malformation.

Neurocutaneous Syndromes

COMMON

Neurofibromatosis
Tuberous sclerosis

UNCOMMON

Sturge-Weber syndrome
Klippel-Trenaunay-Weber syndrome
von Hipple-Lindau disease
Ataxia-telangiectasia (Louis-Bar syndrome)

RARE

Hereditary hemorrhage telangiectasia
   (Osler-Weber-Rendu disease)
Epidermal nevus syndrome

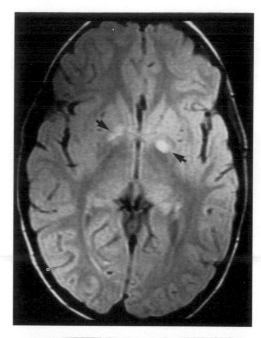

Fig. 6-21 Neurofibromatosis 1 and glial dysplasia. Axial proton-density MRI demonstrates bilateral nodular high intensities involving the basal ganglia and deep capsular tracts (*arrows*) characteristic of neurofibromatosis 1.

ischemic or infectious origin (e.g., TORCH). It may also be seen in children with metabolic disorders (phenylketonuria). CT or MRI may demonstrate a small but formed brain, a small but malformed brain, or in the encephaloclastic type caused by a later insult, encephalomalacia or atrophy.

Megalencephaly Megalencephaly may be anatomic or caused by metabolic disorders such as a leukodystrophy or the mucopolysaccharidoses. The unilateral type may be considered a hemispheric form of lissencephaly with polymicrogyria and heterotopias. These children often have intractable seizures, hemiplegia, and developmental delay.

Hydranencephaly Hydranencephaly, that is, severe hypoplasia or destruction of the telencephalon, occurs secondary to absence of, or occlusion of, the internal carotid or anterior and middle cerebral arteries. Predisposing factors include TORCH infection, radiation, and trauma. There may be microcephaly or macrocephaly with only a brain stem, diencephalon, and cerebellum present. The falx is usually present in some form, but the cortical mantle is deficient. The condition is often fatal.

Disorders of histogenesis Neurocutaneous syndromes are characterized by the simultaneous occurrence of CNS abnormalities and skin lesions (see box). MRI is the preferred modality for definitive evaluation of the dysplastic, neoplastic, or vascular lesions associated with these syndromes.

Neurofibromatosis Type 1 neurofibromatosis (peripheral form; NF1) is the most common type encountered in children (90%) and represents the classic von Recklinghausen disease, including optic gliomas, hamartomas of the brain, and café-au-lait spots. The incidence of NF1 is 1:3500, and the gene defect is

located on chromosome 17. There is autosomal dominant inheritance in 50%, whereas the remainder occur spontaneously. Clinical manifestations of CNS involvement may or may not be related to identifiable neuropathology. Short-segment kyphoscoliosis, prominent vertebral body scalloping, ribbon rib deformity, thinned pedicles, and a widened canal (dural ectasia) are characteristic conventional radiographic findings of the mesodermal dysplasia of NF1. There may be a characteristic lytic defect at the lambdoid suture (left side more often than right), often associated with deficient mastoid pneumatization. MRI identifies increased signal intensity of the dysplastic glial foci within the basal ganglia, brain stem, cerebellum, and cerebrum as characteristic of NF1 (Fig. 6-21). CT and MRI both delineate the sphenoorbital dysplasia of NF1 with associated plexiform neurofibroma and buphthalmus. This process produces the "empty orbit" appearance on AP skull radiographs. The most common associated intracranial tumor of NF1 is the optic glioma (Fig. 6-22). Spinal neurofibromas and schwannomas are common, and plexiform neurofibromas are characteristic of NF1.

Type 2 neurofibromatosis (central form; NF2) most commonly appears during adult life, with patients presenting with acoustic neuromas, meningiomas, subcutaneous neurofibromas, multiple spinal neurofibromas, and spinal cord gliomas. Bilateral and multilevel tumors are more characteristic of NF2, especially nerve

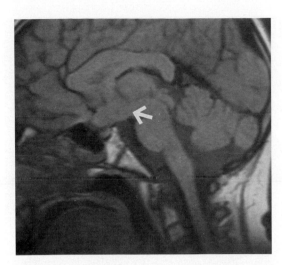

Fig. 6-22 Neurofibromatosis 1 and optic glioma. Sagittal T1-weighted MRI demonstrates isointense tumor involvement of the optic chiasm and hypothalamus (*arrow*).

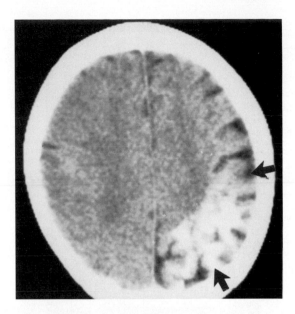

Fig. 6-23 Sturge-Weber syndrome. Axial CT demonstrates calcifications and cerebral cortical atrophy (*arrows*).

sheath tumors (neuromas) and meningiomas. Its incidence is 1:50,000, with the gene defect located on chromosome 22. Skin changes are less common than in patients with NF1.

Tuberous sclerosis An autosomal dominant lesion (chromosome 9) with variable penetrance (although 60% of cases are sporadic), tuberous sclerosis (Bourneville disease) classically is seen in a child with seizures, mental retardation, and facial adenoma sebaceum (70%). Hamartomas occur in the brain, skeleton, skin, and viscera. Brain "tubers" are present in all patients, and these lesions contain giant cells, spindle cells, and glial cells. Most commonly located subependymally in the wall of the lateral ventricles, they may also be present in the cortex and subcortically. They often calcify. Prominent contrast enhancement on either CT or MRI may indicate neoplastic degeneration (giant cell tumor). US may demonstrate renal hamartomas in 50% to 80% of these patients.

Sturge-Weber syndrome Sturge-Weber syndrome, or encephalotrigeminal angiomatosis, is characterized by a capillary malformation of the face in a V_1 distribution (facial port-wine stain or nevus flammeus) and by leptomeningeal venous malformations of the ipsilateral or bilateral cerebrum, most often occurring in the occipital, temporal, and parietal regions. Gyriform subpial (tramline) calcifications may be seen on conventional radiographs and CT (Fig. 6-23). These dystrophic calcifications are located in the pericapillary region of the fourth layer of the cerebral cortex and appear in a child between 5 and 15 years of age. CT and MRI demonstrate atrophy with ventricular dilation. MRI may demonstrate associated cortical dysplasias.

von Hippel-Lindau disease von Hippel-Lindau disease (CNS angiomatosis) is of autosomal dominant inheritance (chromosome 3) and classically consists of retinal, cerebellar, and visceral angiomatous lesions. MRI reveals characteristic retinal and cerebellar hemangioblastomas and occasional spinal cord or brain stem lesions.

Other, much more rare lesions include *Klippel-Trenaunay-Weber* (*angioosteohypertrophy* syndrome), which occurs sporadically and manifests as capillary and cavernous malformations and varicosities of the trunk or limbs that may occur unilaterally or bilaterally and cause hemihypertrophy. Associated CNS vascular malformations may occur. It may occur as a variant of the Sturge-Weber syndrome.

Ataxia-telangiectasia (*Louis-Bar syndrome*) is of autosomal recessive inheritance and manifests as facial and conjunctival capillary telangiectasias, cerebellar atrophy, and demyelination. There is cellular immunodeficiency with recurrent infections and neoplasia (e.g., lymphoma, sarcoma).

Hereditary hemorrhagic telangiectasia (*Osler-Weber-Rendu syndrome*) is of autosomal dominant inheritance and manifests as cutaneous and mucous membrane telangiectasias. There is only occasional brain involvement that may include an aneurysm, vascular malformation, cerebral infarction, or abscess.

Disorders of sulcation and migration Neuroblasts migrate from the periventricular germinal matrix and undergo proliferation to form neurons of the gray matter (neurogenesis), which precedes the migration and proliferation of glioblasts to form the glia of the white

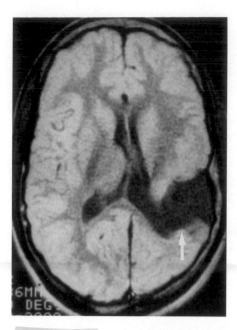

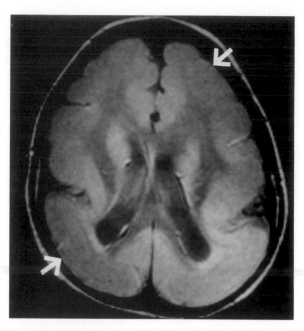

Fig. 6-24 Schizencephaly. Axial proton-density MRI demonstrates cerebrospinal fluid intensity cleft lined by gray matter intensities and extending from the lateral ventricle through the cerebral cortex (*arrow*).

Fig. 6-25 Agyria. Axial proton-density MRI demonstrates a bilaterally thick and flat cortex (agyria and pachygyria; *arrows*) with dysmorphic sylvian fissures, hypoplastic white matter, and lateral ventricular dilation.

matter (gliogenesis). Cortical organization with the formation of gyri and sulci is the final stage of the neuronal migration process. Any insult to the developing brain during this period can result in a disturbance of development, including schizencephaly, neuronal heterotopias, lissencephaly, pachygyria, or polymicrogyria.

Schizencephaly Schizencephaly (a "cleft" in the brain) probably results from an early insult to the germinal matrix that produces a gray matter-lined parasylvian and paracentral full-thickness cleft that extends from the lateral ventricle to the pial surface. It may be unilateral or bilateral and symmetric. The cleft may be narrow or closed (type 1) or wide and open (type 2) and is frequently associated with complete or partial absence of the septum pellucidum or with other anomalies. Associated heterotopias and polymicrogyria may also occur. MRI differentiates schizencephaly from encephaloclastic porencephaly by demonstrating gray matter intensities along its entire course (Fig. 6-24).

Neuronal heterotopias Neuronal heterotopias result from focal arrest of neuroblast migration with subsequent proliferation of gray matter in abnormal locations. Neuronal heterotopias may be of the nodular type or the laminar type and occur in a subpial location (nodular type), a subependymal location (nodular type), or a subcortical location (laminar type). Seizures are a common manifestation. Nodular subependymal

heterotopias must be distinguished from the subependymal neuroglial hamartomas of tuberous sclerosis.

Agyria Agyria (lissencephaly) is characterized by hypoplasia of the brain with lack of formation of cerebral sulci and gyri caused by failure of neuronal migration. These children are developmentally delayed and often have microcephaly. Agyria may be associated with a number of dysgenetic syndromes (e.g., Miller-Dieker, Walker-Warburg). CT and MRI show a smooth brain, ventriculomegaly, white matter hypoplasia, poor gray-white matter differentiation, wide sylvian fissures, and wide central sulci. A figure-eight appearance may be seen on axial images (Fig. 6-25).

Pachygyria Pachygyria (macrogyria) is characterized by a few broad gyri and shallow sulci with short fingers of white matter extending into them. The neuronal migration arrest is thought to occur somewhat later than in children with agyria and thus may be considered a milder form.

Polymicrogyria Polymicrogyria (cobblestone-like gyri) results from a later insult to cortical organization. Numerous tiny gyri are apparent and give a serrated or striated appearance to the cortex. This appearance may be diffusely distributed or more focal in occurrence. It is often associated with schizencephaly and is the major component of the cortical dysplasias, both of

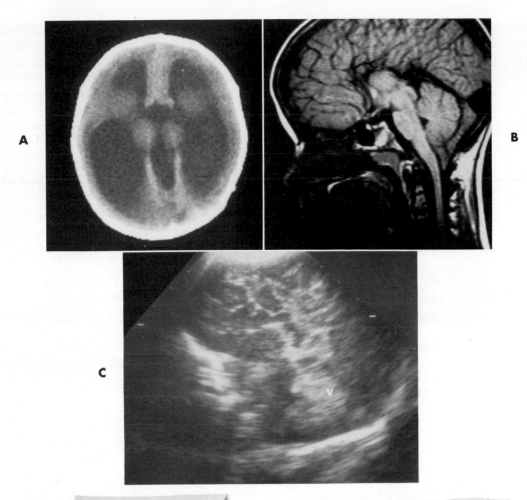

Fig. 6-26 Agenesis of the corpus callosum. A, Axial CT illustrating the parallel separated and dilated lateral ventricles. **B**, Agenesis of the corpus callosum on MRI. **C**, US demonstrating radiating linear markings (Probst bundles) (*v*, cerebellar vermis).

which may be associated with focal seizures.

Agenesis or dysgenesis of corpus callosum Callosal agenesis or dysgenesis occurs when there is failure of the commissural plate to facilitate interhemispheric axonal passage either primarily (by being absent) or by creating a glial barrier to passage. These primordial axonal fibers either degenerate or line the ventricular walls as Probst bundles. Callosal agenesis or dysgenesis is often associated with other intracranial abnormalities (Dandy-Walker complex, Chiari II malformation, holoprosencephaly, basal encephaloceles). Seizures, developmental delay, and mental retardation may be noted early in infancy. Because the intact corpus callosum can be thought of as the "anchor" of the two hemispheres, its absence leads to four characteristic CT and MRI findings: parallel and separated lateral ventricles; U-shaped frontal horns; elevation of the third ventricle

with elongation of the foramina of Monroe; and dilated occipital horns (colpocephaly) (Fig. 6-26). Radially oriented sulci may be seen on US and MRI.

Callosal or pericallosal lipomas and interhemispheric cysts are not infrequently associated with corpus callosum agenesis or dysgenesis.

Arachnoid cysts Arachnoid cysts are developmental or acquired collections of CSF. They are located more often in the middle cranial fossa (60%), quadrigeminal plate region (10%), or the posterior fossa (5%). Seizures or headache is often the presenting symptom. If midline in location, these cysts can cause hydrocephalus. Differential diagnosis may include a cystic tumor, schizencephaly, Dandy-Walker complex, or a vein of Galen aneurysm. CT or MRI is the modality of choice (CSF characteristics); in infancy cranial US often delineates this lesion (Fig. 6-27).

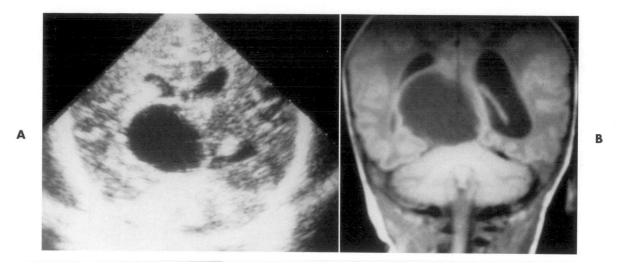

Fig. 6-27 Arachnoid cyst. A, Coronal US and, **B**, coronal MRI illustrate an arachnoid cyst of the quadrigeminal plate region producing hydrocephalus.

Metabolic and Degenerative Disorders

Metabolic and neurodegenerative disorders are characterized by progressive brain deterioration and are classified according to the type of metabolic defect (e.g., enzymatic deficiency), the clinical features (including inheritance), and the anatomic pattern of involvement. Definitive diagnosis, when possible, is usually obtained by metabolic assays or biopsy of CNS or other tissues. In some cases, the imaging findings are characteristic (Fig. 6-28).

These disorders include amino acid disorders (e.g., phenylketonuria or homocystinuria), carbohydrate metabolism disorders (e.g., galactosemia), disorders of lysosomal enzymes (e.g., mucopolysaccharidoses and sphingolipidoses), respiratory oxidative disorders (i.e., Leigh disease or necrotizing encephalopathy), disorders of peroxisomes (e.g., adrenoleukodystrophy complex), and diseases that predominantly involve gray matter (e.g., lipofuscinosis, Alpers syndrome), white matter (e.g., Canavan disease), the basal ganglia (e.g., Wilson disease), or the cerebellum, brain stem, and spinal cord (e.g., olivopontocerebellar degenerative disease).

Clinical features that assist in the differential diagnosis include microcephaly (e.g., phenylketonuria), macrocephaly (e.g., Hunter-Hurler syndrome), acidosis (e.g., maple syrup urine disease), hyperammonemia (e.g., defects in the urea cycle enzymes), food intolerance (e.g., galactosemia), familial clustering, systemic disease, and dysmorphia. Imaging findings that may be helpful include characteristic anatomic distribution (e.g., basal ganglia), calcification, atrophy, white matter degeneration, meningeal involvement, migrational

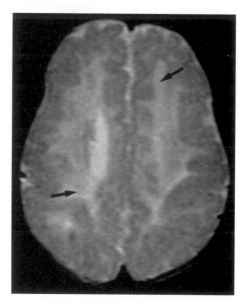

Fig. 6-28 Zellweger syndrome. Axial T2-weighted MRI demonstrates abnormal cerebral white matter hyperintensities (*arrows*) and cortical polymicrogyria.

anomalies, bony involvement, or vascular occlusive disease.

Basal ganglia mineralization (e.g., calcium, iron) may occur in children with tuberous sclerosis, Down syndrome, parathyroid disorder, the TORCH infections (see "Viral Infections" on p. 214), and AIDS (Fig. 6-29). Other causes include anoxia, carbon monoxide toxicity, lead poisoning, radiation, methotrexate therapy, and renal tubular acidosis. *Basal ganglia lesions without mineralization* (i.e., edema, necrosis) are seen in chil-

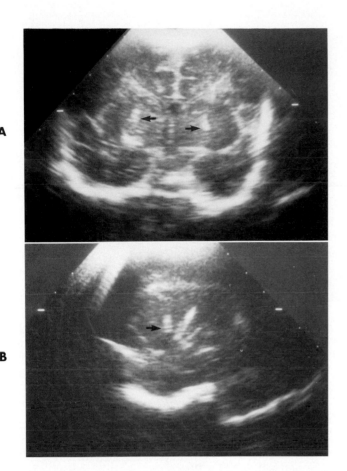

Fig. 6-29 Linear echogenic striations in the basal ganglia in the coronal (**A**) and sagittal (**B**) planes (*arrows*) in a patient with AIDS.

dren with anoxic brain damage, encephalitis, and acute insults such as carbon monoxide inhalation and cyanide poisoning.

Infections and Inflammatory Processes

Inflammation of the immature nervous system differs in its manifestations from that of the mature nervous system in two aspects: (1) in the first two trimesters of fetal life, malformations are the likely result of inflammation; and (2) the fetal nervous system has the capacity to repair damaged neurons and thus compensate, unlike the developed nervous system. Bacteria and viral infections are the most common causes of intracranial inflammation in infants and children.

Bacterial infections Meningitis is the most common result of bacterial infection of the immature nervous system. In the first month of life *Enterobacter*, *Listeria*, and β-streptococci are the most common agents, whereas *H. influenzae*, *Neisseria* meningitides, and pneumococcus are the most common in subsequent years. Acutely, the result of infection is cerebral edema that may be difficult to appreciate on US. CT and MRI may reveal hypodensities and T2 hyperintensities, respectively, that may not be indistinguishable from the high water content of the developing brain. Meningeal enhancement may occur. Complications of meningeal infection include cerebral infarction, ventriculitis, subdural collections, hydrocephalus, and atrophy (Fig. 6-30). Intracerebral abscesses are rare but may complicate *Citrobacter* meningitis in neonates.

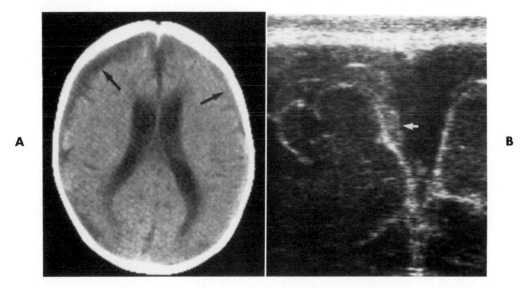

Fig. 6-30 Meningitis and effusion. A, Axial CT demonstrates bilateral low-density extracerebral collections (*arrows*) and ventricular dilation consistent with subdural effusions and hydrocephalus complicating Haemophilus influenzae meningitis. **B**, US confirming exudate (*arrow*) within the extraaxial collection.

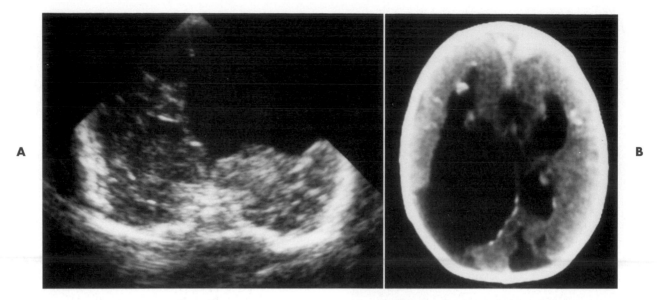

Fig. 6-31 Toxoplasmosis. A, Coronal US demonstrates ventriculomegaly with porencephaly. **B,** Unenhanced axial CT also demonstrates the periventricular calcifications.

Childhood brain abscesses (and empyemas) are often bilateral and of hematogenous origin. Abscesses usually arise at cerebral gray-white junctions, rarely in the cerebellum. They are more likely to occur in patients with uncorrected cyanotic congenital heart disease (CHD), sinus infection, or trauma and in immunocompromised hosts (HIV, after transplants). The CT and MRI appearance evolves from an ill-defined area (cerebritis) to a mass with a well-defined ring that enhances.

Viral infections Most viral infections in infancy result from transplacental transmission except for herpes simplex, which is contracted during passage through the infected birth canal. Perinatally acquired viral infections belong to the TORCH group (*toxoplasmosis; other* enteroviruses, varicella, mumps, measles; *rubella; cytomegalovirus; herpes* simplex and *HIV*).

CMV infection is the most common. Periventricular calcification is the hallmark, with resulting atrophy and encephalomalacia often identified (see box). Migrational disorders are associated with first trimester infections.

Toxoplasmosis Toxoplasma gondii infection is appearing with increased frequency in the perinatal period and is also part of the AIDS epidemic. Transplacental passage of the parasite usually occurs in the third trimester. If the infection occurs early in pregnancy, enlargement of the third and lateral ventricles, often marked, is characteristic. Periventricular calcifications are multiple and often symmetric, lining the ventricles and occurring in the basal ganglia. Porencephalic cysts may develop subsequently (Fig. 6-31).

Herpes simplex encephalitis Herpes simplex type 2 is responsible for the acute perinatal encephalitis. Herpes simplex type 1 usually occurs in older children and adults. It preferentially involves the frontal and temporal lobes. Generalized encephalitis is manifested by cerebral edema that may be accompanied by multifocal necrosis.

HIV encephalitis is manifested in up to half of HIV-positive patients with a progressive encephalopathy. CT demonstrates diffuse atrophy with ventriculomegaly and bilateral basal ganglia calcification. CMV infection commonly complicates this disease.

Leukoencephalitis Acute disseminated encephalomyelitis (ADEM) is the most common viral related encephalopathy of childhood. MRI is the imaging modality of choice, revealing multifocal white matter lesions that occasionally mimic those of multiple sclerosis and are often responsive to steroid therapy (Fig. 6-32).

Progressive multifocal leukoencephalopathy (PML) caused by the papovavirus is a common demyelinating disorder occurring in immunocompromised patients. Subacute sclerosing panencephalitis (SSPE) is a progressive encephalitis that produces demyelination and atrophy.

Subacute and chronic infections Subacute and chronic infections include tuberculosis and those of fungal etiology. Tuberculous meningitis is rare in infancy, occurring more commonly around age 5 years. Mycoses include aspergillosis, histoplasmosis, and coccidiomycosis and those caused by *Candida* or *Cryptococcus*. Basal cistern enhancement, hydro-

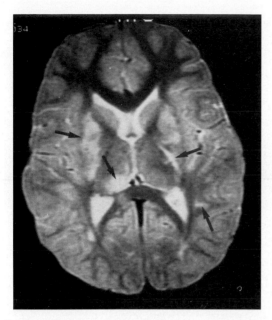

Fig. 6-32 Acute disseminated encephalomyelitis. Axial T2-weighted MRI demonstrates multiple hyperintensities involving the brain stem, basal ganglia, and capsular and periventricular white matter (*arrows*) characteristic of postviral acute disseminated encephalomyelitis.

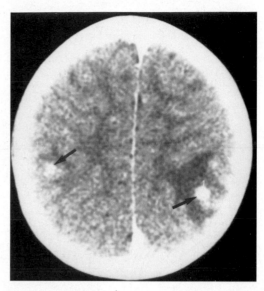

Fig. 6-33 Cysticercosis. Axial CT demonstrates high-density calcified and nodular-enhancing lesions (*arrows*) characteristic of

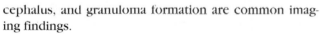

cephalus, and granuloma formation are common imaging findings.

Parasitic infections *Hydatid disease* occurs more frequently in children than in adults. The brain cysts grow slowly and usually are associated with cysts in the liver.

Cysticercosis is caused by the *Taenia solium* parasite. Its larvae have a predilection for the CNS. The lesions are cystic and often calcify (Fig. 6-33).

Lyme disease is caused by the spirochete *Borrelia burgdorferi* and manifests as an encephalopathy and a neuropathy associated with meningitis after the child is bitten by a tick. MRI and CT findings may mimic those of ADEM.

Vascular Disease, Hemorrhage, and Trauma

Hemorrhage Intracranial hemorrhage is a common occurrence in newborns less than 32 weeks gestation. Another risk factor is multiple gestation.

US screening for intracranial hemorrhage in infants less than 32 weeks gestation should occur routinely between 4 and 7 days of life unless there are earlier clinical indications (Fig. 6-34). More than 90% of neonatal hemorrhage occurs in the first week of life. If perinatal trauma is a consideration, CT may be needed to evaluate for subdural, epidural, or subarachnoid hemorrhage.

Intracranial Calcification (Conventional Radiograph)
PHYSIOLOGIC CAUSES
Choroid plexus
Habenula
Pineal gland (in older children)
ABNORMAL CAUSES
Infection (TORCH, HIV)
Metabolic disorders (hyperparathyroidism)
Tumors (craniopharyngioma, oligodendroglioma)
Phakomatosis (von Hippel-Lindau disease, Sturge-Weber syndrome, tuberous sclerosis)

Germinal matrix hemorrhage Germinal matrix hemorrhage, the most common type of hemorrhage, occurs in preterm infants of less than 32 weeks gestation who weigh less than 1500 g. It occurs rarely in term infants. The germinal matrix remnant is located near the head of the caudate nucleus at 28 weeks of gestation. It is richly vascularized, has little supporting stroma, and drains into the deep venous system (Fig. 6-35). Additional factors associated with germinal

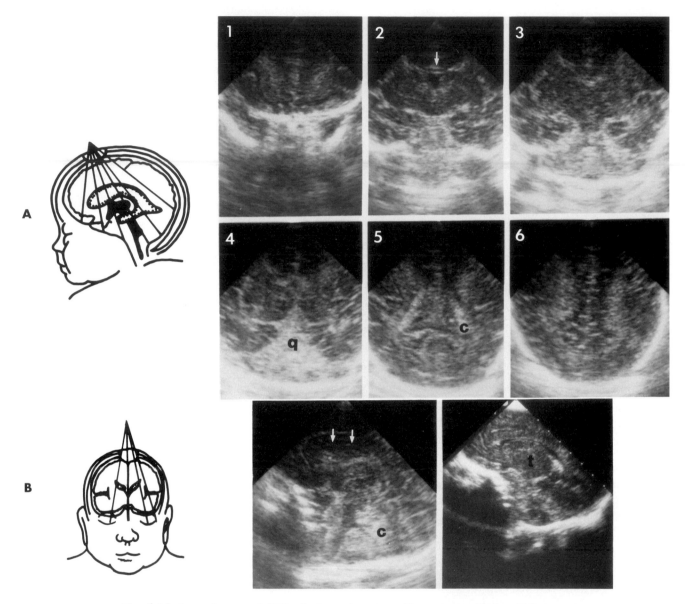

Fig. 6-34 Screening cranial US. **A**, Coronal sections. Note corpus callosum (CC) (*arrow*) on section 2; the "Christmas tree" (*q*), representing the quadrigerminal plate on section 4; the "moustache" of the choroid plexus (*c*) on section 5; and the symmetric centrum semiovale on section 6. **B**, Sagittal sections. Note the CC (*arrows*) in the same plane as the cerebellar vermis (*c*) in the midline section; the thalamus (*t*) is "hugged' by the (slitlike) occipital horns.

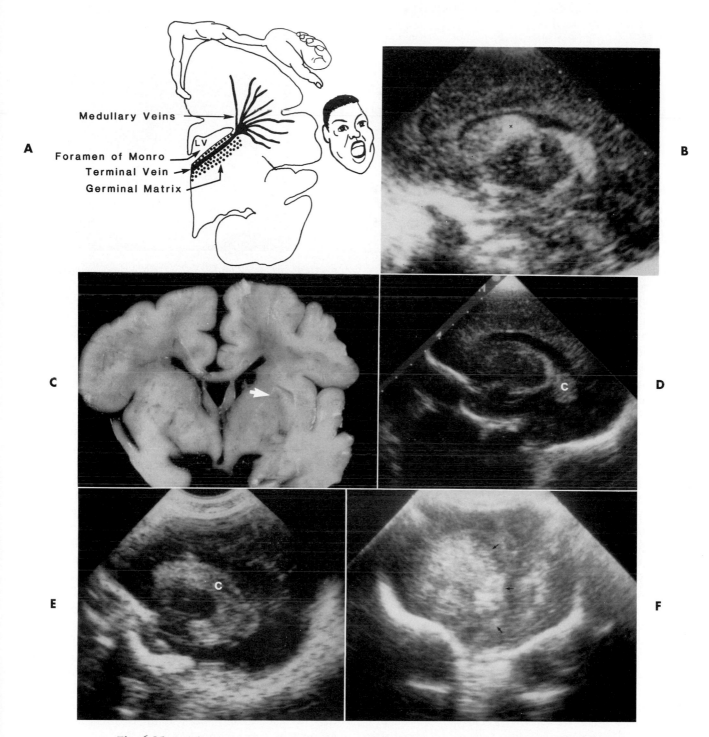

Fig. 6-35 **A**, Schematic representation of the germinal matrix. Periventricular veins and cortical representation of motor functions (*LV*, lateral ventricle). **B**, Grade 1 hemorrhage in the germinal matrix (*x*) on sagittal US. **C**, Gross specimen of same (*arrow*). **D**, Grade 2 hemorrhage with minimal ventricular dilation and clot (*c*) abutting the choroid plexus. **E**, Grade 3 hemorrhage (*c*) filling the entire ventricle. **F**, Grade 4 hemorrhage causing mass effect across the midline (*arrows*).

Grading of Germinal Matrix Hemorrhage

Grade 1: confined to subependymal germinal matrix
(see Fig. 6-35, *B* and *C*)
Grade 2: extends into ventricles but is not associated
with ventricular dilation (see Fig. 6-35, *D*)
Grade 3: fills the ventricle, causing ventricular dilation
(see Fig. 6-35, *E*)
Grade 4: intracerebral extension of grade 3 hemorrhage
(see Fig. 6-35, *F*)

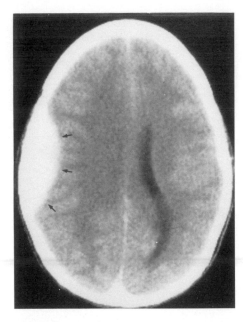

Fig. 6-36 Epidural hemorrhage. CT demonstrates a biconvex acute hemorrhage (*arrows*).

matrix hemorrhage include respiratory distress (hyaline membrane disease), fluctuations in systemic blood pressure and cerebral blood flow, and hypercarbia and hypoxia. Males are affected twice as often as females.

A grading system has been devised as shown in the box.

Whether grade 4 hemorrhage represents direct extension of the subependymal hemorrhage into the cerebrum or results from hemorrhagic venous infarction is subject for debate.

Grades 3 and 4 hemorrhages are associated with increased morbidity and mortality. Hydrocephalus occurs in approximately 70% of patients with intraventricular hemorrhage. In one third of patients ventriculoperitoneal shunting may be required.

Intracerebral hemorrhage In term infants coagulopathy, use of heparin therapy during ECMO, and vitamin K deficiency may be predisposing factors to intracerebral hemorrhage. Most commonly, however, intracerebral hemorrhage occurs in the presence of subependymal or intraventricular hemorrhage (choroid plexus or thalamic origin). US and CT reveal an echogenic and hyperdense lesion, respectively, that gradually becomes less echogenic and less dense during the first week. MRI may reveal dural venous sinus thrombosis. Porencephaly may develop, especially if the hemorrhage extends from the ventricle.

Epidural hemorrhage Commonly, epidural hemorrhage occurs in older children as a result of trauma and can occur infratentorially or supratentorially. These hemorrhages are caused by an arterial tear, often the result of calvarial fractures extending across the course of the anterior or posterior branches of the middle meningeal artery. Venous bleeding also may occur, particularly in the posterior fossa, from tearing of the dural venous sinuses. CT classically demonstrates a biconvex high-density lesion between the brain and the skull, occasionally limited by the attachment of the dura to the sutures (Fig. 6-36). Acute, active hemorrhage may appear mixed in density. More chronic hemorrhage may be isodense or low density.

Subdural hemorrhage Subdural hemorrhage occurs as a result of tearing of the falx or tentorial veins or the bridging veins. It may occur as a result of severe head molding during delivery or with trauma in the older infant and child as a result of severe head injury. If the subdural hemorrhage is of arterial origin, clinical manifestations occur earlier in the course. If it is of venous origin, the accumulation may be slow and take weeks. The possibility of child abuse must always be kept in mind. CT characteristically demonstrates an extracerebral high-density lesion in the acute phase, usually crescentic, and occasionally extending into the interhemispheric fissure. MRI is sensitive and more specific than CT in both the subacute and the chronic stages. The chronic lesion is often hyperintense on both T1 and T2 images because of the methemoglobin or high protein content (Fig. 6-37).

Benign extracerebral collections of infancy Benign extracerebral collections of infancy are associated with macrocephaly and are often noted incidentally on cranial US as an echofree extracerebral fluid collection (Fig. 6-38) or on CT as nonspecific low densities that may be bilateral and may vary in size. The collections are usually subarachnoid and may be associated with ventriculomegaly, which represents a type of transient external hydrocephalus caused by immaturity of the arachnoid villi. MRI may be needed to differentiate these collections from chronic subdural hematomas. There is often little or no mass effect, and the condition is characterized by gradual resolution to normal.

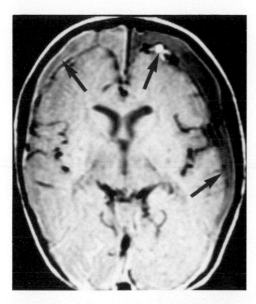

Fig. 6-37 Child abuse and subdural hematomas. Axial proton-density MRI demonstrates bilateral subdural collections and intensity findings (*arrows*) consistent with hemorrhages of varying age.

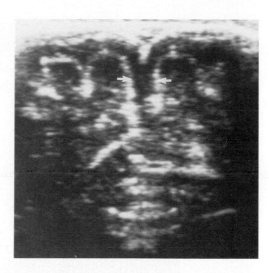

Fig. 6-38 Benign extracerebral collection of infancy. Coronal US reveals the echofree extracerebral fluid collection (*arrows*).

Subarachnoid hemorrhage is more easily detected on CT in the acute phase.

An *intracerebral hematoma* is not a frequent occurrence in infants and children. MRI is more sensitive than CT in demonstrating this in the subacute and chronic stages after trauma.

Contusions and shear injury Contusion is the result of microscopic hemorrhage within the brain. Local trauma to the static skull may create a depressed skull fracture and underlying bruising. An acceleration-deceleration force causes movement of the brain within the confines of the calvaria, producing bruising on the contralateral aspect of the brain (contracoup injury). This most commonly occurs in the frontal and anterior temporal lobes. CT may demonstrate an ill-defined area of increased density with surrounding edema, but MRI shows the extent of the contusion and gliosis better. Acceleration-deceleration forces may also produce shearing injury at gray-white matter junctions. Such injury may only be detected by MRI as T2 hyperintensities.

Ischemia

Hypoxic-ischemic brain injury Hypoxic-ischemic brain injury is a major cause of morbidity and mortality in the perinatal period and may result in developmental delay as a static encephalopathy. The causes include intrauterine factors, hyaline membrane disease (HMD), cyanotic CHD, and meconium aspiration. The common denominator is alteration of cerebral blood flow. Autoregulation allows constant cerebral blood flow, but in

the newborn infant this reflex has not been fully developed. The subsequent injury depends on the severity of the insult and the gestational age of the infant. In the preterm infant periventricular leukomalacia is the most common sequella, whereas in the term infant cortical and subcortical cerebral injury or basal ganglia injury is more common.

Periventricular leukomalacia Periventricular leukomalacia is defined as ischemic injury to the periventricular white matter in the preterm infant or preterm fetus. It results from diminished cerebral perfusion caused by hypotension. The white matter of the periventricular border zone is most vulnerable to this decreased flow, and because of the lack of autoregulation, infarction often occurs in the deep cerebral white matter adjacent to the lateral ventricles. The most common sites of ischemia are at the level of the occipital radiations at the trigones of the lateral ventricles and at the level of the cerebral white matter around the foramen of Monro. US is rather sensitive in the neonatal period, initially demonstrating areas of increased echogenicity. This then progresses to cystic lesions resembling Swiss cheese (Fig. 6-39). CT becomes more sensitive when ventriculomegaly and encephalomalacia have occurred. MRI may demonstrate white matter involvement to a greater extent (Fig. 6-39). There may be hemorrhage within areas of periventricular leukomalacia. With more profound asphyxia, there may be more extensive basal ganglia, thalamic, and brain stem or cerebellar injury.

Ischemic cerebral cortical and subcortical injury Focal or multifocal cerebral necrosis may result from hypoxia, hypotension, or either venous or arterial

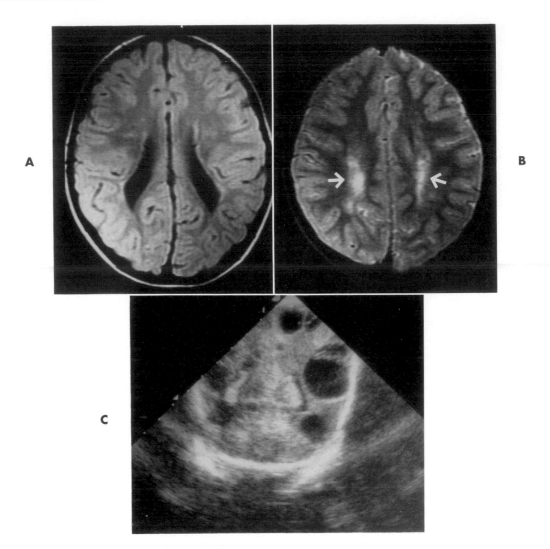

Fig. 6-39 Periventricular leukomalacia. Axial proton-density and T2-weighted MRIs (**A, B**) demonstrate lateral ventricular dilation and periventricular white matter hyperintensities (*arrows*) characteristic of periventricular leukomalacia. **C,** Characteristic Swiss-cheese appearance on coronal US.

occlusion. In the term infant or term fetus, asphyxia may result in border zone cortical and subcortical injury, whereas with more profound asphyxia more extensive injury may occur as described previously. In term infants the middle cerebral artery distribution is often involved in arterial occlusive disease, and the lesions tend to become cystic and may develop into porencephaly. The most common recognizable causes of arterial or venous occlusion in infancy include thromboembolism of placental or umbilical venous origin, disseminated intravascular coagulation (DIC), and neonatal polycythemia.

Vascular occlusive diseases Vascular occlusive disease may be arterial or venous in origin and related to stenosis, thrombosis, or embolization. The result may be ischemic edema, ischemic infarction, or hemorrhagic infarction. Vascular occlusion may occur with

known disease such as infection (e.g., meningitis with arteritis or thrombophlebitis), cardiovascular disease (e.g., CHD with polycythemia, hypoxemia, or embolism), hematologic disease (e.g., sickle cell disease with thrombosis), or trauma (e.g., penetrating oropharyngeal injury). Other *arterial* causes include metabolic disease (homocystinuria, mitochondrial cytopathies), moyamoya disease, vasculitis (systemic lupus erythematosis), migraine, fibromuscular disease, neurofibromatosis, familial lipid disorders, and chromosomal anomalies (Down syndrome). Cerebral infarction may occur after cardiac surgery or cardiac catheterization; with ECMO; in association with systemic disease (e.g., hemolytic-uremic syndrome); with hypertensive encephalopathy, cardiopulmonary arrest, carbon monoxide toxicity, radiation therapy, or near-sudden infant death syndrome (SIDS); or with neoplastic vascu-

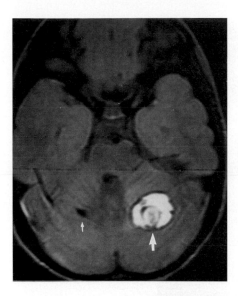

Fig. 6-40 Cavernous angioma. Axial proton-density MRI demonstrates a left cerebellar mass with central hyperintensities (methemoglobin) and concentric laminated ringlike hypointensities (hemosiderin) characteristic of a cavernous angioma (*large arrow*). A second hypointense lesion (hemosiderin) is demonstrated in the right cerebellum (*small arrow*).

lar invasion. Conditions associated with or known to produce *venous* occlusive disease include infection, dehydration, cyanotic CHD, leukemia, chemotherapy (L-asparaginase), venous catheters, neoplastic invasion, polycythemia, DIC, and use of oral contraceptives.

US or CT is done initially to detect or confirm the infarction as hemorrhagic or nonhemorrhagic and to distinguish it from hematoma. Often the initial imaging satisfies the clinical request. However, MRI has proved more sensitive and often more specific for vascular occlusive conditions, including multiple infarction, hemorrhagic infarction, and dural venous sinus occlusion. When infarction is associated with known disease (e.g., perinatal hypoxic-ischemic brain injury, infection, CHD, metabolic disorder, systemic disease), no further imaging may be necessary. The use of angiography may be considered for infarction of unknown cause only after MRI evaluation. In a substantial proportion of children with stroke syndrome, no cause is apparent after extensive clinical evaluation. The results of angiography are commonly negative or nonspecific as to causation or therapeutic significance. Commonly, these are children who previously were well, often have minimal or nonspecific imaging findings, and frequently recover without further episode. Because the clinically significant yield in this single-event group is quite low, angiography often is not done. However, angiography is considered for children with repeated unexplained episodes or for others with disease processes warranting more specific medical or surgical treatment. They include children with moyamoya disease, vasculitis, or traumatic arterial injury (e.g., carotid dissection, carotid-cavernous fistula).

Vascular anomalies, malformations, and aneurysms These lesions most often appear in a patient with a hemorrhagic event, seizures, headaches, or a progressive neurologic deficit. The majority become apparent during the second or third decade of life.

Acute spontaneous hemorrhage may be subarachnoid, intracerebral, or rarely intraventricular, subdural, or epidural and is readily detected by CT (or US in the neonate and young infant). The pathogenesis includes abnormal vessels (e.g., vascular malformation, aneurysm, neovascularity, hypoxic-ischemic injury) or abnormal blood (e.g., coagulopathy, hypertension). Vascular malformations of the CNS include arteriovenous shunts (AVM), cavernous angiomas, venous malformations, and telangiectasias (Fig. 6-40). Aneurysms are very rare in childhood but may be congenital; associated with Ehlers-Danlos syndrome, coarctation of the aorta (Turner syndrome), or polycystic kidney disease; or related to trauma or infection (mycotic aneurysm).

Congenital aneurysms of the circle of Willis rarely occur in infants or children (3% of all aneurysms). The underlying cause is a congenital defect in the media in up to 80% of patients, and many are giant aneurysms in contradistinction to those in adults. Mycotic aneurysms are often associated with bacterial endocarditis. The vessel wall is invaded by infected emboli, with subsequent degeneration and focal expansion. A classic type of aneurysm in infancy associated with congestive heart failure and hydrocephalus is the vein of Galen aneurysm. It may represent a direct arteriovenous shunt or the venous component of a separate AVM. Headaches and seizures may be the presenting symptoms in adolescents. Color-flow doppler US and MRI will demonstrate the enlarged vein and flow turbulence (Fig. 6-41).

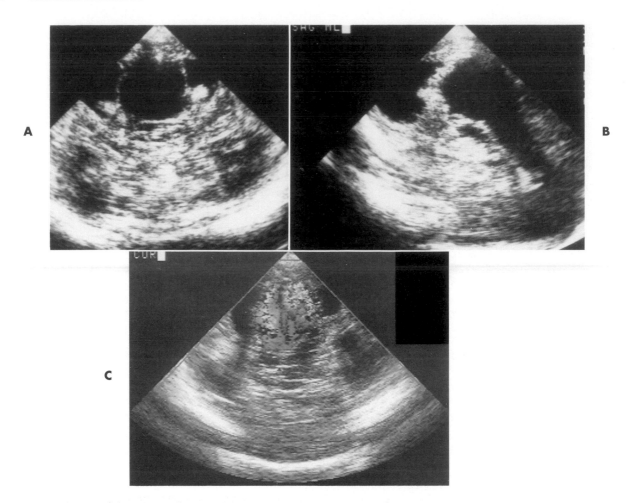

Fig. 6-41 Vein of Galen aneurysm. A, Transverse and, **B,** sagittal US reveals a dilated cystic structure in the region of the vein of Galen. **C,** Color-flow Doppler image corresponding to **A** (see Color Plate 3).

Neoplasms

US or CT detects the majority of intracranial masses in childhood, particularly in infancy, mainly because of their large size at presentation. Definitive evaluation, including treatment planning and follow-up of tumor response and treatment effects, is done with MRI. For the evaluation of tumor seeding, gadolinium enhancement is necessary.

Cerebral hemispheric tumors Cerebral hemispheric tumors often manifest in children as seizures or hemiparesis. The vast majority are of neuroepithelial origin. Meningeal, vascular, and lymphoreticular tumors and metastatic neoplasms rarely occur in childhood. In infancy most intracranial masses are nonneoplastic and cystic (Dandy-Walker cyst, arachnoid cyst, porencephaly), and neoplasia is rare (PNET, astrocytomas and germ cell tumors, choroid plexus tumors).

Neuroepithelial tumors Neuroepithelial tumors include gliomas (astrocytoma, ependymoma, oligoden-

droglioma), neuronal and mixed neuronal-glial tumors (ganglioglioma), embryonal tumors (PNET), and choroid plexus and pineal cell tumors.

Astrocytomas are a heterogeneous group that comprise 40% to 50% of all brain tumors in childhood. They can occur anywhere within the CNS (e.g., optic glioma, brain stem glioma, thalamic glioma). Only the hemispheric gliomas are more common in adults. Depending on the classification, there are grades of malignancy including astrocytoma, anaplastic astrocytoma, and glioblastoma.

Oligodendrogliomas are developed from the myelin-forming cells of the CNS. They are uncommon and may contain astrocytic components (mixed glioma). Calcification occurs more frequently than in other gliomas. Edema and mass effect are often lacking.

Choroid plexus papillomas arise from the papillary secretory epithelial cells of the choroid plexus. They are classic tumors of infancy and seldom appear beyond childhood. The lateral ventricle is the most frequent location, especially in the region of the trigone,

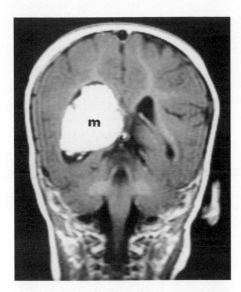

Fig. 6-42 Choroid plexus papilloma. Gadolinium-enhanced coronal T1-weighted MRI demonstrates a markedly enhancing right lateral intraventricular tumor (*m*).

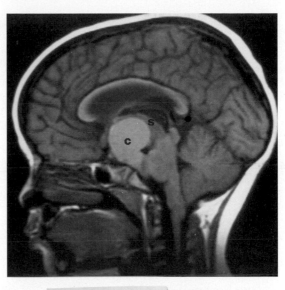

Fig. 6-43 Craniopharyngioma. Sagittal T1-weighted MRI demonstrates a hyperintense suprasellar cyst (*c*) and isointense solid tumor (*s*) characteristic of a craniopharyngioma.

and hydrocephalus is almost always present in children with these lesions (Fig. 6-42). The majority are benign and slow growing. Occasionally there is anaplastic change (carcinoma), and seeding may occur. Surgical excision of choroid plexus papillomas leads to excellent survival.

Neuronal tumors include gangliocytoma and ganglioglioma. Gangliocytomas lack a glial component and may actually represent hamartomas. Gangliogliomas are slow growing and often calcified.

The primitive neuroectodermal tumor (PNET) resembles the cerebellar medulloblastoma, is a generic term for an undifferentiated CNS tumor with neurectodermal features in any location, and often contains small round (blue) cells. Calcification and cyst formation are common, and enhancement occurs on CT and MRI.

Tumors near the third ventricle Tumors near the third ventricle may be subdivided into lesions that arise in the suprasellar region (anterior third ventricle), the pineal region (posterior third ventricle), or in an intraventricular or paraventricular location. Children with these lesions may have hydrocephalus, a neuroendocrine disorder (precocious puberty, failure to thrive, diabetes insipidus), or visual impairment (optic pathway involvement).

Craniopharyngioma Craniopharyngiomas represent epithelial proliferations of Rathke's pouch origin. They are considered benign and are slow growing. Characteristically, they are cystic suprasellar tumors with calcifications and are more common in boys. Rathke's cyst has a similar appearance except calcification is rare (Fig. 6-43).

Optic hypothalamic glioma Astrocytomas arising from the optic pathways or hypothalamus can lead to visual disturbances, neuroendocrine disorders, or seizures. Gliomas arising along the optic chiasm, the optic nerves, or the optic tracts are especially common in patients with neurofibromatosis 1. Calcification or cyst formation is unusual. Ependymomas, oligodendrogliomas, and choroid plexus tumors rarely occur in this region.

Dermoid or epidermoid tumors Dermoid or epidermoid tumors usually are cystic and probably result from inclusion of epithelial rest elements at the time of neural tube closure. Epidermoid tumors contain keratin debris ("pearly tumor" or cholesteatomas) and often show CSF characteristics on CT and MRI imaging. Dermoids may contain skin appendages, sweat glands, and their breakdown products, resulting in an oily, often calcified midline lesion with T1 hyperintensity.

Germ cell and pineal cell tumors Germ cell tumors commonly occur in the suprasellar and pineal regions. Histologically, pineal region tumors include both germ cell tumors (germinomas, teratomas, choriocarcinoma, embryonal carcinoma, endodermal sinus tumors) and pineal cell tumors (pineoblastoma, pineocytoma). Because pineal region tumors often obstruct the aqueduct, hydrocephalus is a common presenting symptom. Calcification occurs commonly, and seeding is fre-

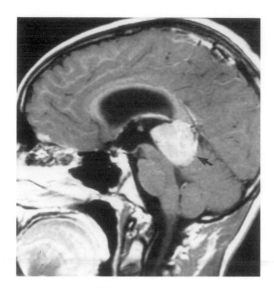

Fig. 6-44 Pineal germinoma. Gadolinium-enhanced sagittal T1-weighted MRI demonstrates a markedly enhancing pineal region tumor (*arrow*) characteristic of a germinoma.

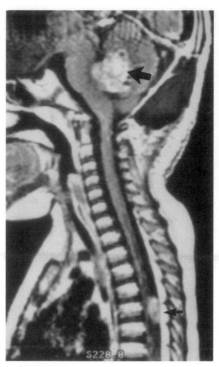

Fig. 6-45 Medulloblastoma. Gadolinium-enhanced sagittal T1-weighted MRI demonstrates a midline enhancing posterior fossa tumor (*upper arrow*) and an enhancing intradural nodule (*lower arrow*) characteristic of medulloblastoma with spinal seeding.

quently seen. Partial excision may be possible; however, radiotherapy or chemotherapy is often needed to control tumor growth (Fig. 6-44).

Posterior fossa tumors Posterior fossa tumors of childhood often present with hydrocephalus, ataxia, cranial nerve palsies, or head tilt.

Cerebellar astrocytoma Often eccentric lesions in the posterior fossa, cerebellar astrocytomas comprising 30% of posterior fossa tumors are derived from astrocytic glial cells and are often cystic with solid tumor nodules. They are frequently benign, and the cystic component may be large. Symptoms often are related to those of hydrocephalus. CT and MRI characteristically reveal a cyst with an enhancing mural nodule or nodules. The cystic component of the tumor is often more dense or intense than CSF because of its high protein content. Treatment involves surgical resection, often with excellent results.

Medulloblastoma Twenty-five percent of posterior fossa tumors are medulloblastomas. These highly malignant and invasive tumors are often classified as PNETs. They classically are rapidly growing midline posterior fossa lesions, although they may be eccentrically located. The appearance may simulate that of an ependymoma or an astrocytoma. Often hyperdense on unenhanced CT images, there is marked enhancement after IV contrast administration. MRI defines the extent of the tumor to better advantage, especially with gadolinium enhancement. Seeding of the CNS is a common occurrence, and hematogenous metastases rarely extend to bone or lung (Fig. 6-45).

Ependymoma Arising from the ependymal lining of the ventricles, most commonly the floor of the fourth ventricle, ependymomas (15% of posterior fossa tumors) are usually slow-growing lesions producing hydrocephalus. Seeding of the subarachnoid space rarely occurs. Often there is a well-circumscribed eccentric posterior fossa mass of heterogeneous density or intensity, with frequent calcification, edema, and necrosis. A lobular contour is characteristic, with extension into the adjacent cisterns around the brain stem and upper cervical cord.

Brain stem tumors Brain stem tumors are almost always astrocytomas. These lesions most commonly occur in the pons or less often in the midbrain or medulla and upper cervical spinal cord. Multiple areas may be involved, and the presenting symptoms usually relate to involvement of the cranial nerves or pyramidal tracts. It is unusual for increased ICP to develop until late. Most lesions are inhomogeneous in appearance, and some have a cystic component. Enhancement is often modest.

The conventional radiograph of the spine remains the most important initial test, and it serves as a guide to further, more definitive imaging. Evaluation of cran-

THE SPINE

Normal Spinal Column and Its Variants
Developmental Abnormalities
    Myelodysplasias
        Meningomyelocele
        Meningocele
        Hydromyelia
        Lipomyelomeningocele
        Tethered cord syndrome
        Anterior meningocele
        Diastematomyelia
        Neurenteric cyst
        Caudal dysplasias
        Developmental tumors
    Spondylodysplasias
        Scoliosis and kyphosis
        Scheuermann "disease"
        Spinovascular anomalies
        Craniocervical anomalies
Acquired Abnormalities
    Inflammatory lesions
    Trauma
        Spondylolysis and spondylolisthesis
    Neoplasms
        Intramedullary lesions
        Intradural lesions
        Extradural lesions
            Benign lesions
            Aggressive lesions

iocervical anomalies and trauma requires conventional radiographs in the frontal and lateral projections and an open-mouth frontal view to evaluate the atlantoocciptal and atlantoaxial relations. Oblique views occasionally are helpful to evaluate the facet joints and the intervertebral foramina. Fluoroscopy helps evaluate both soft tissue contours and mobility or instability. In both instances, further imaging (CT or MRI) then can be appropriately directed.

CT is useful in evaluating bony traumatic, dysplastic, or neoplastic changes (e.g., spondylolysis, diastematomyelia, osteoid osteoma), but MRI is the ideal modality for definitive imaging of neural, vascular, and CSF-containing structures.

US is a useful screening modality in the neonate and young infant to document normal conus level (above L2-3), especially in infants who have a sacral dimple or equivocal spine radiographs. Intraoperative US may assist in guiding neurosurgical procedures (e.g., hydrosyringomyelia).

Normal Spinal Column and Its Variants

Each vertebral segment develops separately from the ones above and below it by a process of condensation of the sclerotome on the notochord. Resegmentation then results in a membranous vertebra. At 4 weeks gestation, three separate mesenchymal centers develop in each vertebral unit: the centrum (surrounding the notochord) and the neural processes (neural arches). Chondrification starts at 6 to 8 weeks gestation (Fig. 6-46).

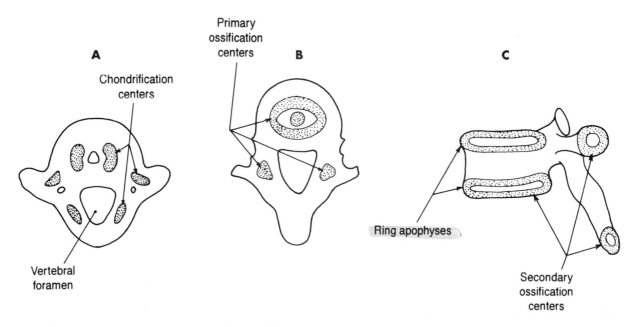

Fig. 6-46 A through C, Vertebral body development.

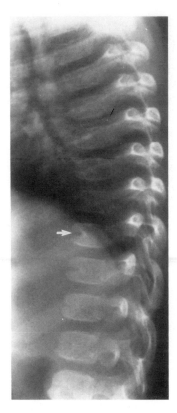

Fig. 6-47 "Hamburger" appearance of a 2-year-old child's ovoid vertebral body. Note the vascular channels anteriorly (*arrow*).

There are two *chondrification centers* in each half of the vertebral body and in each half of the neural arches (posterior elements). These centers in each half of the neural arches appear first in the cervical region. At 8 to 9 weeks, they have fused and become the primary *ossification centers*, the anterior and posterior ossification centers of the vertebral body. The arches ossify from the cervical region caudally, and the laminae ossify from the lumbar region cephalad. The notochordal remnants, located between the two vertebral body chondrification centers, coalesce to become the nucleus pulposus. Fusion of the vertebral arch and the centrum occurs anterior to the pedicles at the neurocentral synchondroses. Between 3 and 6 years of age, these synchondroses ossify to unite the centrum and neural arches. Before 3 years of age, the vertebrae appear ovoid, with anterior and posterior vascular clefts visible ("hamburger appearance") (Fig. 6-47). There may be a "bone-within-bone" appearance of the vertebral bodies up to approximately 1 month of life. This is a normal "growth spurt" phenomenon. Anterior and posterior vascular channels are often evident. The latter disappear in infancy; the anterior channels may persist through adolescence. End-plate (secondary ossification center) ossification appears between 6 and 9 years, forms a ring by 12 years, and fuses to the vertebral body at maturity.

Developmental landmarks peculiar to C1 and C2 include the following. The subdental synchondrosis may make the dens appear separated from the axis body. This line consists of a disk-shaped cartilaginous plate that may persist to age 6 years. Likewise, on the anterior "open mouth" view, the odontoid may appear split into halves as a result of the unfused lateral ossification centers. At the tip of the dens, the ossiculum terminale may be identified between 6 and 12 years of age. Finally, the anterior arch of the atlas (C1) also has a separate (sometimes multiple) ossification center. This is exquisitely visible on CT at birth in 25% of patients. The synchondroses may not fuse until 6 years of age.

Vertebral body height changes with age and is influenced by gravitational forces. Square in the neonate and more rectangular with advancing age, vertebral body height is accentuated in patients who cannot maintain the erect position (e.g., cerebral palsy). Vertebral body shape in these patients resembles rabbit or canine vertebral bodies.

The *vertebral disk* is composed of the annulus fibrosus, attached to the vertebral body, and the nucleus pulposus. As large as the ossified vertebral body at birth, the disk "shrinks" because of gravitational forces as the child starts to ambulate. Calcification occurring in the nucleus pulposus is rare but can be seen in the cervical and thoracic regions. Symptoms are rare but may include pain, and the calcifications often are associated with anterior or posterior disk protrusions. Prognosis is favorable. The differential diagnosis includes disk space infection (diskitis).

Disorders of end-plate chondrification and ossification may provide the explanation for Schmorl's nodules and Scheuermann "disease" because both conditions can be brought about by persistent notochordal remnants interfering with these processes (see Scheuermann "Disease" on p. 231).

The *normal alignment of the craniocervical junction* can be established by McGregor's line, which is drawn from the hard palate to the inferior occiput. The tip of the dens should not be more than 4.5 mm above this line; 7 mm is definitely abnormal. The anterior arch-dens interval varies from 3 mm to 5 mm with flexion and extension in children up to age 12 years. The posterior dens–posterior arch (spinal canal) should be greater than 15 mm (19 mm in adults).

The normal alignment of the cervical spine may vary slightly from that in adults (Fig. 6-48, *A*). Normally, a line (1) through the anterior inferior aspect of the cervical vertebral bodies and along the posterior aspect of same (2) should be a smooth continuum. Likewise a line (3) drawn through the anterior aspects of the spin-

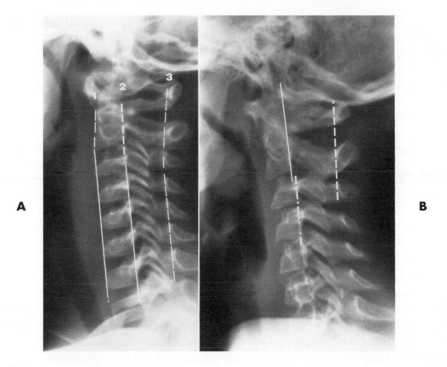

Fig. 6-48 Pseudosubluxation. A, Normal alignment of vertebral bodies. **B**, Pseudosubluxation of C2 with regard to C3 in a flexed cervical spine.

ous processes is smoothly convex anteriorly. Because the fulcrum of cervical motion in children is centered at and above C4 (as opposed to C5-6 in adults), C2 may appear anteriorly subluxed with regard to C3 in a slightly flexed cervical spine. Line 3 remains undisturbed in this condition. Ligamentous laxity and apophyseal joint orientation (more horizontal in children) have been implicated (Fig. 6-48, *B*). This is called *pseudosubluxation*.

Developmental Abnormalities

Myelodysplasias *Dysraphic myelodysplasia* refers to any incomplete midline closure of the neural tube, including the vertebral column and associated soft tissues. It may be overt or occult. Overt posterior myelodysplasias are anomalies of the spinal column and neuraxis that result when the posterior elements have failed to fuse completely (i.e., defects of primary neurulation). Clinical findings include an obvious dorsal defect plus scoliosis, gait disturbances, paresis, and/or bladder or bowel dysfunction. Primary neurulation defects include meningomyelocele, Chiari II malformation, and hydromyelia. Secondary neurulation defects or occult myelodysplasias are skin-covered malforma-

---

Spinal Dysraphism

PRIMARY NEURULATION DEFECTS

Meningomyelocele
Meningocele
Hydrosyringomyelia

SECONDARY NEURULATION DEFECTS

Lipomyelomeningocele
Tethered cord with thickened filum
Anterior meningocele
Diastematomyelia
Neurenteric cyst
Caudal dysplasias
Developmental tumors

---

tions and include lipomyelomeningocele, dermal sinus, or tethered cord syndrome. Anterior dysraphism includes anterior meningocele, diastematomyelia, and neurenteric cyst. The caudal dysplasia spectrum (e.g., sacral agenesis) and developmental mass lesions (e.g., lipomas, dermoids, epidermoids) are also included in the occult dysraphism category. Often they occur in combination (see box).

In the evaluation of anterior dysraphic changes, the plain film findings may include congenital scoliosis or kyphosis caused by formation anomalies (e.g., butterfly vertebra, hemivertebra, wedge vertebra) or segmentation anomalies (e.g., block vertebra, pedicle bar). Associated myelodysplasia occurs in 15% to 20% of patients with these anomalies, especially the neurenteric spectrum (e.g., diastematomyelia). Posterior dysraphic changes are related to defective spinolaminal development that results in spina bifida and dural ectasia, most often at the lumbosacral level. Myelodysplasias occur in more than 90% of these patients and include the primary and secondary neurolation defects listed in the box on p. 227.

Meningomyelocele Myelomeningocele is the most common primary neurulation defect (1:1000 live births). The neural tube remains approximated to the ectoderm for some distance, and the spinal cord and/or nerve roots are incorporated within a sac and exposed externally. These abnormalities are associated with the Chiari II malformation and often with hydrocephalus and hydrosyringomyelia. Seventy percent occur below the level of L2. Conventional radiographs of the spine reveal characteristic widening of the spinal canal (interpediculate distance). Hemivertebra, fused vertebrae, and fused pedicles all may be seen, and there may be an associated kyphoscoliosis in up to one third of patients. Skull radiographs may show a lacunar skull (lückenschädel), a dysplasia of the membranous calvaria. Cranial CT and craniospinal MRI may further delineate extent and involvement of the neural dysplasias, the postsurgical appearance, and any sequelae. Tethering or scarring of the cord/placode and dural sac stenosis are sequelae that may be difficult to define with imaging.

Meningocele A meningocele is a protusion of the meninges through a defect of the posterior bony elements, with the spinal cord often in its normal position within the spinal canal. Dura and arachnoid form the wall of this CSF-filled sac.

Hydromyelia Hydromyelia is the dilation of the central canal of the spinal cord. If a cavitation of the spinal cord also has occurred, it is called *syringomyelia*. Since these conditions often occur together, the commonly used term is *hydrosyringomyelia*. Hydrosyringomyelia occurs most frequently with the Chiari malformations. It may also occur after trauma, with neoplasia, or after surgery. MRI is the imaging modality of choice.

Lipomyelomeningocele Lipomyelomeningoceles are probably the most common of the occult dysraphic myelodysplasias. Similar to myelomeningoceles, they incorporate fat into the defect. They may appear with a lipoma that is located subcutaneously and extends into the spinal canal (Fig. 6-49). There is usually no associated Chiari II malformation or hydrocephalus. Symptoms and signs eventually develop in all patients with this condition. The mildest form of incomplete separation of the dorsally closing neural tube from the overlying ectoderm is probably represented by a dermal sinus or a dimple.

Tethered cord syndrome Tethering of the cord is caused by primary shortening of the filum terminale or is secondary to dysraphic changes preventing the normal "ascent" of the conus medullaris above L2-3. It can also be the sequela of the surgical repair of these entities. The ischemic tension of the spinal cord leads, depending on severity, either to neurologic symptoms and signs or to muscle weakness and gait disturbance caused by scoliosis or foot deformities. Bladder and bowel dysfunction are the most common presenting symptoms in the older children. Physical examination may reveal a hairy patch, a dorsal dimple, or a sinus tract in more than 50% of these children. In an infant US may demonstrate *low* termination of the conus medullaris below L2 or L2-3, a *thick*(>2 mm) filum terminale, or a tethering mass (e.g., lipoma). MRI confirms the findings.

Anterior meningocele An anterior meningocele is most often found in the sacral region. It is a relatively infrequent anomaly that consists of absence of part of the sacrum, producing a characteristic semicircular or sickle-shaped bony defect. Bladder or bowel dysfunction is the most common presentation, along with an occasional presacral pelvic mass. MRI exquisitely delineates the protruding CSF-containing sac communicating with the lumbar subarachnoid space.

Diastematomyelia Diastematomyelia ("cleft" or "split" spinal cord) is an abnormality of spinal development in which there is longitudinal splitting of the spinal cord. This may be accompanied by a dividing bony septum or fibrous band that extends from the posterior spinous process toward the midline of the vertebral body. This transfixes the spinal cord and may be identified on plain films as a midline bony density at the widest part of the spinal canal. The split cord may extend for several vertebral bodies and usually reconstitutes above and below the split. It usually occurs in the lower thoracic and upper lumbar regions and presents with a clinical picture similar to that for tethered cord. Cutaneous abnormalities of the back may include a dimple or a hairy nevus. Girls are affected much more commonly than boys. Early diagnosis and treatment may preserve spinal cord function. Although it can be imaged by US in the newborn and demonstrated well on CT, MRI is the modality of choice for definitive demonstration of this abnormality (Fig. 6-50). Hydromyelia is seen in approximately half of these patients.

Neurenteric cyst A neurenteric cyst may result from

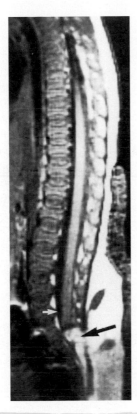

Fig. 6-49 Tethered cord syndrome and lipoma. Sagittal T1-weighted MRI demonstrates low position of the caudal spinal cord (*white arrow*) and a tethering intradural lipoma (*black arrow*) continuous with a dorsal subcutaneous lipoma (lipo-myelomeningocele).

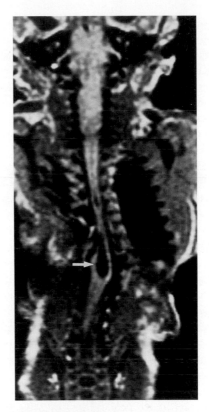

Fig. 6-50 Diastematomyelia. Coronal T1-weighted MRI demonstrates longitudinal splitting of the spinal cord with a bony septum (*arrow*).

persistent connection of the endoderm to the noto-chord. A thoracic mass is often identified on the chest radiograph in the posterior mediastinum and is associated with vertebral anomalies and occasionally an intraspinal component. In infants meningitis often occurs. Gastric mucosa has been demonstrated in neurenteric cysts that may ulcerate and bleed. Conventional radiographs illustrate multiple hemiverte-bra, block vetrebrae, or butterfly vertebrae, and there is associated widening of the spinal canal. Cross-sectional and axial imaging by MRI provides definitive anatomic delineation. With a meningocele, the cord and nerve roots are often deviated toward the opening; the reverse occurs in a child with neurenteric cyst.

Caudal dysplasias Caudal regression syndrome is a broad spectrum of abnormalities characterized by hypoplasia or agenesis of the lower lumbar and sacral spine (lumbosacral agenesis or dysgenesis) that may be associated with absence or underdevelopment of the lower extremities (sirenomelus). Maternal diabetes as a risk factor and a familial incidence have been described. The incidence is 1:7500 live births. If the sacral hypoplasia is mild, the symptoms may include gastrointestinal (GI), genitourinary (GU), or motor impairment later in life. If it is severe, anorectal and urogenital malformations are seen at birth, as well as anomalies or absence of the lower limbs. Absence of the spine above T12 is incompatible with life. Severity of hypoplasia ranges from mild (type 1) to severe (type 4). Patients with either a type 1 or 2 sacral hypoplasia or agenesis only can ambulate and sit. Types 3 and 4 include variable involvement of the lumbar spine with or without iliac fusion. Conventional radiographs often suggest the diagnosis. Associated myelodysplasias may include presacral meningocele, dysplastic conus, lipomyelomeningocele, or myelocystocele.

Developmental tumors Developmental tumors other than lipomas include (epi)dermoid cysts, teratomas, and vascular malformations.

(Epi)dermoids are developmental cysts that occur occasionally with dysraphism. Twenty percent are associated with a dermoid sinus. They account for approximately 10% of all intraspinal lesions, and 80% occur in the lumbar region.

Teratomas (involving all three germinal layers) occur in approximately one of every 40,000 live births. The sacrococcygeal region is the most frequent site of occurrence, and Hensen's node the site of origin. Teratomas occur more frequently in girls (4:1). When identified at birth, the neoplasms are more aggressive in boys. Because these tumors have a high incidence of malignant elements in older patients, probably as a result of malignant transformation with age, any delay in diagnosis and treatment should be avoided. In infants more than 2 months of age, 90% of sacrococcygeal teratomas contain some malignant tissue. Type 1 tumors are primarily external in location; type 2 tumors have intrapelvic components; and type 3 tumors are primarily intrapelvic in location. Type 4 tumors are presacral in location and are the most difficult to detect. An intraspinal component is infrequent. Conventional radiographs may reveal a soft tissue mass, scoliosis, canal or foraminal widening, pedicle erosion, and abnormal calcification (Fig. 6-51). Calcification is present in two thirds of patients and can occur in a variety of shapes. US assists in determining cystic or partially cystic lesions and their extent. These patients are treated by surgical excision of the entire coccyx. Differential diagnostic possibilities include an anterior meningocele, neuroblastoma, rectal duplication, and ovarian pathology. MRI or occasionally CT is useful to define the extent of the lesion.

Spondylodysplasias Spondylodysplasia is the term used for developmental abnormalities of the spinal column.

Scoliosis Scoliosis is the presence of one or more lateral curvatures of the spine. *Kyphosis* refers to increased posterior angulation of the spine, whereas *lordosis* denotes increased anterior angulation of the spine. Scoliosis in children is most often idiopathic (85%) and is usually painless. The remaining 15% of cases are congenital (abnormal bone development—e.g., hemivertebra, pedicle bar), neuromuscular (e.g., poliomyelitis, cerebral palsy) due to neurofibromatosis, or are posttraumatic or inflammatory (e.g., tuberculosis, juvenile rheumatoid arthritis), dysplastic, or associated with neoplasia.

In the idiopathic group a strong genetic component has been implicated and is transmitted as an autosomal dominant trait. There is a strong family occurrence (80%), and girls outnumber boys 8 to 9:1. There are three major groups: infantile (<3 years of age); juvenile (4 to 9 years); and adolescent (10 years to skeletal maturity). Typically there is a convex right thoracic curve. Congenital scoliosis often is associated with spinal dysraphism (20%), GU anomalies (20%), and CHD (20%). Rib fusion, absence, or hypoplasia is also common. Klippel-Feil syndrome and Sprengel's deformity comprises a subgroup of children with congenital scoliosis.

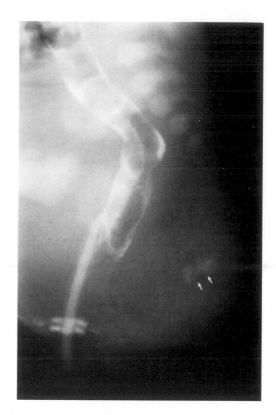

Fig. 6-51 Sacrococcygeal teratoma. Lateral radiograph demonstrates contrast medium in the rectum and a large soft tissue mass containing calcifications (*arrows*).

Imaging depends on patient age and the cause of the curvature. Initial examination includes standing frontal and lateral radiographs of the entire spine obtained in association with a bone age evaluation. Findings on this examination determine the need for MRI or CT and the occasional skeletal survey in patients with suspected skeletal dysplasias or other syndromes. Posterior anterior radiographs are suggested to reduce the radiation to developing breasts and gonads (since girls significantly outnumber boys). Bending films may be obtained to determine the degree of mobility and potential for correction. Measuring the magnitude of the curve may be necessary, and the method of Cobb is used most often. This is achieved by using perpendiculars constructed to a line tangential to the upper border of the most cephalad body and a similar line related to the lower border of the most caudal body; this will measure the angle of scoliosis. Angles less than 20 degrees are often neither clinically noted nor treated.

In 25% of cases of idiopathic scoliosis, the most common type, the curve may progress. Surgical correction of the scoliosis often is not contemplated until the Cobb angle exceeds 40 degrees after skeletal maturity. In children with lesser degrees of scoliosis, initial treatment includes the use of a brace to counteract progression. Operative treatment may include internal fixation

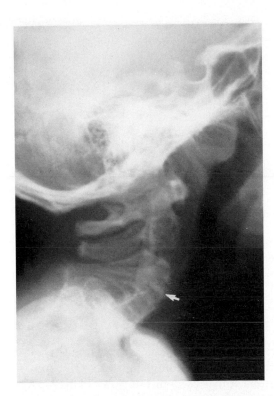

Fig. 6-52 Klippel-Feil syndrome. Lateral cervical spinal plain film demonstrates bony fusion (failure of segmentation) of multiple segments (*arrow*) characteristic of Klippel-Feil syndrome

(e.g., with Harrington rods, Dwyer apparatus) and bony fusion.

In congenital scoliosis, the bony anomalies may occur in isolation, may be part of the VATER or VACTERL association, or may be associated with the neurenteric spectrum of malformations. Short neck, low hairline, and lack of neck motion associated with cervical spinal segmentation anomalies are characteristic of children with the Klippel-Feil syndrome, radiographically evident as fusion of one or two pairs of cervical vertebrae (Fig. 6-52). There may be underlying myelodysplasias, including diastematomyelia or hydrosyringomyelia. Associated GU, GI, CNS, and cardiovascular anomalies occur. One third of these patients also have Sprengel deformity, which is failure of descent of one or both scapulae. A fibrous or bony connection between the scapula and the cervical spine may persist (omovertebral bone).

Kyphosis Kyphosis, increased posterior angulation of the spine, most commonly is congenital and is caused by formation-segmentation anomalies, but it may also be caused by Scheuermann "disease," neurofibromatosis, skeletal dysplasias, neuromuscular disorders, osteopenia, or trauma.

Lordosis Excessive lordosis is often congenital, but it may be acquired. In the latter group of patients

skeletal dysplasias or neuromuscular causes may be implicated, as may spondylolysis and/or spondylolisthesis (see "Spondylolysis and Spondylolisthesis" pp. 232-233).

Scheuermann "disease" Herniation of the nucleus pulposus into an adjacent vertebral body (Schmorl's node) usually occurs in the central portion of the vertebral body. When it occurs eccentrically and the patient is a teenager (commonly male) with back pain and thoracic kyphosis, Scheuermann "disease" (juvenile kyphosis or "round-back" syndrome) is diagnosed. Imaging criteria include narrowing of the intervertebral spaces of at least three adjacent vertebral bodies, with irregularities and/or Schmorl's nodes in the lower thoracic (most commonly T6-10) and upper lumbar region that may be lead to anterior wedging and kyphosis. A genetic weakness of the vertebral end plates (notochordal remnant?) has been suggested as a cause. Possible contributory factors are stress spondylodystrophy caused by traumatic growth arrest and/or end-plate fractures during the adolescent growth spurt.

Spinovascular anomalies Spinovascular anomalies occur infrequently and are due to maldevelopment during the second stage of vascular formation (6 weeks gestation). They can be classified as vascular malformations (e.g., AVM), vascular tumors (i.e., hemangioma), and angiodysplastic syndromes (e.g., Sturge-Weber).

Vascular malformations are congenital. AVMs are the most common. Patients with intramedullary, dural, or metameric AVMs often initially have pain or myelopathy. These AVMs are demonstrated best by MRI and angiography. Less common are vascular anomalies such as telangiectasias, venous malformations, hemangiomas, and lymphatic malformations. Angiodysplastic syndromes (neurocutaneous syndromes) are discussed earlier in this chapter.

Craniocervical anomalies Important anomalies include basilar invagination, occipitalization of the atlas, odontoid hypoplasia, os odontoideum, and atlantoaxial and occipitoatlantal instability (e.g., Down syndrome). Conventional radiographs may be sufficient for detecting these anomalies (Fig. 6-53). Flexion and extension filming, CT, and MRI may be necessary for evaluating unstable anomalies.

Acquired Anomalies of the Spine and Neuraxis

Inflammatory lesions Inflammatory lesions of the vertebral column, especially hematogenously borne spondylitis (i.e., diskitis, osteomyelitis), are uncommon. Vertebral disk and body destruction with collapse can result in kyphosis. *Diskitis* occurs when the infection is contained in the intervertebral disk with minimal contiguous spread. *Osteomyelitis* is present when there is vertebral body involvement. Spondylitis is

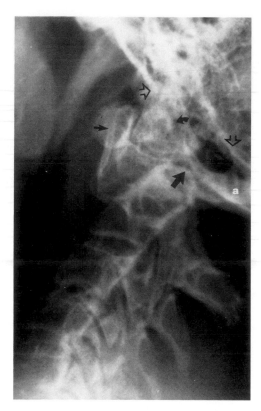

Fig. 6-53 Down syndrome with atlantoaxial dislocation. Lateral cervical spinal plain film demonstrates atlantoaxial dislocation with hypoplastic dens (*large black arrow*), os odontoideum (*curved black arrow*), hypertrophied anterior atlas arch (*small black arrow*), and bifid posterior atlas arch (*a*). Open black arrows delineate the anterior and posterior margins of the foramen magnum. There is marked compromise of the upper cervical spinal canal between the dislocated, hypoplastic dens and the posterior atlas arch and posterior foramen magnum.

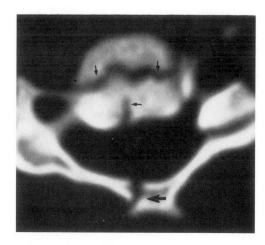

Fig. 6-54 Cervical spinal trauma. Axial CT demonstrates coronal and sagittal plane fractures of the vertebral body and neural arch (*arrows*).

most common in children 6 months to 6 years of age and 10 to 14 years of age. The most common sites are L2-3 and L3-4. In both instances the offending organism most commonly is *Staphylococcus aureus*, which is treated by either antibiotics or surgical drainage.

Juvenile rheumatiod arthritis uncommonly (<10% of all cases of juvenile rheumatiod arthritis) involves the diarthroidal joints (cervical more than lumbar), especially in girls. Atlantoaxial subluxation may result. Ankylosis of the apophyseal joints occurs only in children with long-standing juvenile rheumatiod arthritis.

Ankylosing spondylitis rarely is seen in childhood. Symptoms of back pain occur in 10% of patients. HLA-B27 antigen is positive, as is the bone scan, whereas conventional radiographs reveal bilateral sacroiliac sclerosis, paraspinal ossification, or synovial inflammation with erosion.

Trauma Spinal trauma is best understood by the fundamental three-column approach. The bony and ligamentous spinal column consists of three parts: the posterior, middle, and anterior columns. The neural arch, ligamenta flava, and interspinous ligaments comprise the *posterior* column; the *middle* column is composed of the posterior vertebral body, anulus fibrosis, and posterior longitudinal ligament and is the pivot between the posterior and *anterior* column, which consists of the anterior longitudinal ligament, anulus fibrosis, and vertebral body. Hyperflexion produces anterior column compression and posterior column distraction; a hyperextension injury produces the reverse. The fulcrum of flexion and extension is above C4 in the infant and young child and is below C4 in the adolescent and adult. Compression (burst injuries), extension, and rotational forces form the basis of the hangman's, Jefferson (C1), and teardrop (C2) fractures (Fig. 6-54). In the thoracic and lumbar spine, a Chance fracture caused by hyperflexion (classically with a loop seat belt as the fulcrum) consists of a horizontal fracture of the body and neural arch with posterior element separation.

Spinal injuries occur less commonly in children than in adults. Extension of the injury is the most common cause of transsection or hematoma of the spinal cord. Spinal cord injury in the newborn may be due to traction forces during a difficult delivery. Other causes include motor vehicle accidents and sports-related trauma. Conventional radiographs are essential as the initial imaging modality, followed by US in the newborn or CT or MRI. Myelomalacia or focal syrinx as sequelae are best shown on MRI.

Spondylolysis and spondylolisthesis The weakest part of the vertebral arch is the pars interarticularis. If

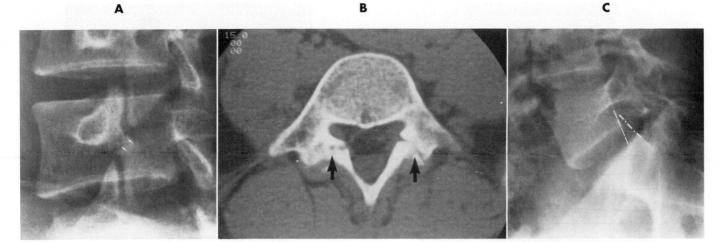

Fig. 6-55 Spondylolysis and spondylolisthesis. **A**, Conventional radiograph and, **B**, axial CT demonstrate bilateral neural arch defects (*arrows*) and reactive bony changes characteristic of spondylolysis, resulting in (**C**) grade 1 spondylolisthesis.

it breaks (spondylolysis or fatigue fracture) as a result of gravitational or biomechanical forces, it may cause pain. If it breaks bilaterally, it may lead to subluxation (spondylolisthesis), most commonly at L5-S1 and less frequently at L4-5. The risk of slippage is greater in girls during adolescence. Conventional radiographs in the lateral projection identify four grades of severity (Fig. 6-55). The anteroposterior view is less specific but may demonstrate the "upside-down Napoleon hat" sign. Scintigraphy or oblique views may localize the defect; CT is more specific.

Neoplasms Spinal tumors in children arise within the spinal cord (intramedullary), within the dura but outside the spinal cord (intradural-extramedullary), or outside the dura (extradural), originating from the bony column or paraspinal tissues. MRI and CT have replaced myelography in the precise evaluation of these lesions. Conventional radiographs suggest a lesion in only half of the patients.

Intramedullary lesions The vast majority (95%) of all intramedullary lesions are gliomas. The most common of these primary neoplasms are astrocytomas and ependymomas. Focal or long-segment cord involvement is the rule, often with expansion and syrinx or cyst formation. Conventional radiographs may show scoliosis and widening of the spinal canal. The lesion shows characteristic enhancement on gadolinium-enhanced MRI (Fig. 6-56).

Intradural lesions Intradural lesions include nerve sheath tumors, neoplastic seeding, and developmental tumors (e.g., dysraphism). The most common benign lesions include schwannomas and neurofibromas that may occur sporadically or as part of neurofibromatosis (Fig. 6-57).

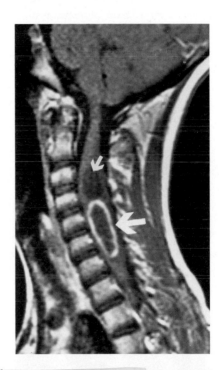

Fig. 6-56 Spinal cord astrocytoma. Gadolinium-enhanced sagittal T1-weighted MRI demonstrates a ring-enhancing intramedullary tumor of the cervical spinal cord (*large arrow*) with cord expansion and an associated nonenhancing tumor cyst (*small arrow*).

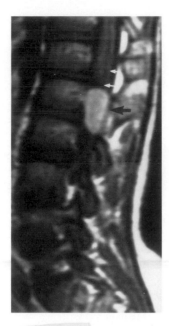

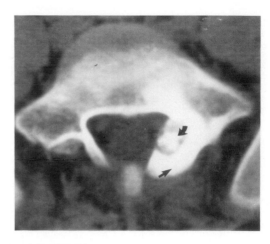

Fig. 6-58 Osteoid osteoma. Axial CT demonstrates a hyperdense sclerotic nidus (*curved arrow*) with a lucent collar and markedly sclerotic reactive changes (*straight arrow*) characteristic of osteoid osteoma.

Fig. 6-57 Spinal neurofibroma. Gadolinium-enhanced sagittal T1-weighted MRI of the lumbar spine demonstrates a markedly enhancing intradural, extramedullary tumor (*black arrow*) compressing the central canal (*white arrows*) characteristic of a neurofibroma associated with neurofibromatosis.

Neoplastic seeding of the subarachnoid space occurs most commonly with medulloblastoma, germ cell tumors, ependymoma, and pineal neoplasms. Gadolinium-enhanced MRI is the imaging procedure of choice and shows laminar or nodular enhancement along the cord surfaces and nerve roots (see Fig. 6-45).

Extradural lesions Tumors of the spinal column or paraspinal tissues may encroach on the spinal canal directly, extend by epidural venous spread, or disseminate by hematogenous or lymphatic routes.

Benign lesions Osteoid osteoma is a sclerotic lesion that contains a radiolucent nidus that often has a central calcification within it. Less than 10% of all osteoid osteomas occur in the spine. Most commonly, they become evident in children 10 to 12 years of age. The most common location is a pedicle in the lumbar region. Clinically the child has pain and tenderness that is worse at night but relieved with aspirin (Fig. 6-58). Associated scoliosis is common.

Aneurysmal bone cysts are nonneoplastic solitary lesions that are filled with nonclotted blood. Up to 30% arise within the axial skeleton, most often in the spinous or transverse processes of the lumbar and sacral region. They commonly are associated with other lesions, including osteoblastoma and giant cell tumor.

Aggressive lesions Neuroblastoma and other neural crest tumors most often are found in the abdomen and thorax. Involvement of the spine may occur with or without bone erosion or neurologic signs (Fig. 6-59). MRI is the modality of choice for evaluating this invlovement.

Ewing sarcoma and osteosarcoma are rare primary lesions of the bony spine. Involvement of the spinal

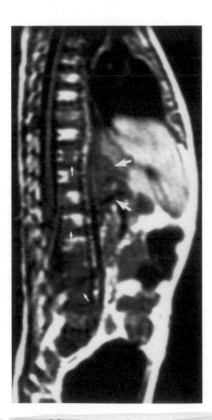

Fig. 6-59 Neuroblastoma and marrow involvement. Sagittal T1-weighted MRI demonstrates a large abdominal mass (*large arrows*) plus extensive hypointense tumor replacement (*small arrows*) of the normally hyperintense spinal vertebral marrow.

cord marrow is seen in children with histiocytosis, leukemia, metastatic tumor, and hematologic conditions (e.g., hemosiderosis). Chloromas (leukemic masses) may arise as epidural, intraspinal, or paraspinal masses, usually associated with acute myelocytic leukemia.

AML

SUGGESTED READINGS
Texts

Barkovich A: *Pediatric Neuroimaging*, New York, 1990, Raven Press.

Harwood-Nash D, Fitz CR: *Neuroradiology in Infants and Children*, St. Louis, 1976, Mosby.

Healy G, editor: *Common Problems in Pediatric Otolaryngology*, St Louis, 1990, Mosby.

Kirks DR, editor: *Practical Pediatric Imaging*, Boston, 1992, Little, Brown and Co, pp 62-183 (skull), 197-257 (spine).

Kleinman PK: *Diagnostic Imaging of Child Abuse*, Baltimore, 1987, Williams & Wilkins, pp 91-102, 159-200.

Siegel MJ, editor: *Pediatric Sonography*, New York, 1991, Raven Press, pp 9-63.

Silverman FM, Kuhn JP, editors: *Caffey's Pediatric X-Ray Diagnosis*, ed 9, vol 1, St Louis, 1992, Mosby, pp 1-344.

Sty JR, Wells RG, Starshak RJ et al: *Diagnostic Imaging of Infants and Children*, vol 2, 1992, Aspen Publisher.

Swischuk LE: *Imaging of the Newborn, Infant and Young Child*, ed 3, Baltimore, 1989, Williams & Wilkins, pp 893-1034.

Teele RL, Share JC: *Ultrasonography of Infants and Children*, Philadelphia, 1991, WB Saunders, pp 1-72.

Wolpert SM, Barnes PD: *MRI in Pediatric Neuroradiology*, St Louis, 1992, Mosby.

Articles

Babcock DK: Sonography of congenital malformations of the brain, *Neuroradiology* 28:428, 1986.

Bowerman RA, Donn SM, DiPietro MA et al: Periventricular leukomalacia in the pre-term newborn infant: sonographic and clinical features, *Radiology* 151:383, 1984.

Buetow PC, Smirniotopolous JG, Done S: Congenital brain tumors: a review of 45 cases, *AJR* 155-587, 1990.

Funk KC, Siegal MJ: Sonography of congenital midline brain malformations, *Radiographics* 8:11, 1988.

Kirks DR, Bowie JD: Cranial ultrasonography of neonatal periventricular/intraventricular hemorrhage: who? how? why? and when? *Pediatr Radiol* 16:114, 1986.

Nadich TP, Yousefzadeh DK, Gusnard DA: Sonography of the normal neonatal head: supratentorial structures—state-of-the-art imaging, *Neuroradiology* 28:408, 1986.

Rubin J, DiPietro M, Chandler W et al: Spinal ultrasonography: intraoperative and pediatric applications, *Radiol Clin North Am* 26:1, 1988.

Thornbury JR, Masters SJ, Cambell JA: Imaging recommendations for head trauma: a new comprehensive strategy, *AJR* 149:781, 1987.

VanderKnaap M, Valk J: Classification of congenital abnormality of the CNS, *AJNR* 9:315, 1988.

Volpe J: Current concepts of brain injury in the premature infant, *AJR* 153:243, 1989.

Index

236

Sclerosis, "physiologic," 151, *152*
Scoliosis, 230-231
Scrotum, 146
  masses in, 146-147
Scurvy, 163
Septic arthritis, 171
Short stature, asymmetric, 154
Shortening
  acromelic, 154-155
  mesomelic, 154, *155*
Sickle cell disease, 164-165
Sinding-Larson-Johansson "disease," 182
Sinuses, paranasal, 200
Skeletal dysplasias, 153-158
Skeletal system, 149-191; *see also* Bone
  congenital abnormalities of, 153-161
  development of, normal, 149-151
  disorders of
    metabolic, 161-163
    systemic and generalized, 161-168
  infection of, 168-172
  ossification centers in, 150-151
  trauma to, 181-188; *see also* Fractures
  variants in, normal, 151-153
Skeleton, thoracic, 14, *15*, 16
Skull, 194-199
  congenital and developmental anomalies of, 197
  convolutional markings of, 194-195
  development of, normal, 194-196
  infections involving, 198
  molding of, 196
  sutures of, 195-196
  systemic diseases involving, 197-198
  trauma to, 198-199
  tumors of, 199
  vascular lesions of, 198
  vascular markings of, 195
Slipped capital femoral epiphysis (SCFE), 185
Soavé pull-through procedure for Hirschsprung disease, 90
Sphenoidal cephaloceles, 205
Spine, 225-235
  acquired anomalies of, 231-235
  developmental anomalies of, 227-231
  inflammatory lesions of, 231-232
  neoplasms of, 233-235
  normal, 225-227
  trauma to, 232-233
Spinovascular anomalies, 231
Spleen, 103-104
  cysts of, 104, *105*
  trauma to, 107, *108*, 109
Spondylitis, ankylosing, 190
  spine in, 232
Spondylodysplasias, 230-231
Spondylolisthesis, 232-233
Spondylolysis, 232-233
Staphylococcal pneumonia, 29
Stein-Leventhal syndrome, 144
Still disease, 189-190
Stomach, 76-81
  acquired conditions of, 79-80
  air distention of, 79
  anomalies of, 77-79
  embryogenesis of, 77-78
  inflammation of, 79
  neoplasms of, 80-81

Stomach—cont'd
  ulceration of, 79-80
  volvulus of, 77-78
Stress fracture, 186
Sturge-Weber syndrome, 209
Subarachnoid hemorrhage, 219
Subdural hemorrhage, 218, *219*
Subglottic region, 11-12, *13*
Supraglottic area, 8, *9-10*, 10-11
Supraglottic hypermobility syndrome, 8
Sutures of skull, 195-196
Swenson operation for Hirschsprung disease, 90
Swyer-James syndrome, 33
Synostoses, 158-159
Synovitis, toxic, 171
Syphilis, skeletal manifestations of, 171, *172*

T

Tachypnea of newborn, transient, 26-27
Telangiectasia, hereditary hemorrhagic, 209
Temporal bone, petrous, 200-201
Teratomas, 39
  ovarian, 144-145
  spinal, 230
Testicle, undescended, 146
Tethered cord syndrome, 228, *229*
Tetrad of Fallot, 47-48
Thalassemia, 165
Thoracic skeleton, 14, *15*, 16
Thymoma, 39
Thymus, 37-38
Thyroglossal duct remnant, 202
Toddler's fracture, 186
Tomography
  of chest, 4
  computerized; *see* Computerized tomography (CT)
Total anomalus pulmonary venous return (TAPVR), 46-47
Toxic synovitis, 171
Toxoplasmosis, 214
Trachea
  development of, 4
  stenosis of, 11-12
  vascular lesions between esophagus and, 74
Tracheal impressions, 73-74
Tracheobronchomegaly, 7
Tracheoesophageal fistula (TEF), 70-72
Tracheomalacia, 11
Transposition of great arteries (TGA), 44-46
Trauma
  abdominal, 107-109
  to genitourinary tract, 140-141
  to skeletal system, 181-188; *see also* Fractures
    birth, 188
    nonaccidental, 186, 188
  to skull, 198-199
  to spine, 232-233
Tricuspid atresia, 48
Trigonocephaly, 197
Tuberculosis, 30, *31*
Tuberculous meningitis, 214
Tuberous sclerosis, 209
Tuboovarian abscess, 144
Tumor(s); *see* Neoplasm(s)
Typhlitis, 94